International Studies on Childhood and Adolescence 3

# International Studies on Childhood and Adolescence (ISCA)

The aim of the ISCA series is to publish theoretical and methodological studies on the social, cultural, economic, and health situation of children and adolescents.

Almost all countries worldwide report increased risks and problems in the development of children and adolescents. Many pedagogic, psychosocial, and medical institutes as well as education and training centers are trying to help children and adolescents deal with problematic situations. They step in to help with existing difficulties (intervention) or to avoid problems in advance (prevention). However, not enough is known about the causes and backgrounds of the difficulties that arise in the life course of children and adolescents. There is still insufficient research on the effectiveness and consequences of prevention measures and intervention in families, pre-school institutions, schools, youth service, youth welfare, and the criminal justice system.

The ISCA series addresses these issues. An interdisciplinary team of editors and authors focusses on the publications on theoretical, methodological, and practical issues in the above mentioned fields. The whole spectrum of perspectives is considered: analyses rooted in the sociological as well as the psychological or medical and public health tradition, from an economic or a political science angle, mainstream as well as critical contributions.

The ISCA series represents an effort to advance the scientific study of childhood and adolescence across boundaries and academic disciplines.

## Editorial Board

Prof. Klaus Hurrelmann (Coord.), Faculty of Health Sciences, University of Bielefeld, Postfach 10 01 31, D-33501 Bielefeld, Tel.: (49-521)-106-3834, Fax: (49-521)-106-2987; Prof. Günter Albrecht, Faculty of Sociology; Prof. Michael Brambring, Faculty of Psychology; Prof. Detlev Frehsee: Faculty of Law; Prof. Wilhelm Heitmeyer, Faculty of Pedagogics; Prof. Alois Herlth, Faculty of Sociology; Prof. Dietrich Kurz, Faculty of Sports Sciences; Prof. Franz-Xaver Kaufmann, Faculty of Sociology; Prof. Hans-Uwe Otto, Faculty of Pedagogics; Prof. Klaus-Jürgen Tillmann, Faculty of Pedagogics; all University of Bielefeld, Postfach 10 01 31, D-33501 Bielefeld

## Editorial Advisors

Prof. John Bynner, City University, Social Statistics Research, London, Great Britain; Prof. Manuela du Bois-Reymond, University of Leiden, Faculty of Social Sciences, Leiden, The Netherlands; Prof. Marie Choquet, Institut National de la Santé, Paris, France; Prof. David P. Farrington, University of Cambridge, Institute of Criminology, Cambridge, Great Britain; Prof. James Garbarino, Erikson Institute, Chicago, USA; Prof. Stephen F. Hamilton, Cornell Human Development Studies, Ithaca, USA; Prof. Rainer Hornung, University of Zurich, Institute of Psychology, Zurich, Switzerland; Prof. Gertrud Lenzer, Graduate School CUNY, New York, USA; Prof. Wim Meeus, University of Utrecht, Faculty of Social Sciences, Utrecht, The Netherlands; Prof. Ira M. Schwartz, University of Pennsylvania, School of Social Work, Philadelphia, USA; Prof. Giovanni B. Sgritta, University of Rome, Department of Demographic Sciences, Rome, Italy; Prof. Karl R. White, Utah State University, Logan, USA

# Eating Disorders in Adolescence

Anorexia and Bulimia Nervosa

Edited by

Hans-Christoph Steinhausen

Walter de Gruyter · Berlin · New York 1995

*Hans-Christoph Steinhausen*
M.D., Ph.D., Professor, Psychiatrische Universitäts-Poliklinik für Kinder und Jugendliche, Zürich, Switzerland

With 25 figures and 43 tables

*Library of Congress Cataloging-in-Publication Data*

Eating disorders in adolescence ; anorexia and bulimia nervosa / edited by Hans-Christoph Steinhausen,
XVIII, 374 p. 17 × 24 cm. -- (International studies on childhood and adolescence ; 3)
   Includes index.
   ISBN 3-11-014347-X (alk. paper)
   1. Eating disorders in adolescence.   I. Series.
   [DNLM: 1. Eating Disorders -- in adolescence. WM 175 E14819 1995]
RJ506.E18E28  1995
616.85′26′00835--dc20
DNLM/DLC
for Library of Congress                                              95-547
                                                                      CIP

*Die Deutsche Bibliothek − Cataloging-in-Publication Data*

**Eating disorders in adolescence** : anorexia and bulimia nervosa / ed. by Hans-Christoph Steinhausen. − Berlin ; New York : de Gruyter, 1995
   (International studies on childhood and adolescence ; 3)
   ISBN 3-11-014347-X
NE: Steinhausen, Hans-Christoph [Hrsg.]; GT

∞ Printed on acid-free paper which falls within the guidelines of the ANSI to ensure permanence and durability.

© Copyright 1995 by Walter de Gruyter & Co., D-10785 Berlin
All rights reserved, including those of translation into foreign languages. No part of this book may be reproduced or transmitted in any form or by any means, electronic or mechanical, including photocopy, recording or any information storage and retrieval system, without permission in writing from the publisher. Printed in Germany Printing: WB-Druck GmbH, Rieden am Forggensee. Binding: D. Mikolai GmbH, Berlin. Cover Design: Johannes Rother, Berlin.

# Contents

Preface .................................................................................................. vii

Foreword
G. Russell ........................................................................................... ix

Contributors ......................................................................................... xv

## Part I: Epidemiological and Cultural Issues

**The Incidence of Anorexia Nervosa in Adolescent Residents of Rochester, Minnesota Over Fifty Years**
A. R. Lucas ......................................................................................... 3

**A Population Study of Bulimia Nervosa and Subclinical Eating Disorders in Adolescence**
M. Flament, S. Ledoux, P. Jeammet, M. Choquet and Yves Simon ................. 21

**Transcultural Comparisons of Adolescent Eating Disorders**
H.-C. Steinhausen, K.-J. Neumärker, and S. Boyadjieva .............................. 37

## Part II: Clinical and Psychological Issues

**Individual and Familiy Factors in Adolescents with Eating Symptoms and Syndromes**
H. Steiger and S. Stotland .................................................................... 49

**Social Avoidance, Social Negativism and Disorders of Empathy in a Subgroup of Young Individuals With Anorexia Nervosa.**
M. Råstam, C. Gillberg, and I. C. Gillberg ............................................... 69

**Risk Factors for the Development of Early Onset Bulimia Nervosa**
U. Schmidt, J. Tiller, M. Hoades, and J. Treasure ...................................... 83

**Precursors and Risk Factors of Juvenile Eating Disorders**
H. Steiner, M. Sanders, and E. Ryst ....................................................... 95

**Anorexia Nervosa and Depression: Results of a Longitudinal Study**
B. Herpertz-Dahlmann and H. Remschmidt .............................................. 127

**How Specific are Body Image Disturbances in Patients With Anorexia Nervosa?**
H. Flechtner, C. Eltze, and G. Lehmkuhl ................................................. 145

**Sexual Abuse and Psychological Dysfunctioning in Eating Disorders**
J. Vanderlinden and W. Vandereycken .......................................................... 161

**Neurobiology of Eating Disorders in Adolescence**
K.M. Pirke and P. Platte ................................................................................. 171

**Psychophysiology of Anorexia Nervosa**
A. Rothenberger, C. Dumais-Huber, G. Moll, and W. Woerner ..................... 191

## Part III: Management and Treatment

**Medical Assessment and the Initial Interview in the Management of Young Patients with Anorexia Nervosa**
P.J.V. Beumont, K. Lowinger, and J. Russell ................................................ 221

**The Inpatient Management of Adolescent Patients With Anorexia Nervosa**
S.W. Touyz, D.M. Garner, and P.J.V. Beumont ............................................ 247

**Psychopharmacology in Adolescents With Eating Disorders**
D.M. Heebink and K.A. Halmi ...................................................................... 271

**The Place of Family Therapy in the Treatment of Eating Disorders**
W. Vandereycken ............................................................................................ 287

## Part IV: Course and Outcome

**Comparative Studies on the Course of Eating Disorders in Adolescents and Adults. Is Age at Onset a Predictor of Outcome?**
M. Fichter and N. Quadflieg .......................................................................... 301

**The Utrecht Prospective Longitudinal Studies on Eating Disorders in Adolescence: Course and the Predictive Power of Personality and Family Variables**
H. van Engeland, Th. van der Ham, E.F. van Furth, and D.N. van Strien ...... 339

**The Outcome of Adolescent Eating Disorders in Two Different European Regions**
H.-C. Steinhausen, M. Amstein, M. Reitzle, and R. Seidel ........................... 359

**Subject Index** ............................................................................................. 371

# Preface

In the recent past the eating disorders have received considerable attention both among experts and the lay public. The multitude of facets of these disorders have been the object of an increasing number of scientific studies and continue to be so. However, the great majority of research activities, as reflected by monographs and journal publications, has so far concentrated on issues that deal with adult patients suffering from anorexia or bulimia nervosa. In contrast, rather less emphasis has been given to the younger patients. This is surprising considering that, in a large proportion of the eating disordered patients, onset of the disorder occurs in adolescence.

The observation that adolescence as a critical age period for the development of eating disorders has not received sufficient attention in the expert community served as an incentive for creating the present monograph. With the help of a group of international contributors who are distinguished both for their clinical expertise and their research in the field of eating disorders, it was possible to tentatively close a gap in the current literature on anorexia and bulimia nervosa.

With a variety of contributions that make up the four main parts of this monograph—namely epidemiological and cultural issues, clinical and psychological aspects, management and treatment, and course and outcome—the specific aspects of the eating disorders in adolescence are well covered. In the editor's perception, the authors of the present monograph did extremely well in contributing to a synthesis of scientific rigor and clinical practice. For all these efforts the sincerest thanks are devoted to the contributors of the present book. However, the production of this camera-ready book would also not have been possible without the enormous assistance provided by Ms. R. Maly, Ms. B. Fechtig, and Ms. C. Rauss-Mason, who were extremely supportive in the process of editing and producing this monograph.

This book is dedicated foremost to the increasing number of adolescents with eating disorders, who will hopefully profit from well-informed experts. Certainly, it is the task of the reader to go beyond the individual chapters with their compilation of current research and clinical expertise and to integrate all this information into a comprehensive synthesis of our understanding of the eating disorders in adolescents.

# Foreword

The editor of this book commissioned the authors to review aetiological, clinical, therapeutic and prognostic aspects of eating disorders, but to focus their task on their occurrence during adolescence. Adolescence is that ill-defined developmental period between childhood and maturity. Its beginning may be defined more closely as the onset of the pubertal period of development. Its end is more imprecise and fades into full adult maturity. The relevance of adolescence to eating disorders is evident. After all, anorexia nervosa is an illness with an onset most commonly between 14 and 17 years, soon after the completion of puberty. It is sometimes viewed as a failure of adaptation to the biological demands of puberty and the required psychosocial adjustment of adolescence. Bulimia nervosa has a peak onset at the age of 18, and thus commonly begins in late adolescence or early maturity.

In this book therefore, the authors have endeavoured to describe those aspects of eating disorders that are more characteristic of their occurrence in adolescent patients. Some of the chapters lend themselves more to this focussed approach. In others the authors have wisely broadened their scope in order to embrace a wider field of knowledge when this is appropriate. In this foreword I shall indicate some of the signposts pointing to the specific features of eating disorders in adolescence. But this book should be read in its entirety to do justice to the wide-ranging material which has been ably assembled by each contributor.

Perhaps the most specific clinical manifestations of anorexia nervosa in early adolescence are those that result from the disruption of the normal physical and emotional development of puberty. The normal sequence of pubertal events spans at least three years (Tanner 1962). In girls the completion of puberty is usually marked by the first menstrual period. Premenarchal anorexia nervosa refers to the illness in girls when it strikes during early adolescence. The associated malnutrition frequently disrupts physical development. Growth in stature is delayed, and there may be other signs of pubertal arrest, depending on the timing of the illness in relation to puberty. The appearance of secondary sex characteristics is delayed: in girls the breasts remain undeveloped, in boys the penis and scrotum remain infantile. By definition this early form of anorexia nervosa leads to primary amenorrhea in girls (Russell, 1985, 1992).

At the heart of this book on eating disorders in adolescence is the chapter on the neurobiology of eating disorders during this period of development (Pirke and Platte). It describes most directly the mechanisms whereby anorexia nervosa causes a regression to an infantile stage of function of the hypothalamic-pituitary axis. This regression leads not only to impaired gonadal function but also to reduced adrenal function. Thus the biological clock is set back to a stage before the menarche, and indeed before the adrenarche. When the patient recovers, there occurs a staged reversal of these regressive changes with a progressive return to normal gonadotropin function. The infertility that often complicates bulimia nervosa is now better understood in the light of a failure of ovulation and an over production of cortisol. It remains uncertain, however, whether patients with bulimia nervosa during their recovery repeat the development of hypothalamic-pituitary-gonadal function, as do younger patients with anorexia nervosa.

The chapters on epidemiology confirm that anorexia nervosa is predominantly an illness afflicting adolescent girls. Moreover, its incidence in 15 to 19 year old girls has shown an increasing trend during the fifty years from 1935 to 1984. The incidence of premenarchal anorexia nervosa has also increased since 1965 (Lucas and Holub). Preoccupation's with weight, body shape and dieting are widespread among teenage girls. By the age of 12 years, small numbers of adolescents have already induced vomiting or taken laxatives or diet pills in order to reduce their weight. In girls the frequency of these behaviours increases with age after 14 years. The prevalence rate for bulimia nervosa in adolescents was found to be 1.1% in girls and 0.2% in boys, confirming that bulimic behaviour develops during adolescence (Flament and colleagues).

Eating disorders in adolescence were compared in four European cities with widely differing political and socio-cultural conditions (Steinhausen and colleagues). In spite of these differences, the patients displayed very similar clinical features. The clinics in the four centres (West and East Berlin, Sofia, and Zurich) saw populations of patients which varied in the age of onset of the illnesses. In Sofia the patients were admitted for treatment after a longer delay than in the other centres, probably because of a relative lack of psychiatric facilities for children and adolescents in that city. Thus, the availability of medical services may introduce a selection bias in the populations under study.

# Foreword

Several chapters in this book provide information on psychosocial causes of eating disorders more specific to adolescence, while stressing that the causes and clinical manifestations are usually very similar irrespective of the age of onset. For example, Steiger and Stotland indicate that deficits in family functioning are more likely to be predictive of personality disturbances and their severity than the severity of the eating disturbance.

In the chapter on risk factors leading to early onset bulimia nervosa, lack of parental care is described as being nearly twice as common in an early onset group (age of 15 or below) as in a group with an older age of onset (Schmidt and colleagues). Parents who are unavailable to their teenage daughter may not provide her with regular meals. Once rigid dieting or an eating disorder has set in, these parents may fail to act appropriately.

The review on sexual abuse in eating disorders succeeds in clarifying this sad and emotive subject (Vanderlinden and Vandereycken). Sexual abuse is reported by a substantial number of female patients with an eating disorder. The frequency is higher than in the general female population, but no higher than in patients with other psychiatric disorders. The rate of reported sexual abuse seems to be higher in patients with bulimic symptoms than in those with classical anorexia nervosa who simply restrict their food intake. Sexual abuse was more often reported by patients with a borderline personality disorder and dissociative symptoms.

An interesting multifactorial model is provided in the chapter on precursors and risk factors of juvenile eating disorders (Steiner and colleagues). The precipitating cause of the eating disorder is considered to be the stress of adolescence, but there are several antecedents to the disorder that accumulate over the years and lead to the "stacking of risk factors". There follows an extensive list of different factors, any of which may contribute to the disorder but few of which can yet be said to be necessary or specific. We are reminded, however, that the biology of being female confers a more important risk than societal expectations in terms of gender-related roles.

An interesting association of empathy disorder and anorexia nervosa of early onset is described in the chapter by Råstam and her colleagues. Thus 29% of the anorexic patients were found to have an empathy disorder, among whom 12% met the criteria for Asperger syndrome and 8% for autistic-like conditions. The authors recognise that some clinicians rarely diagnose autistic-like problems in anorexia nervosa but suggest they might do so more readily if they considered the diagnosis in anorexic patients who manifest alexithymia (an inability to verbalise their feelings).

This book contains excellent contributions on the general assessment and management of patients with eating disorders (Beumont and colleagues) and their inpatient management (Touyz and colleagues). A search for treatments more specific for eating disorders in adolescents is undertaken in two chapters. In the first, Heebink and Halmi enquire whether there are pharmacological treatments that are particularly effective in adolescent patients. They make the startling observations that there have been no controlled trials of psychotropic drugs in adolescents with eating disorders, nor trials comparing their response with that of adults. Nevertheless, these authors have done their best to analyse their own research data. In their conclusions they cautiously recommend the use of antidepressants that have been shown to be effective in adult patients with bulimia nervosa (e.g., tricyclic antidepressants and fluoxetine). They are rightly even more cautious about the use of psychotropic drugs in anorexia nervosa. The chapter on family treatments by Vandereycken is the other contribution in which specific benefits for adolescents are examined. Here the guidance can be more precise in view of the published controlled trials. The evidence to date is that in anorexia nervosa formal family therapy is more useful than individual supportive therapy, and this is particularly so in patients with a younger age of onset. The age factor is important because, among younger patients, family therapy is a more acceptable treatment than individual therapy. Preliminary studies also suggest that the simpler family treatment of family counselling is as effective as the more complicated and classical family therapy.

The book ends with chapters on the course of eating disorders and their outcome, containing surprising findings. Researchers at the Utrecht Clinic have followed up juvenile patients suffering in the main from anorexia nervosa. In contrast with previous studies in older patients they found that demographic and behavioural variables were unhelpful in predicting outcome. Instead, psychological and personality variables, as well as the occurrence of maternal criticism, turned out to be more powerful predictors of outcome in adolescent patients (van Engeland and colleagues).

The hitherto widely accepted view that anorexia nervosa of early onset carries a good prognosis is challenged by the impressive German Anorexia and Bulimia Nervosa Study (Fichter and Quadflieg). The investigators were unable to confirm an association between an onset before or at the age of 16 and a more favourable outcome. Moreover, they could not confirm the findings of other investigators who had suggested a worse outcome in bulimia nervosa of early onset.

In conclusion, the editor deserves warm congratulations for gathering within this book current clinical opinion and the latest research findings on Eating Disorders in Adolescence. The material is well focussed on this age group and has the additional merit of covering broader aspects of anorexia and bulimia nervosa.

Gerald Russell
Emeritus Professor of Psychiatry

### References

Tanner J. M. (1962) *Growth at adolescence*: (2nd ed.) Oxford: Blackwell Scientific Publications.
Russell G. F. M. (1985) Premenarchal anorexia nervosa and its sequelae. *Journal of Psychiatric Research, 19*, 363-369.
Russell G. F. M. (1992) Anorexia nervosa of early onset and its impact on puberty. In: (Eds.) P. J. Cooper & A. Stein. *Feeding problems and eating disorders in children and adolescents.: Monographs in Clinical Paediatrics, 5 (pp. 85-112)*. Chur: Harwood Academic Publishers.

# Contributors

**Margret Amstein**, M.D., Department of Child and Adolescent Psychiatry, University of Zurich, 8032 Zürich, Switzerland

**Pierre J.V. Beumont**, M.D., Professor and Head of the Department of Psychiatry, University of Sydney, Lynton Hospital, Sydney NSW 2006, Australia

**Svetlana Boyadjieva**, M.D., Adolescent Psychiatric Clinic, University of Sofia, 1619 Sofia, Bulgaria

**Marie Choquet**, Ph.D., Unité de Recherche 169, Institut National de la Santé et de la Recherche Médical, 94807 Villejuif, France

**Claude Dumais-Huber**, Dr. sc.hum., Cell Physiology Laboratory, Central Institute of Mental Health, J5, 68159 Mannheim, Germany

**Christin Eltze**, M.D., University of Cologne, Department of Child and Adolescent Psychiatry and Psychotherapy, 50931 Köln-Lindenthal, Germany

**Manfred M. Fichter**, M.D., Department of Psychiatry, University of Munich, 80336 Munich, Germany

**Martine Flament**, M.D., Unité de Recherche 302, Institut National de la Santé et de la Recherche Médical, Hôpital de la Salpêtre 47, 75651 Paris, France

**Henning Flechtner**, M.D., University of Cologne, Department of Child and Adolescent Psychiatry and Psychotherapy, 50931 Köln-Lindenthal, Germany

**David M. Garner**, Ph.D., Executive Director, Neurobehavioral Associates, Okemos Minnesota 48864, USA

**Christopher Gillberg**, M.D., Ph.D., Professor and Head of the Section of Child and Adolescent Psychiatry, Department of Clinical Neuroscience/Child Neuropsychiatry, University of Göteborg, Annedals Clinics, 41345 Göteborg, Sweden

**I. Carina Gillberg**, M.D., Ph.D., Associate Professor, Section of Child and Adolescent Psychiatry, Department of Clinical Neuroscience/Child Neuropsychiatry, University of Göteborg, Annedals Clinics, 41345 Göteborg, Sweden

**Katherine A. Halmi**, M.D., Professor, Department of Psychiatry, The New York Hospital, Cornell Medical Center, Westchester Division, White Plains, N.Y. 10605, USA

**Denise Heebing**, M.D., Department of Psychiatry, Cornell University College of Medicine, New York, NY 10025, USA

**Matthew Hodes**, M.D., Academic Department of Child and Adolescent Psychiatry, St. Mary's Hospital, London W2 1NY, United Kingdom

**Mark. I. Holub**, M.D., Senior Staff Child and Adolescent Psychiatrist, Brainard Regional Human Services Center, Minnesota 56401, USA

**Philippe Jeammet**, M.D., Professor, Hôpital International de l'Université de Paris, 75674 Paris, France

**Sylvie Ledoux**, Ph.D., Unité de Recherche 169, Institut National de la Santé et de la Recherche Médical, 94807 Villejuif, France

**Gerd Lehmkuhl**, M.D., University of Cologne, Professor and Head, Department of Child and Adolescent Psychiatry and Psychotherapy, 50931 Köln-Lindenthal, Germany

**Kitty Lowinger**, M.D., Family Physician, Lynton Hospital, Sydney NSW 2067, Australia

**Alexander R. Lucas**, M.D., Professor and Head, Division of Child and Adolescent Psychiatry, Mayo Clinic and Mayo Foundation, Rochester Minnesota 35905, USA

**Gunther H. Moll**, M.D., Department of Child and Adolescent Psychiatry, Central Institute of Mental Health, J5, 68159 Mannheim, Germany

**Klaus-Jürgen Neumärker**, M.D., Professor and Head of the Department of Child and Adolescent Psychiatry, Humbolt University, Charité Hospital, 10098 Berlin, Germany

**Norbert Quadflieg**, Department of Psychiatry, University of Munich, 80336 Munich, Germany

**Maria Råstam**, M.D., Ph.D., Section of Child and Adolescent Psychiatry, Department of Clinical Neuroscience/Child Neuropsychiatry, University of Göteborg, Annedals Clinics, 41345 Göteborg, Sweden

**Matthias Reitzle**, Ph.D., Department of Developmental Psychology, University of Jena, 07743 Jena, Germany

**Aribert Rothenberger**, M.D., Professor and Head of the Department of Child and Adolescent Psychiatry, University of Göttingen, 37075 Göttingen, Germany

**Janice D. Russell**, M.D., Senior Lecturer, Department of Psychiatry, University of Sydney, Sydney NSW 2006, Australia

**Erika Ryst**, B.A., Division of Child Psychiatry, Stanford University School of Medicine, California 94305-5540, USA

**Mary Sanders**, Ph.D., Division of Child Psychiatry, Stanford University School of Medicine, California 94305-5540, USA

**Ulrike Schmidt**, M.D., Consultant Psychiatrist, Department of Psychiatry, St. Mary's Hospital, London W2 1NY, United Kingdom

**Reinhold Seidel**, M.D., Child and Adolescent Psychiatric Service Neukölln, 12043 Berlin, Germany

**Yves Simon**, M.D., Hôpital Erasme, 1070 Bruxelles, Belgium

**Howard Steiger**, Ph.D., Associate Professor, Eating Disorders Unit, Douglas Hospital Centre, Montreal (Verdun) Quebec H4H 1R3, Canada

**Hans Steiner**, M.D., Associate Professor, Division of Child Psychiatry, Stanford University School of Medicine, California 94305-5540, USA

**Hans-Christoph Steinhausen**, M.D., Ph.D., Professor and Head of the Department of Child and Adolescent Psychiatry, University of Zurich, 8032 Zurich, Switzerland

**Stephen Stotland**, Ph.D., Eating Disorders Unit, Douglas Hospital Centre, Montreal (Verdun) Quebec H4H 1R3, Canada

**Jane Tiller**, M.D., Senior Registrar, Maudsley Hospital, London SE5 8AF, United Kingdom

**Stephen W. Touyz**, Ph.D., Clinical Professor in Psychiatry and Head of the Department of Medical Psychology, University of Sydney, Westmead Hospital, New South Wales, Australia

**Janet Treasure**, M.D., Consultant Psychiatrist, Maudsley Hospital, London SE5 8AF, United Kingdom

**Thecla van der Ham**, Ph.D., Eating Disorders Unit, Robert-Fleury Stichting, 2260 AK Leidschendam, The Netherlands

**Herman van Engeland**, M.D., Ph.D., Head of the Department of Child and Adolescent Psychiatry, Utrecht University Hospital, 3508 GA Utrecht, The Netherlands

**Din C. van Strien**, M.D., Department of Child and Adolescent Psychiatry, Utrecht University Hospital, 3508 GA Utrecht, The Netherlands

**Walter Vandereycken**, M.D., Ph.D., Professor, Alexian Brothers Psychiatric Hospital, Catholic University of Leuven, 3300 Tienen, Belgium

**Johan Vanderlinden**, Ph.D., Department of Behavior Therapy, University Center St. Joseph, 3070 Kortenberg, Belgium

**Wolfgang Woerner**, Ph.D., Child and Adolescent Psychiatry, Central Institute of Mental Health, 68159 Mannheim, Germany

# Part I

# Epidemiological and Cultural Issues

# The Incidence of Anorexia Nervosa in Adolescent Residents of Rochester, Minnesota, During a 50-Year Period

*Alexander R. Lucas and Mark I. Holub*

## 1 Introduction

Although anorexia nervosa can begin at any time between the ages of 8 or 9 and middle age, it is predominantly a disease of pubertal girls. The process of puberty typically extends over several years and leads into adolescence. Anorexia nervosa may delay or even forestall puberty. Premenarchal anorexia nervosa has been described in patients in whom the onset is early in the process of puberty and before menstruation has begun. Powerful biological changes triggered by the hormonal surge at puberty cause increased fat deposition. These changes may lead to dieting in vulnerable girls and are among the multifactorial determinants of anorexia nervosa.

It generally has been assumed that the incidence of anorexia nervosa in Western countries has increased markedly, particularly since the 1960s. Few epidemiologic studies investigated population groups before 1960 (Brems, 1963; Innes & Sharp, 1962; Kidd & Wood, 1966), and only one, with the exception of ours, included subjects in whom the diagnosis was made before 1950 (Lucas, Beard, O'Fallon, & Kurland, 1988; Theander, 1970). Our population-based study of anorexia nervosa in Rochester, Minnesota, spanning the 50-year period from 1935 through 1984, revealed that incidence trends differed between female and male patients with anorexia nervosa and also among different age groups in female patients. The incidence rates in 15- through 24-year-old female residents of Rochester increased steadily from 1935 through 1984, but the rates for female subjects 25 years or older at onset and the rates for male subjects did not increase over time. It was especially surprising that anorexia nervosa existed in significant numbers during the 1930s and early 1940s, even among the youngest age group identified, those children 10 through 14 years of age at onset (Lucas, Beard, O'Fallon, & Kurland, 1991). Other studies differed in their diagnostic criteria and in their methods of case ascertainment. Some used hospital admissions (Brems, 1963; Kidd & Wood, 1966; Theander, 1970; Willi & Grossmann, 1983) and others used psychiatric case registers as their sources of data (Hoek & Brook, 1985; Jones, Fox, Babigian, & Hutton, 1980; Kendell, Hall, Hailey, & Babigian, 1973; Szmukler, McCance, McCrone, & Hunter, 1986). We were able to study a population-based sample spanning 50 years because of the unique nature of the Mayo Clinic epidemiologic archive. We did not set arbitrary upper or lower age limits for identifying cases of anorexia nervosa but objectively applied standard diagnostic criteria to possible cases regardless of age. Nor did we confine the study to female patients, as did some other reports (Theander, 1970; Willi & Grossmann, 1983). These methods permitted us to calculate incidence rates for all age groups and for both sexes.

## 2  Background of the Rochester Study

Rochester is a Midwestern U.S. city located on the 44th parallel of latitude, about 75 miles southeast of Minneapolis and St. Paul, the nearest urban areas. Its population was approximately 23,000 in 1935 and 60,000 in 1985. Although the local economy once was based chiefly on farming and light industry, the Mayo Medical Center and International Business Machines (IBM) became the largest employers in the city. The homogeneous population is primarily of northern European origin. In 1980, the racial composition was 98% white. Compared with the U.S. population as a whole, there was a relatively greater proportion of female residents between the ages of 15 and 25 years. Population-based epidemiologic research is possible in Rochester because medical care is virtually self-contained within the community and is delivered by a small number of providers. Most of the health care is provided by the Mayo Clinic, which has maintained a common medical record system with its two large affiliated hospitals (Saint Marys and Rochester Methodist) during the past 85 years. Although best known as a referral center, the Mayo Clinic has always provided much of the primary care and almost all of the specialty care in the area.

The Mayo Clinic dossier-type medical record contains both inpatient and outpatient data and is easily retrievable for review. By 1985, the records of nearly 4 million patients, including referral patients from outside the local area, had been collected and preserved. The diagnoses and surgical procedures entered into these records are indexed. The index includes the diagnoses made for outpatient office or clinic consultations, emergency room visits, nursing home care, hospitalizations, autopsy examinations, and death certification (Kurland & Molgaard, 1981). The medical records of the other medical care providers in the area who serve the local population and surrounding Olmsted County are also indexed and are retrievable. Thus, all details of the medical care provided to the residents of Olmsted County are available for study through this archive (the Rochester Epidemiology Project), which links the medical records of patients seen at the Mayo Clinic and its affiliated hospitals with the records from the Olmsted Medical Group, Olmsted Community Hospital, and other health care providers in the surrounding area.

## 3 Methods

Using this unique database, we screened for approximately 30 diagnostic terms, particularly for amenorrhea, oligomenorrhea, starvation and weight loss from any cause, and anorexia nervosa (Table 1) (Lucas et al., 1991). From 13,559 medical records that were screened, 213 patients were identified who had been residents of Rochester for at least 1 year and who met the criteria of the *Diagnostic and Statistical Manual of Mental Disorders* (DSM-III) and of the Pathology of Eating Group report (American Psychiatric Association, 1980; Garrow et al., 1976). At the time that most records were reviewed, the third edition of the *Diagnostic and Statistical Manual of Mental Disorders* (DSM-III) was in use. Its criteria specified a weight loss of at least 25%. The broader criterion of a weight loss of 15% specified in the 1987 revision of the DSM criteria (DSM-III-R) (American Psychiatric Association, 1987) was adopted before record review was completed, and this standard was applied to the records that had already been reviewed, before the final identification of cases was made. The broader standard specified in DSM-III-R seemed more appropriate for adolescent subjects. Our criteria approximated those established by Russell (1970), whose three cardinal features formed the basis of the Pathology of Eating Group criteria. Thus, our inclusion criteria were also similar to those specified by Szmukler and co-workers (Szmukler, McCance, McCrone, & Hunter, 1986), and our patient group was diagnostically similar to theirs.

Table 1. Diagnostic Categories Reviewed to Identify All Cases of Anorexia Nervosa in Rochester, Minnesota, 1935 Through 1984

| Diagnostic category | Number of records screened | Cases of anorexia nervosa identified N | % |
|---|---|---|---|
| Anorexia nervosa | 231 | 97 | 42.0 |
| Anorexia | 826 | 15 | 1.8 |
| Amenorrhea | 3,789 | 70 | 1.8 |
| Oligomenorrhea | 878 | 14 | 1.6 |
| Anovulation, irregular menstruation, menstrual dysfunction | 2,120 | 5 | 0.2 |
| Ovarian dysfunction, hypo-ovarianism | 607 | 3 | 0.5 |
| Delayed puberty, delayed menarche | 428 | 1 | 0.2 |
| Delayed menstruation | 181 | 2 | 1.1 |
| Starvation, weight loss, underweight, malnutrition | 1,483 | 51 | 3.4 |
| Inadequate diet | 1,775 | 4 | 0.2 |
| Nutritional disturbance, marasmus | 377 | 0 | 0.0 |
| Anasarca, edema, hydrops | 138 | 0 | 0.0 |
| Addison's disease | 54 | 0 | 0.0 |
| Simmonds' disease | 52 | 1 | 1.9 |
| Malaise | 61 | 0 | 0.0 |
| Nervous exhaustion | 344 | 1 | 0.3 |
| Nervous stomach, psychogenic gastrointestinal disorder | 12 | 0 | 0.0 |
| Vomiting | 203 | 0 | 0.0 |
| Total | 13,559 | 264[a] | 1.9 |

Note. Data are from Mayo Clinic records and other sources
[a] 213 incidence and prevalence cases were identified; some appeared in more than one diagnostic category
From Lucas et al. 1988. By permission of Mayo Foundation

By carefully reviewing the original medical records retrospectively, we could consistently apply modern diagnostic criteria to the recorded signs and symptoms throughout the 50-year period, when standards for the diagnosis of anorexia nervosa were continually changing. Because the amount of data specified in the medical records was not always complete, we categorized the records as representing definite, probable, or possible cases of anorexia nervosa, as defined in Table 2.

Table 2. Diagnostic Criteria for Definite,[a] Probable,[b] and Possible[c] Cases of Anorexia Nervosa

1. Self-imposed weight loss of at least 15% from prior weight, or weight 15% less than that projected for those still actively growing
2. Amenorrhea in female patients; suggestive evidence of endocrine dysfunction in male patients
3. Psychologic disorder manifested by fear of fatness or loss of control of eating, expressed or implied
4. No physical illness to account for the weight loss

[a] Definite cases: presence of all four criteria
[b] Probable cases: presence of three criteria, including criteria 1 and 4 (either 2 or 3 unknown or absent)
[c] Possible cases: presence of criteria 1 and 4 (both 2 and 3 unknown or absent)

From Lucas et al., 1988. By permission of Mayo Foundation

## 4 Results

In the community-based study of the incidence and prevalence of anorexia nervosa spanning the 50-year period from 1935 through 1984, we found that the disorder began as early as 10 years of age and as late as 57 years of age. It occurred much more commonly in female than in male subjects. By far the most common age at onset in girls was between 15 and 19 years, as shown in the age distribution graph (Figure 1). A smaller number of subjects had onset before age 15. Half the subjects had onset before 20 years of age, and these are the subjects described herein. This chapter focuses on incidence in the adolescent and preadolescent patients, those in whom anorexia nervosa began from 10 through 19 years of age. Thus, premenarchal subjects are included, as are those in the adolescent age group.

Because the upper age of adolescence is not clearly demarcated, some subjects whose onset was in their early 20s might have legitimately been included among the adolescents; however, they were not. Age 20 years was used as the arbitrary upper limit of adolescence.

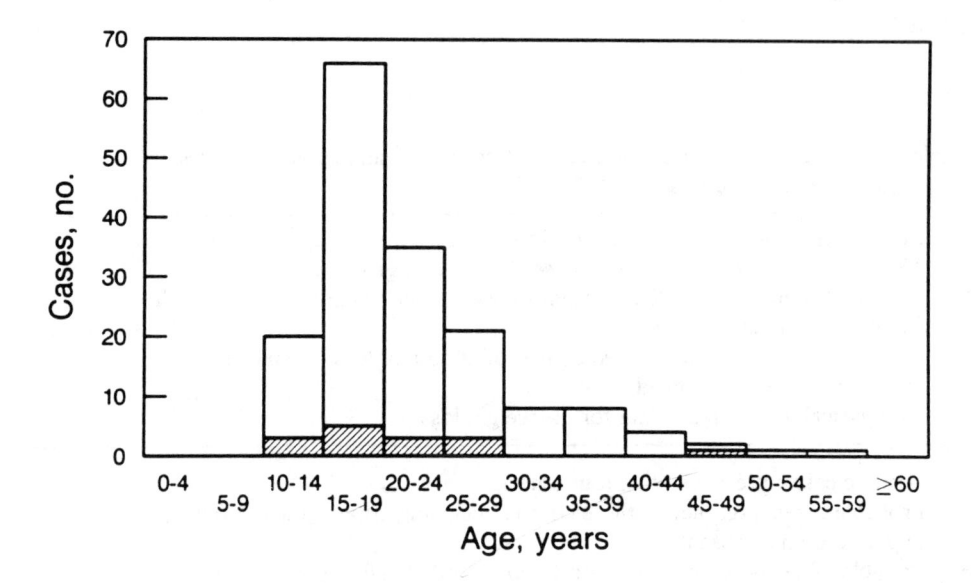

Figure 1. Age at diagnosis of anorexia nervosa from 1935 through 1984 among female and male residents of Rochester, Minnesota. Hatched bars, male subjects. (From Lucas et al., 1988. By permission of Mayo Foundation.)

Ninety-four subjects (86 female and 8 male) were younger than 20 years when anorexia nervosa developed. The incidence for female and male subjects by quinquennia is shown in Table 3, and the trend in incidence for female subjects is shown in Figure 2. In the few male patients with anorexia nervosa, the diagnoses were made sporadically during the study period.

Table 3. Age- and Sex-Specific Incidence Rates (per 100,000 Person-Years[a]) for Anorexia Nervosa Among 10- Through 19-Year-Old Residents of Rochester, Minnesota

| | Age 10-14 years | | | | Age 15-19 years | | | |
|---|---|---|---|---|---|---|---|---|
| | Female | | Male | | Female | | Male | |
| Years | N | Incidence | N | Incidence | N | Incidence | N | Incidence |
| 1935-39 | 5 | 104.2 | 2 | 45.5 | 1 | 17.1 | 0 | 0 |
| 1940-44 | 1 | 25.3 | 0 | 0 | 3 | 50.3 | 1 | 23.8 |
| 1945-49 | 1 | 27.8 | 0 | 0 | 5 | 78.3 | 0 | 0 |
| 1950-54 | 0 | 0 | 1 | 21.2 | 2 | 27.2 | 0 | 0 |
| 1955-59 | 0 | 0 | 0 | 0 | 3 | 34.2 | 0 | 0 |
| 1960-64 | 0 | 0 | 0 | 0 | 5 | 48.0 | 0 | 0 |
| 1965-69 | 1 | 8.7 | 0 | 0 | 11 | 92.4 | 0 | 0 |
| 1970-74 | 3 | 23.7 | 0 | 0 | 7 | 54.1 | 1 | 9.6 |
| 1975-79 | 4 | 33.8 | 0 | 0 | 10 | 75.1 | 1 | 8.5 |
| 1980-84 | 5 | 51.8 | 0 | 0 | 19 | 155.9 | 2 | 17.9 |
| 1935-84 | 20 | 25.7 | 3 | 3.7 | 66 | 69.4 | 5 | 7.3 |

[a] Same as cases per year per 100,000 population

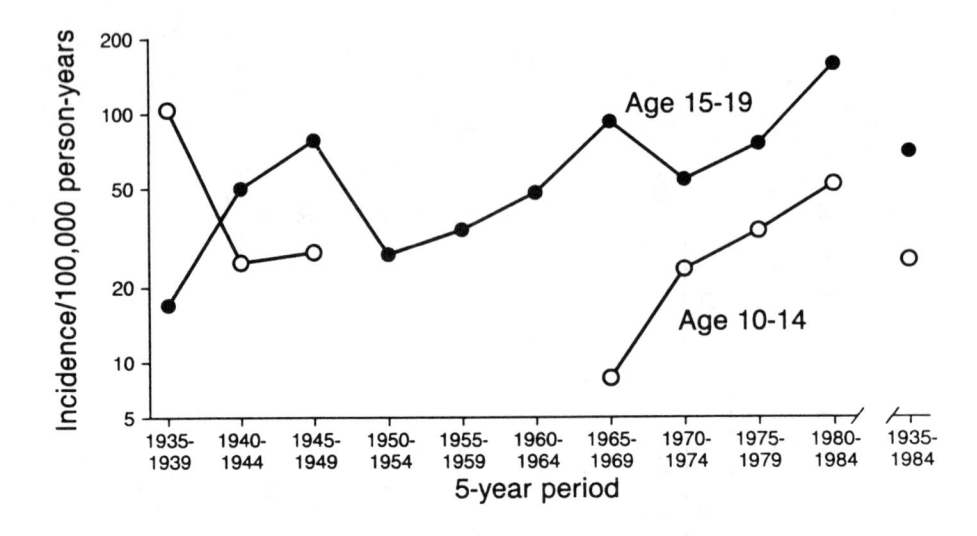

Figure 2. Incidence of anorexia nervosa for female subjects, ages 10 through 19 years, from 1935 through 1984 in Rochester, Minnesota.

There was an increasing trend for female subjects 15 through 19 years of age from 1935 through 1984 and for female subjects 10 through 14 years of age after 1965. A relatively large number of female subjects and male subjects 10 through 14 years of age were identified in the early years of the study--1935 through 1949. Because this group of young subjects with anorexia in the first 15 years of the study did not follow the typical increasing trend and were overly represented in the early years of the study, we scrutinized their medical histories more closely to determine whether they had any features in common and whether they differed from other subjects with anorexia nervosa. The group was composed of nine young subjects with anorexia nervosa, seven girls and two boys.

## 5 The Atypical Subgroup (1935 - 1949)

In the seven female subjects, the diagnostic certainty was definite in one, probable in five, and possible in one. In the two male subjects, the diagnostic certainty was probable in one and possible in one. Diagnostic certainty in the early years of the study was less definite than in the more recent years, when it was more likely that the patients would have been seen by a psychiatrist and information about psychological features of the illness was available. In the pre-World War II years, subjects in our study had not been seen by psychiatrists. Thus, there was less description about attitudes toward weight and body image.

### 5.1 Case Histories (Table 4)[1]

### 5.1.1 Patient One

Poor appetite and sluggish bowels developed in this patient at age 6 years, 2 weeks after she had had mumps. She was 44 inches tall and weighed 37 pounds, a weight considered 5 pounds below normal. By age 11 years, she had grown to 54 inches but weighed only 56 pounds, below the 5th percentile for age. She was considered 15 pounds underweight by her pediatrician and described as "poorly nourished [with] poor appetite and rather apprehensive." It was then that her condition was diagnosed as undernourished. The pediatrician noted, "Appetite has been poor this spring. Some better since receiving medication for appetite." By age 17 years she was 64 inches tall (50th percentile) and weighed 107 pounds (15th percentile). Results of her physical examination were normal, but she reported dizziness on rising. She was doing poorly in school and had frequent absences, but she was obsessed with exercise, walking up the stairs to the 10th floor for her doctor's appointment. Her weight remained near 100 pounds until age 35, when she began gaining weight rather rapidly. During the next 2 years she gained 40 pounds. At age 46 she weighed 164 pounds, and obesity was diagnosed. At age 50 she was 65 1/2 inches tall and weighed 170 pounds. She had graduated from high school and completed 3 years of college. She was married for 23 years and widowed at age 62. She had two children and worked for almost 40 years as a bookkeeper.

---

[1]Height and weight data are given in the U.S. system of inches and pounds, as originally recorded in the medical records of the 1930s and 1940s.

Table 4. Demographic Characteristics of 10- Through 14-Year-Old Residents of Rochester, Minnesota, With Atypical Anorexia Nervosa, 1935 Through 1949

| Patient | Sex | DOB[a] | Date at diagnosis[b] | Age at onset | Original diagnosis | Diagnostic certainty |
|---|---|---|---|---|---|---|
| 1 | F | 6/24 | 8/35 | 11 yr 2 mo | Undernutrition | Probable |
| 2 | M | 12/22 | 8/35 | 14 yr 8 mo | Delayed puberty | Probable |
| 3 | F | 4/25 | 2/37 | 11 yr 10 mo | Anorexia nervosa | Probable |
| 4 | F | 7/26 | 8/37 | 11 yr 1 mo | Malnutrition | Probable |
| 5 | F | 2/25 | 8/38 | 13 yr 6 mo | Starvation | Probable |
| 6 | F | 1/27 | 3/39 | 12 yr 2 mo | Malnutrition | Definite |
| 7 | M | 7/24 | 4/39 | 14 yr 9 mo | Underweight | Possible |
| 8 | F | 2/29 | 12/40 | 11 yr 10 mo | Malnutrition | Probable |
| 9 | F | 1/31 | 1/45 | 14 yr 0 mo | Delayed menstruation | Possible |

[a] Date of birth, month/year
[b] Month/year

## 5.1.2 Patient 2

One of the male subjects was a rachitic infant found to have marked craniotabes of the occipital bones at age 4 1/2 months. Petit mal seizures developed when he was 2 years of age, and these were treated with phenytoin and phenobarbital. At age 5 years he was reported not to be eating well. He was an awkward child who had difficulty learning from the beginning of his schooling. His weight remained adequate until age 12. Then, over an 8-month period, he lost 3 pounds, and his weight category decreased from the 25th to the 5th percentile (71 pounds), and he was considered malnourished with delayed puberty. Psychometric testing revealed an IQ of 75. His weight remained just below the 5th percentile until age 22, when he began steadily to gain weight. His highest recorded weight was 152 pounds at age 43. He completed 11th grade and worked as a bellhop and desk clerk at hotels. He was married for 26 years and had five children. He was widowed at age 67. Eventually he resided in a nursing home.

## 5.1.3 Patient 3

The patient was colicky and a fussy eater as an infant. Her mother reported frequent constipation during the first 5 years of life, and her pediatrician noted that the mother seemed overconcerned about bowel function. When the patient was age 5 years, her mother became concerned about her daughter's poor posture and about her nutrition, although her weight was average. Weight gain then decelerated between age 9 and 11 years, and her weight percentile declined from the 35th to the 15th percentile. Several somatic complaints developed, mostly gastrointestinal. This condition resulted in frequent absences from school. The patient often cried before going to school and became especially upset when a boy became ill at school. Her pediatrician diagnosed anorexia nervosa at that time and described her as emotionally unstable. At age 12, colloid goiter was diagnosed because of an enlarged thyroid gland; it was treated with potassium iodide solution. An endocrinologist recommended subtotal thyroidectomy, which was done at age 13. Subsequently, she was treated with thyroid extract, 2 grains daily, and her weight increased to the 30th percentile. When she graduated from high school, she weighed 117 pounds (30th percentile) and was 67 inches tall (85th percentile). She attended a competitive college and subsequently earned a master's degree at a university. She began a professional career but developed what was called postinfection exhaustion state. She never married and had no children. In adulthood, her weight gradually increased and reached 136 pounds in middle age. At age 65 she retired from a long career. She had continued to gain weight and weighed 202 pounds at age 68.

### 5.1.4 Patient 4

At age 3 1/2 years, this child was noted to have a poor appetite. Nonetheless, her weight was at the 50th percentile, and her pediatrician described her as chubby. At age 11, after returning from camp, she was seen by her pediatrician because of concerns about her weight, which had declined to the 10th percentile. She was reported to have "lost a lot of weight and had a poor appetite." Malnutrition was diagnosed. She was seen and weighed weekly by the pediatrician for the next year and encouraged to gain weight and to restrict her high activity. Her father, a physician, threatened to hospitalize her and feed her through tubes if she did not gain weight. She gradually gained weight to the 20th percentile by age 12. During her teen years she remained thin, between the 10th and 25th percentiles, and healthy. Her weight at age 18 was 110 pounds, and her height was 65 inches. Her parents persisted in their concerns about her appetite and food intake. She married at age 26 and had four children. She completed two years of college and worked in an office until she retired at age 65. She maintained her slender, athletic build throughout life.

### 5.1.5 Patient 5

This patient was described as pale and underweight at the time of a tonsillectomy and adenoidectomy at age 4, although both height and weight were at the 25th percentile. In the following year, concern about her pale and apathetic appearance, poor muscle tone, and poor posture continued. At age 13, her height was 60 1/2 inches (25th percentile), but her weight was only 75 pounds (less than the 5th percentile). She had a 2-week history of enuresis, and she was noted to be very high-strung and nervous. Her pediatrician commented that she was working too hard in school and was overinvolved in her studies and music lessons. Weight loss and starvation were diagnosed. Her pediatrician recommended that she not attend school for 6 to 12 months and that she have rest periods in both the morning and the afternoon. Six months later, she was much less nervous and had gained more than 13 pounds. Her weight was 89 pounds (10th percentile). Her weight improvement continued during the next year. At age 14 1/2 years, she weighed 97 pounds (20th percentile) and was described as much less nervous. She graduated from high school as an honor student and studied economics in college. However, while at college, she had an emotional breakdown, manifested by panic and preoccupation with religious thoughts. Agitated depression requiring psychiatric hospitalization was diagnosed. She responded well to electroconvulsive treatments. Her weight varied between 108 and 117 pounds. She married and had two children, but she had another breakdown at age 31 with religious preoccupation.

### 5.1.6 Patient 6

The patient was seen at age 8 years because of a 2 1/2-month history of poor appetite and loss of weight. She had a high level of activity, riding her bicycle much of each day. Her diet consisted of toast, coffee, and bacon. She refused to eat vegetables or fruit. Her height was at the 85th percentile, but she had lost 6 pounds, and her weight was at the 20th percentile. Her pediatrician prescribed a strict program of rest, discontinuation of coffee, and no school for the following year. By age 12 years, her weight had increased to 71 1/2 pounds, but her weight percentile had declined to the 10th percentile. She was described as nervous, fearful of school, crying a great deal, and eating poorly. It was then that malnutrition was diagnosed, and it was recommended that she be hospitalized for 3 to 4 weeks in order to learn to rest, to eat, and to overcome her morbid fears. She had gained 4 pounds with the threat of hospitalization but lost 2 pounds in the hospital. Despite the recommendations for a longer stay, she left the hospital after 5 days. She graduated from high school and went on to a university. She achieved an adult weight of 125 pounds, was married at age 24, and had three children. Her mother died of liver cancer when the patient was 22 years of age. At age 27 her weight decreased to 114 pounds, attributed to emotional stress associated with financial difficulties. By age 30 she had regained weight to 127 pounds. She died at age 41 of cancer.

### 5.1.7 Patient 7

At age 14 years 9 months, this male patient lost 6 pounds during a 2-week period while attending scout camp. He was tall for his age, at the 75th percentile. His pediatrician diagnosed him as underweight (weight was at the 20th percentile). He had previously lost 3 pounds at age 13 but had increased his weight to the 50th percentile by the age of 14 years. He was seen for weekly weighing during the next 3 months and managed to gain weight rapidly. Within 6 months his weight had increased to the 30th percentile. He continued to grow and gain weight (to around the 25th percentile), weighing somewhat more than 130 pounds as he reached adulthood, and attaining a height of 71 inches. At age 30 years he again lost a significant amount of weight, to 118 pounds, and was seen by an internist expert in the diagnosis and treatment of anorexia nervosa, who did not regard the weight loss as pathological.

### 5.1.8 Patient 8

The patient was examined 2 months before her 12th birthday, presenting with the complaint of abdominal pain after meals. She was 21 pounds underweight. Her height was near the 50th percentile, and her weight was at the 10th percentile. Her pediatrician, who diagnosed malnutrition, recommended that she eat more and that she take daily rest periods for 2 hours before lunch and again after lunch until mid-afternoon. It is not known whether she followed these instructions, but 10 months later she had gained only 3 1/2 pounds, which was a decline to the 5th weight percentile. At age 18 years she was hospitalized for lower abdominal pain and nocturia, but her weight was not recorded. Little is known about her subsequent weight history or adjustment until age 31 years, at which time she weighed 106 pounds and had had four children. She presented with left lower quadrant pain. Her adult height was 67 inches. She had two more children, and at age 43 years she weighed 137 pounds. By age 62 her weight had increased to 149 1/2 pounds.

### 5.1.9 Patient 9

The patient was examined at age 14 years with symptoms of tiredness, headache, and dizzy spells, having lost 12 pounds, to a weight of 102 pounds, in 4 months. She had had one menstrual period, lasting only 1 day, almost 2 years before. She had secondary sexual characteristics but an infantile uterus. Delayed menstruation was diagnosed. No treatment was given. When she was next seen again at age 15 years 10 months, she weighed 123 pounds, was 66 inches tall, and was menstruating. She had completed the 11th grade and was married at age 17 years.

At age 18 years, her first child was born. Her young adult weight fluctuated between 130 and 140 pounds. At age 28 years she was seen by a psychiatrist because of premenstrual irritability and temper outbursts. She lived on a farm and had four children. Character neurosis with underlying hostility and psychosexual conflicts was diagnosed. She weighed 155 pounds at age 43 years, and at age 60 she weighed 147 pounds. Two malignancies had developed: colon cancer and basal cell carcinoma. Both were successfully treated.

## 5.2 Summary of Patients

These nine patients, in whom onset of disease was before age 15 years and who had the condition before 1950, were reviewed in detail because they stood out as an overrepresentation of this age group in the early years of the study. What did these young subjects have in common? Considerable clinical diversity was present in this small group. Depression may have played a role in some. Most notably, however, in several cases, the pediatricians who treated the children and the parents of the children seemed overconcerned about dietary habits and apparent poor appetite from an early age, even at times when these children were within the normal range for height and weight. When the children's weight decreased slightly below norms, a great deal of concern was expressed. The pediatric recommendation invariably was for lengthy rest periods and improved nutrition. At times the children were even taken out of school in order to relearn how to rest and to eat. One wonders whether the overconcern expressed by adults in the 1930s and early 1940s may not have reinforced food refusal, which might have resolved with a less rigid attitude about nutrition.

Two women became obese. Three women and one man became normal in weight. Two women and one man remained slender, but none became chronically anorexic.

Infertility was not a common outcome in this group. On the contrary, one woman had six children and one man fathered five. Two women each had four children. Three other women each had two or three children. Only one woman and one man remained single and childless.

In some of these patients, the two who became obese and the ones who remained slender in adulthood, we had the sense that there was biologic pressure to gain weight, which these children were resisting. We have seen a subgroup of pubertal anorexic children among our clinical referral cases whose intense desire to diet, and whose fear of gaining weight, was realistically based on their awareness that their weight gain was accelerating and that they were at risk of becoming obese. These children and young adolescents may legitimately be identified as having a realistic fear of fatness.

It is of interest that none of the nine patients in the atypical subgroup received the intense psychological treatment that is now considered necessary. Several were exhorted by their pediatricians to eat, and at least one was threatened by her parents. One was hospitalized on a pediatric unit but refused to stay. Others received little or no formal treatment, but they probably did receive benign encouragement to gain weight. Weight outcome in this group of cases was better than that reported in most clinical series of anorexia nervosa. In two patients, psychiatric conditions (most likely depressive disorders) developed when they were adults.

## 6 Conclusions

The incidence of anorexia nervosa in 15- through 19-year-old female adolescent residents of Rochester, Minnesota, showed an increasing trend over the 50-year period from 1935 through 1984. The incidence increased from 17.1 per 100,000 person-years in 1935 through 1939 to 155.9 in 1980 through 1984. A similar increasing trend was found for 10- through 14-year-old female subjects from 1965 through 1984; the lower incidence rates in this age group increased from 8.7 per 100,000 person-years in 1965 through 1969 to 51.8 in 1980 through 1984. A group with an atypical decreasing trend in incidence was identified in 10- through 14-year-old girls from 1935 through 1949. That group was heterogeneous in clinical presentation and in the clinical course after diagnosis. It was apparent that during the 1930s and 1940s physicians and parents were acutely attuned to and concerned about even minor changes in children's eating habits.

The overall incidence in 15- through 19-year-old female subjects during the 50-year period was 69.4 per 100,000 person-years. In 15- through 19-year-old male subjects it was 7.3. The overall incidence in 10- through 14-year-old girls during the 50-year period was 25.7 per 100,000 person-years. In 10- through 14-year-old boys it was 3.7.

The study confirmed the general assumption that anorexia nervosa is predominantly a disorder of adolescent girls and that the incidence of anorexia nervosa in adolescent girls has increased over time since 1935. Since 1965 the incidence of premenarchal anorexia nervosa also has increased. A relatively large number of female and male patients with mild anorexia nervosa were identified in the early years of the study, 1935 through 1949, when physicians and parents were very concerned about minor deviations in weight and eating habits of children.

## References

American Psychiatric Association. (1980). *Diagnostic and statistical manual of mental disorders* (3rd ed.). (pp. 67-69). Washington, DC: American Psychiatric Association.
American Psychiatric Association. (1987). *Diagnostic and statistical manual of mental disorders* (3rd ed. rev.). (pp. 65-67). Washington, DC: American Psychiatric Association.
Brems, O. (1963). Anorexia nervosa. *Ugeskrift For Laeger, 125*, 821-828.
Garrow, J.S., Crisp, A.H., Jordan, H.A., Meyer, J.-E., Russell, G.F.M., Silverstone, T., Stunkard, A.J., & Van Itallie, T. B. (1976). Pathology of Eating Group report. In T. Silverstone (Ed.), *Appetite and food intake: Report of the Dahlem Workshop on Appetite and Food Intake* (pp. 405-416). Berlin: Abakon.
Hoek, H.W., & Brook, F.G. (1985). Patterns of care of anorexia nervosa. *Journal of Psychiatric Research, 19*, 155-160.
Innes, G., & Sharp, G. A. (1962). A study of psychiatric patients in North-East Scotland. *Journal of Mental Science, 108*, 447-456.
Jones, D.J., Fox, M. M., Babigian, H.M., & Hutton, H.E. (1980). Epidemiology of anorexia nervosa in Monroe County, New York: 1960-1976. *Psychosomatic Medicine, 42*, 551-558.
Kendell, R.E., Hall, D.J., Hailey, A., & Babigian H.M. (1973). The epidemiology of anorexia nervosa. *Psychological Medicine, 3*, 200-203.
Kidd, C.B., & Wood, J.F. (1966). Some observations on anorexia nervosa. *Postgraduate Medical Journal, 42*, 443-448.
Kurland, L.T., & Molgaard, C.A. (1981). The patient record in epidemiology. *Scientific American, 245*, 54-63.
Lucas, A.R., Beard, C.M., O'Fallon, W.M., & Kurland, L.T. (1988). Anorexia nervosa in Rochester, Minnesota: A 45-year study. *Mayo Clinic Proceedings, 63*, 433-442.
Lucas, A.R., Beard, C.M., O'Fallon, W.M., & Kurland, L.T. (1991). 50-Year trends in the incidence of anorexia nervosa in Rochester, Minn.: A population-based study. *American Journal of Psychiatry, 148*, 917-922.
Russell, G.F.M. (1970). Anorexia nervosa: Its identity as an illness and its treatment. In J. H. Price (Ed.). *Modern trends in psychological medicine* (Vol. 2) (pp. 131-164). London: Butterworth.
Szmukler, G., McCance, C., McCrone, L., & Hunter, D. (1986). Anorexia nervosa: A psychiatric case register study from Aberdeen. *Psychological Medicine, 16*, 49-58.
Theander, S. (1970). Anorexia nervosa: a psychiatric investigation of 94 female patients. *Acta Psychiatrica Scandinavica, 214 Suppl*, 1-194.
Willi, J., & Grossmann, S. (1983). Epidemiology of anorexia nervosa in a defined region of Switzerland. *American Journal of Psychiatry, 140*, 564-567.

# A Population Study of Bulima Nervosa and Subclinical Eating Disorders in Adolescence

*Martine F. Flament, Sylvie Ledoux, Philippe Jeammet, Marie Choquet, and Yves Simon*

Bulimic behaviors have been reported in the psychiatric and psychoanalytic literature for more than a century. However, it was only in the late 1970s that "bulimia nervosa" was identified and described as a distinct clinical disorder occurring mainly in young women (Russell, 1979; Igoin, 1979). Most clinicians now agree on three core features of the disorder: bulimia is characterized by uncontrolled and recurrent eating binges in subjects who are, nevertheless, overly concerned about their weight and body shape; as a result, they are led to adopt extreme compensatory weight control strategies of purging type (self-induced vomiting, use of laxatives or diuretics) and/or restricting type (dieting, fasting, rigourous exercise).

Clinical experience has shown that bulimic and associated problematic behaviors are often kept secret for many years, and patients only seek help when the disorder has reached unmanageable levels. By that time, the symptomatic behaviors are well entrenched, and associated difficulties and social incapacitation have begun to develop. Most patients come for treatment in their mid-twenties, whereas the disorder had started, on average, at around 18 years of age (Flament et al., in press).

Therefore, the study of clinical and subclinical forms of bulimia nervosa in the general adolescent population should bring important information on the prevalence and clinical features of the disorder in its early stage.

## 1  Studies of the Epidemiology of Bulimia Nervosa in Adolescents

We reviewed eighteen published studies on the prevalence and clinical features of bulimia nervosa in adolescents from the community. All have been conducted among secondary school students. Table 1 summarizes the results obtained.

The first group of studies (Pope et al., 1984; Lachenmeyer & Muni-Brander, 1988; Gross & Rosen, 1988; Whitaker et al., 1990; Dacey et al., 1990; Raich et al., 1992; De Azevedo & Ferreira, 1992), defining bulimia according to either DSM-III criteria (American Psychiatric Association, 1980) or Russell criteria (Russell, 1979), do not include any frequency criterion for bulimic binges. As shown, the obtained prevalence rates vary greatly and are sometimes surprisingly high for a pathology that was previously almost "unknown": 1% to 10% of the girls, 0% to 5% of the boys.

In the second series of studies (Crowther et al., 1985; Maceyko & Nagelberg, 1985; Greenfeld et al., 1987; Mumford & Whitehouse, 1988; Johnson et al., 1984; Johnson et al., 1989; Timmerman et al., 1990; Szabo & Tury, 1991; Ledoux et al., 1991), the diagnosis includes a frequency criterion of at least one binge a week--two binges a week for DSM-III-R criteria (American Psychiatric Association, 1987). Prevalence rates obtained are lower but still heterogeneous: 0.6% to 4.7% of all adolescent girls surveyed.

These studies, carried out in high school populations, have the advantage of obtaining, with a few exceptions, excellent response rates (over 80% in two-thirds of the studies), but they exclude institutionalized adolescents and school dropouts, who might be expected to have higher rates of emotional disorders in general.

Most studies have relied exclusively upon self-report questionnaires. This is obviously the most feasible procedure for studying relatively rare disorders but, of course, the method carries some uncertainty, especially because several of the central features of bulimia nervosa present some difficulties of definition and interpretation: binge eating might not have a generally accepted specific meaning, and assessing whether subjects have "overvalued" ideas toward shape and weight is difficult. However, in the one study (Whitaker et al., 1990) including a test of the efficiency of the screening instrument, the screening properties of the questionnaire were satisfactory (sensitivity: 87%; specificity: 73%).

Overall, as methodology has improved, sample sizes have increased, and diagnostic criteria for bulimia nervosa have been refined, the obtained prevalence rates have become lower and more consistent across studies.

The wide majority of studies were conducted in the United States. The only study to compare an American sample to a Spanish sample (Raich et al., 1992) shows a lower rate of "symptoms suggestive of bulimia nervosa" (based on the Eating Attitude Test) in Europe. Differences might be related to cultural differences in weight and eating, as well as to less specific factors such as family interactions, the development of adolescent autonomy, etc.

One American study (Rasic Lachenmeyer & Muni-Brander, 1988) attempted to assess bulimic symptoms in the populations of two high schools that differed in their cultural and socio-economic background. One school was attended mainly by minority students from Hispanic, Black, or Asian origin who belonged to lower or middle socio-economic classes. In the other school, students were primarily white American adolescents from upper or upper-middle socio-economic classes. The investigators found no ethnic differences. There was significantly more binge eating and greater use of diuretics and diet pills among subjects of higher socio-economic status, but no significant difference for the diagnosis of bulimia.

Anorexia nervosa and bulimia nervosa are commonly said to be related to western attitudes towards body shape, weight, and dieting behaviour. A study of secondary school students on an island of Azores (De Azevedo & Ferreira, 1992) showed that adolescents living in an isolated, insular community in the middle of the Atlantic, who might be assumed to be relatively free of the socio-cultural pressures to control eating and weight that prevail in western industrialized countries, indeed do have low rates of eating disorders (0.3% of the girls and 0% of the boys received a diagnosis of bulimia nervosa). In the United Kingdom, a study comparing (in very small samples) adolescent girls from western and Asian origin showed a higher prevalence among the Asian girls (Mumford & Whitehouse, 1988). This unexpected finding suggested that immigrants might be rapidly adopting western patterns of reaction to stress.

Contrary to the common assumption that prevalence of bulimia nervosa has been on a rise during the last decade, one study repeated five years apart in the same high school (Johnson et al., 1984; Johnson et al., 1989) did not find an increase -but, rather, a decrease- in bulimic attitudes and behaviors among high school girls

Table 1. Studies of the Epidemiology of Bulimia Nervosa in Adolescents

| Study | Country | No. Subjects surveyed | % Target population | Method | Diagnostic criteria | Prevalence Girls | Prevalence Boys |
|---|---|---|---|---|---|---|---|
| *DSM-III or Russell criteria* | | | | | | | |
| Pope et al., 1984 | US | 262 | 85% | questionnaire | DSM-III | 8.4% | 0% |
| Lachenmeyer & Muni-Brander, 1988 | US | 328 G/ 384 B [a]<br>306 G/ 243 B [b] | nr | questionnaire | DSM-III | 9.7%<br>7.6% | 5.7%<br>2.1% |
| Gross & Rosen, 1988 | US | 677 G<br>653 B | 82% | questionnaire | DSM-III+<br>1 binge/mo | 9.6% | 1.6% |
| Whitaker et al., 1990 | US | 2544 G<br>2564 B | 91% (Q)<br>76% (I) | questionnaire [c]<br>+ interview | DSM-III | 4.2% | 0.2% |
| Dacey et al., 1990 | US | 260 G | 54% | questionnaire<br>+ interview | Russell | 5.8% | - |
| Raich et al., 1992 | US | 713 G/ 660 B | 85% | questionnaire | "bulimic symptoms" | 3.5% | 0.2% |
| | Spain | 1868 G/ 1676 B | 97% | | | 0.9% | 0.1% |
| De Azevedo & Ferreira, 1992 | Azores | 654 G<br>580 B | 81% | interview | DSM-III | 0.3% | 0% |
| *DSM-III criteria + frequency criterion, or DSM-III-R criteria* | | | | | | | |
| Crowther et al., 1985 | US | 363 G | 34% | questionnaire | DSM-III+<br>1 binge/wk | 2.8% | - |
| Maceyko & Nagelberg, 1985 | US | 168 G<br>89 B | nr | questionnaire | DSM-III+<br>1 binge/wk | 4.7% | 0% |

Table 1. continued

| Study | Country | no. Subjects surveyed | % Target population | Method | Diagnostic criteria | Prevalence Girls | Boys |
|---|---|---|---|---|---|---|---|
| *DSM-III criteria + frequency criterion, or DSM-III-R criteria, continued* | | | | | | | |
| Greenfeld et al., 1987 | US | 337 G / 424 B | 86% | questionnaire | DSM-III 1 binge/wk | 4.0% | 0.8% |
| Mumford & Whitehouse, 1988 | UK | 204 G (Asian) / 355 G (white) | 69% (Q) / 75% (I) | questionnaire +interview | DSM-III-R | 3.4% / 0.6% | - / - |
| Johnson et al., 1984 | US | 1268 G [d] | 98% | questionnaire | DSM-III+ 1 binge/wk | 4.9% | - |
| Johnson et al., 1989 | US | 1085 G [d] | 96% | questionnaire | DSM-III+ 1 binge/wk | 2.0% | - |
| Timmerman et al., 1990 | US | 686 G / 705 B | 98% | questionnaire | DSM-III-R | 2.0% | 0.1% |
| Szabo & Tury, 1991 | Hungary | 416 G / 119 B | 42% | questionnaire | DSM-III-R | 0% | 0% |
| Ledoux et al., 1991 | France | 1729 G / 1551 B | 93% | questionnaire | DSM-III-R | 1.1% | 0.2% |

Note. G = girls, B = boys; Q = questionnaire, I = interview; nr = not reported.
[a] From lower/middle socio-economic classes, [b] From upper middle/upper socio-economic classes.
[c] With test of efficiency of the screening instrument.
[d] The two samples were drawn five years apart from the same suburban high school.

from 1981 to 1986, with the estimated prevalence of clinically significant cases decreasing from 4.1% to 2.0%.

We will decribe results from a study conducted in secondary schools of the southern part of the Haute-Marne department in France. The aims of the study were to investigate normal and pathological eating behaviors in adolescents, to estimate the prevalence rate of bulimia nervosa in this age group, and to describe the symptomatic presentation of clinical and, possibly, preclinical forms of the disorder, associated features, and psychosocial impairment.

## 2 The Haute-Marne Study

### 2.1 Methods

The study followed a two-stage design: A self-report questionnaire was first administered to a large, unselected school population; then individual clinical interviews were conducted with subgroups of subjects who were selected on the basis of their answers to the initial questionnaire. The entire procedure took place over two school years.

#### 2.1.1 Stage I: Whole Population Survey

All students (N = 3527) from 153 classes that were randomly selected in the junior high schools, high schools, and vocational schools of the Chaumont and Langres districts in the department of Haute-Marne were asked to participate in the study. We designed a self-report questionnaire including 280 questions on different areas of physical and emotional health, family, school, life events, and treatment seeking (questionnaire Choquet-Ledoux), and about 20 questions concerning the different symptoms and attitudes that define anorexia nervosa and bulimia nervosa (including DSM-III-R diagnostic criteria for both disorders). Depressive symptoms were assessed on the French version of the Kandel Depressive Mood Inventory (Kandel & Davies, 1982).

The students were asked to fill out the questionnaire in a classroom situation under the supervision of the school nurse. Completion time was one to two hours, according to the student's level. Anonymous questionnaires were sealed and sent to INSERM (U169). Nominative lists with sociodemographic data (sex, date, and place of birth) entered in the questionnaires and kept by the school nurses allowed for identification of students for selection to Stage II interviews.

## 2.1.2 Stage II: Clinical Interviews

Based on answers to the self-report questionnaire, three groups of subjects were selected for Stage II clinical examination. Group 1 consisted of students with at least one of the following: (a) binge eating twice a month or more, feelings of guilt or self-depreciation after binges, and/or one or more weight control strategies; (b) body mass index (BMI) less than or equal to the 3rd percentile for age and sex, amenorrhea, and/or feeling of being too fat; (c) self-induced vomiting at least twice a month; (d) hospitalization for an eating disorder during the 12 months preceding completion of the questionnaire. Group 2 included students with a total score of 17 or 18 (maximum score = 18) on the Kandel Depressive Mood Inventory and those hospitalized for a suicide attempt during the previous 12 months. Group 3 was a control group randomly selected from students not fulfilling criteria for either Group 1 or Group 2 but matched to each subject of these two groups for age, sex, and school level.

For practical reasons, however, students who had changed school from the previous year (including those who had finished school) and students from the smaller schools outside the two main towns of the study district were excluded from selection to Stage II.

Semistructured clinical interviews were conducted in the schools by seven psychiatrists and one clinical psychologist, all blind to each student's screening status. The interview (lasting one hour to one and a half hours) included French translations of the Kiddie-SADS (Chambers et al., 1985) and of the Children's Global Assessment Scale (CGAS) (Shaffer et al., 1983), to which were added sections developed by the authors on eating behaviors and other areas of interest for the current study.

All clinicians had been trained for the interviews; interrater reliability for DSM-III-R diagnoses, assessed by exchanging records between pairs of clinicians, was satisfactory.

## 2.2 Results

### 2.2.1 Stage I

In the selected classes, 3311 students aged 11 to 20 years, i.e., 93.9% of the total population, participated in the survey. Reasons for non-participation were either refusal of the student or his family, or absence from school the day the study took place. A total of 3287 students (93.2% of the student body), completed the questionnaire.

The prevalence of each of the different eating behaviors and attitudes that define bulimia nervosa were first estimated separately (Ledoux et al., 1991). Recurrent bulimic binges (9.8% of the girls), overconcern with body weight and shape (37% of the girls), dieting (18.9% of the girls), self-induced vomiting (2.3% of the girls), use of laxatives (3.1% of the girls) or diet pills (2.3% of the girls) were more frequent in the girls, but also occured in the boys (respectively: 7.2%; 12.4%; 4.2%; 1.6%; 1.5%; 1.3%). Incidence of all these behaviors increased with age for the girls but remained stable -or even decreased with age- for the boys.

The current prevalence rate of bulimia nervosa (DSM-III-R criteria) in the French general adolescent population was estimated to: 1.1% in the girls and 0.2% in the boys.

In general, eating symptoms were associated with a higher frequency of somatic complaints, fatigue, sleeping problems, and depressive symptoms. Socio-economic variables such as marital and socio-professional status of the parents, size of sibship, or school level did not differentiate subjects with eating symptoms from those without.

### 2.2.2 Stage II

Depending on selection groups, between 76% and 91% of subjects selected for clinical interviews were actually interviewed (participation rates not statistically different between groups). This is shown on Table 2. Non-participants included: 15 students who had left school, four who refused the interview, and 14 students who were sick or absent for other reasons for at least two consecutive appointments. The responses to various items of the initial questionnaire (questions on school, somatic problems, conduct disorders, family relationships, etc.) did not differentiate the subjects who were interviewed from those who were not.

Table 2.   Haute-Marne Study : Stage II Design and Completion Rate

| Selection groups | Subjects selected N | Subjects selected % of whole population | Subjects interviewed N | Subjects interviewed % of subjects selected[a] |
|---|---|---|---|---|
| Eating symptoms group | 59 | 1.8 | 45 | 76.3 |
| Depressive symptoms group | 62 | 1.9 | 54 | 87.1 |
| Control group | 121 | 3.7 | 110 | 90.9 |
| Total | 242 | 7.4 | 209 | 86.4 |

[a] Completion rates are not significantly different between groups.

Among the 209 adolescents interviewed, several types of eating disorders were identified:

- Three girls met diagnostic criteria for anorexia nervosa, one for a current episode and two for past episodes.

- Seven subjects, all girls, fulfilled DSM-III-R criteria for a curent or past diagnosis of bulimia nervosa. (All had at least some current symptoms at the time of the interview.)

In addition, without meeting criteria for a clinical diagnosis of an eating disorder, a large number of adolescents reported disturbed eating habits:

- Twenty-one subjects had prandial hyperphagia.

- Ninety subjects regularly ate excessive amounts of food between the meals (excessive snacking).

The other adolescents who were interviewed presented no eating disturbances. Among them, 64 were free of any Axis I psychiatric diagnosis and will be considered in the following analyses as normal controls. Excluding the anorexics because of their small number, we compared bulimics to prandial hyperphagics and snackers, and these three groups to normal controls. Intergroup comparisons are summarized in Tables 3 and 4.

Table 3. Haute-Marne Study : Comparisons Between Bulimics, Prandial Hyperphagics, Snackers and Normal Controls

|  | Bulimia Nervosa (N=7) | Prandial Hyperphagia (N=21) | Snacking (N=90) | Normal Controls (N=64) |
|---|---|---|---|---|
|  | Mean±SD | Mean±SD | Mean±SD | Mean±SD |
| *Age and weight :* | | | | |
| Current age (years) | 18.0±1.2 | 17.3±1.2 | 17.2±1 | 17.4±1.9 |
| Current weight (kg) | 58.6±4.7 | 64.1±12.6 [c] | 58.6±10.3 | 58.7±11.0 |
| Current BMI | 18.2±1.1 | 18.8±3.2 | 17.7±2.7 | 17.8±2.9 |
| *Children Global Asessment Scale (CGAS) :* | | | | |
| CGAS score | 64.1±7.6 [a] | 75.9±13.2 [e] | 80.0±11.5 [e] | 83.7±10.6 |

|  | N | % | N | % | N | % | N | % |
|---|---|---|---|---|---|---|---|---|
| *Sex :* | | | | | | | | |
| Girls | 7 | 100 | 15 | 71 | 67 | 74 | 47 | 73 |
| *Body image / Weight and food preoccupations :* | | | | | | | | |
| Negative body image | 6 | 86 [c] | 12 | 57 [c] | 17 | 19 | 19 | 21 |
| Feeling overweight | 6 | 86 [d] | 13 | 62 [d] | 34 | 38 | 29 | 45 |
| Afraid of gaining weight | 6 | 86 [a] | 14 | 67 | 47 | 52 | 44 | 48 |
| Obsessed with weight | 7 | 100 [c] | 15 | 71 [c] | 36 | 40 | 34 | 37 |
| Obsessed with food | 7 | 100 [a] | 10 | 48 | 39 | 43 | 29 | 32 |
| *Weight control strategies (lifetime use) :* | | | | | | | | |
| Dieting | 7 | 100 [b] | 9 | 43 | 27 | 30 | 16 | 25 |
| Fasting | 3 | 43 [b] | 3 | 14 | 7 | 8 | 3 | 5 |
| Diet pills use | 2 | 29 [b] | 0 | 0 | 1 | 1 | 1 | 2 |
| Laxatives use | 2 | 29 [b] | 0 | 0 | 1 | 1 | 1 | 2 |
| Diuretics use | 1 | 14 [b] | 0 | 0 | 2 | 2 | 0 | 0 |
| Self-induced vomiting | 4 | 57 [b] | 2 | 10 | 6 | 7 | 1 | 2 |
| *Associated psychopathology (lifetime prevalence) :* | | | | | | | | |
| Major depressive disorder | 5 | 71 [c] | 7 | 33 | 16 | 18 | 21 | 24 |
| Dysthymia | 3 | 43 [e] | 3 | 14 | 13 | 15 | 13 | 14 |

Note. BMI (Body Mass Index) = weight / height squared.
[a] Significantly different from Hyperphagics, Snackers and Normal Controls ($p<0.05$).
[b] Significantly different from Hyperphagics and Snackers ($p<0.05$).
[c] Significantly different from Snackers and Normal Controls ($p<0.05$).
[d] Significantly different from Snackers ($p<0.05$).
[e] Significantly different from Normal Controls ($p<0.05$).

Table 4. Haute-Marne Study : Characteristics of Eating Episodes for Bulimics, Prandial Hyperphagics, and Snackers

|  | Bulimia Nervosa N | Bulimia Nervosa % | Prandial Hyperphagia N | Prandial Hyperphagia % | Snacking N | Snacking % |
|---|---|---|---|---|---|---|
| *Onset of episodes :* | | | | | | |
| In late afternoon | 5 | 71 | 8 | 42 | 25 | 40 |
| At home | 7 | 100 | 16 | 84 | 26 | 42 |
| *Mode of eating :* | | | | | | |
| Loss of control over eating | 7 | 100 [a] | 6 | 32 | 13 | 19 |
| Eating alone | 7 | 100 [a] | 5 | 26 | 16 | 26 |
| Eating secretly | 4 | 57 [a] | 1 | 5 | 3 | 5 |
| Eating with no hunger | 5 | 71 | 6 | 32 | 17 | 27 |
| Eating with no pleasure | 5 | 71 [a] | 2 | 10 | 12 | 19 |
| Eating more rapidly than usual | 7 | 100 [a] | 3 | 16 | 8 | 13 |
| *Feelings after episodes :* | | | | | | |
| Satiety | 1 | 14 | 6 | 32 | 12 | 19 |
| Shame | 5 | 71 [a] | 2 | 10 | 5 | 8 |
| Remorse | 5 | 71 | 5 | 26 | 10 | 16 |
| Sadness | 6 | 86 [a] | 3 | 16 | 5 | 8 |
| *Interference of eating behaviors with psychosocial functioning :* | | | | | | |
| Emotional distress | 5 | 71 [b] | 6 | 32 | 7 | 11 |
| Family conflict | 3 | 43 [b] | 2 | 10 | 4 | 6 |
| Interference with school | 1 | 14 | 0 | 0 | 1 | 3 |
| Interference with social life | 1 | 14 | 1 | 5 | 0 | 0 |

[a] Significantly different from Hyperphagics and Snackers ($p<0.05$)
[b] Significantly different from Snackers ($p<0.05$)

As shown, all bulimics were girls between 16 and 19 years of age. For the hyperphagics and the snackers, the female:male ratio was 3:1. Mean age ranged from 17.2 to 18.0 years across groups. Although the prandial hyperphagics tended to be heavier, the mean BMI was not significantly different between groups.

All of the bulimics were obsessed with weight and food, all but one felt overweight and had a negative body image. These feelings were also reported by one half to two thirds of the hyperphagics, whereas the snackers did not differ from normal controls on body image, or weight and food preoccupations.

We compared lifetime use of weight control strategies across groups. All of the bulimics used or had used dieting, four out of seven self-induced vomiting, a few had abused diet pills, laxatives or diuretics. Except for current or past dieting (from 25% of the controls to 43% of the hyperphagics) and - to a lesser extent - self-induced vomiting (from 2% of the controls to 10% of the prandial hyperphagics), weight control strategies were rare and not significantly different among the three other groups.

Clinical characteristics of the bulimic binges (for bulimics) and of other types of eating episodes (for prandial hyperphagics and snackers) are compared in Table 4. Bulimic binges appear to be quite specific: the bulimics ate alone, at home, more rapidly than usual, most often in the late afternoon, secretly, with no hunger and no pleasure. Hyperphagics and snackers did not hide for eating and reported hunger and pleasure associated with food intake. Loss of control over eating, characteristic of bulimic subjects, was reported only by 32% of the hyperphagics and 19% of the snackers.

After the eating episodes, feelings of well-being and satiety were rare in all groups; bulimics almost always experienced sadness, shame, and guilt, whereas these feelings were rare or unknown among the hyperphagics and the snackers.

Five of the seven bulimics said that their eating behaviors caused marked emotional distress, whereas only 30% of the hyperphagics and 10% of the snackers were disturbed by their eating habits. Eating patterns were the source of family conflict for half of the bulimics but less than 10% for the hyperphagics or the snackers. All but two subjects (one bulimic, one hyperphagic) said that school and social life were not affected by their eating problem.

Globally, psychosocial functioning (CGAS) was significantly impaired for the bulimics compared to the three other groups, but the prandial hyperphagics and the snackers also had significantly lower CGAS scores than the normal controls. Five out of the seven bulimic girls had already had a major depressive episode (significantly more than in the three other groups); dysthymia was more frequent among bulimics than among normal controls.

It is of interest to note than none of the bulimics had ever been treated for their eating disorder.

## 2.3 Conclusion

Our findings confirm that preoccupations with weight, body image, and dieting are widespread among teenage girls and, to a lesser extent, among teenage boys. By the age of 12 years, small numbers of adolescents have already used self-induced vomiting, laxatives, or diet pills in order to control their weight. In girls, the frequency of these behaviors increases with age after 14 years. In the community, a spectrum of eating disturbances is encountered, eating symptoms in general being associated with various depressive and somatic symptoms.

The frequency of binge eating among adolescents that is reported in many studies indicates that binge eating per se should not necessarily be seen as problematic, unless it occurs frequently and is accompanied by negative emotions and unrelenting preoccupation with weight control and food intake.

The prevalence rates of bulimia nervosa in adolescents estimated in the current study - 1.1% for the girls and 0.2% for the boys - are not as high as earlier epidemiological studies had suggested, but fall within the prevalence range reported in young adult females in the most recent studies (Fairburn & Cooper, 1990). This confirms that bulimic behaviors develop during adolescence and do not accelerate from high school through the college years.

In our high school adolescent population, it appears that the distinction between bulimia nervosa and other disturbed eating patterns is justified, based on very specific clinical characteristics of bulimia nervosa: bulimics eat alone, secretly, in the late afternoon, with no hunger and no pleasure, more rapidly than usual; binges are followed by feelings of sadness, shame, and guilt, and are a source of general emotional distress. Even at a normal weight, bulimic adolescents feel overweight and are obsessed with weight and with food; they have a negative body image. Major depressive episodes develop in two thirds of the cases.

All these characteristics are similar to clinical features of bulimia nervosa in women coming for treatment years later. However, weight control strategies - except for dieting - seem less frequent, probably increasing later in the course of the disorder. If bulimic adolescents suffer from their eating habits, school and social life are still preserved.

Unlike what has been described for older patients (Flament, 1991), studies with bulimic adolescents have generally demonstrated that associated general psychopathology is still moderate. Dacey et al. (1990) have reported that the MMPI profiles of high school adolescent bulimics were not suggestive of psychopathology, although their scale scores tended to be higher than those of peer control subjects. Similar results were obtained by Gross & Rosen (1988) for body dissatisfaction, depression, and social anxiety scores.

The other disturbed eating behaviors described in the current study, prandial hyperphagia and excessive snacking, are more difficult to classify. Overall, prandial hyperphagics are more disturbed than the snackers who, on most measures, are not very different from controls, who have no eating disturbance. However, a number of subjects in each of these ill-defined "eating disturbances" groups resemble bulimics in some aspects, and may suffer from premorbid forms of bulimia nervosa.

Research has demonstrated that persistent food preoccupation and vulnerability to binge eating are common side-effects of restrained eating in humans (Polivy & Herman, 1983). In a 12-month follow-up of abnormal attitudes in London schoolgirls, the relative risk of dieters to develop an eating disorder was eight times that of non-dieters (Patton et al., 1990). It is becoming important to educate young adolescent women that chronic dieting is not a benign process, and health educators should inform the community that an emphasis on thinness or weight control may result for some young women in the development of an eating disorder. Clearly, attempts at early detection of eating disorders must be undertaken with high school students, and educational programs concerned with the consequences of disturbed eating habits should be developed.

The study reported here shows that bulimia nervosa should be recognized in adolescent girls. Compared to other disturbed eating patterns, adolescent bulimia nervosa has severe and specific clinical features similar to those seen in adult women with the disorder. However, the effects of bulimia nervosa may be less pronounced at a younger age and when the illness has been of shorter duration. Early detection would allow for less personality disruption and, consequently, greater treatment success, in addition to preventing a teenager from suffering the intense turmoil associated with bulimia.

## Acknowledgement

The study, directed by M. Choquet (INSERM U169), was supported by grants from the Ministère des Affaires Sociales (Stage I) and the Direction Générale de la Santé (Stage II). We are grateful to the personnel of the 23 schools involved in the local realization of the study under the responsability of the schools' principals and the academic inspector.

The clinical interviews for Stage II of the study reported here were conducted by: Mrs. Suzan Clot, Dr. Nathalie Danon, Dr. Nicolas Dantchev, Dr. Martine Flament, Dr. Jacques Laget, Dr. Brigitte Remy, Dr. Yves Simon, and Dr. Catherine Zittoun.

## References

American Psychiatric Association. (1980). *Diagnostic and Statistical Manual of Mental Disorders* (3d ed.). Washington.
American Psychiatric Association. (1987). *Diagnostic and Statistical Manual of Mental Disorders* (3d ed. Revised). Washington.
Chambers, W.J., Puig-Antich, J., Hirsch, M., Paez, P., Ambrosini, P.J., Tabrizi, M.A., & Davies, M. (1985). The assessment of affective disorders in children and adolescents by semistructured interview: Test-retest reliability of the K-SADS-P. *Archives of General Psychiatry, 42*, 696-702.
Crowther, J.H., Post, G., & Zaynor, L. (1985). The prevalence of bulimia and binge eating in adolescent girls. *International Journal of Eating Disorders, 4*, 29-42.
Dacey, C.M., Nelson, W.M., & Aikman, K.G. (1990). Prevalency rate and personality comparisons of bulimic and normal adolescents. *Child Psychiatry and Human Development, 20*, 243-251.
De Azevedo, M.H.P., & Ferreira, C.P. (1992). Anorexia nervosa and bulimia : a prevalence study. *Acta Psychiatrica Scandinavica, 86*, 432-436.
Fairburn, C.G., & Beglin, S.J. (1990). Studies of the epidemiology of bulimia nervosa. *American Journal of Psychiatry, 147*, 401-408.
Flament, M.F. (1991). La boulimie: Evaluation des critères diagnostiques et aspects séméiologiques. In J.L. Venisse (Ed.), *Les Nouvelles addictions* (pp. 74-86). Paris: Masson.
Flament, M.F., Jeammet, P., Payan, C., Dantchev, N., Venisse, J.L., Bailly, D., Igoin-Apfelbaum, L., & Doublet, S. (in press). DSM-III-R / DSM-IV diagnoses and clinical characteristics of 539 consecutive outpatients with binge eating: A French multicenter study. In American Psychiatric Association (Ed.), *DSM-IV Sourcebook*. Washington, DC: Editor.
Greenfeld, D., Quinlan, D.M., Harding, P., Glass, E., & Bliss, A. (1987). Eating behavior in an adolescent population. *International Journal of Eating Disorders, 6*, 99-111.
Gross, J., & Rosen, J.C. (1988). Bulimia in adolescents : prevalence and psychosocial correlates. *International Journal of Eating Disorders, 7*, 51-61.
Igoin, L. (1979). La Boulimie et son infortune. Paris: Presses Universitaires de France.
Johnson, C., Lewis, C., Love, S., Lewis, L., & Stuckey, M. (1984). Incidence and correlates of bulimic behavior in a female high school population. *Journal of Youth and Adolescence, 13*, 15-26.
Johnson, C., Tobin, D.L., & Lipkin, J. (1989). Epidemiologic changes in bulimic behavior among female adolescents over a five-year period. *International Journal of Eating Disorders, 8*, 647-655.
Kandel, D.B., & Davies, M. (1982). Epidemiology of adolescent depressive mood. *Archives of General Psychiatry, 39*, 1205-1212.
Lachenmeyer, J.R., & Muni-Brander, P. (1988). Eating disorders in a nonclinical adolescent population : Implications for treatment. *Adolescence, 23*, 303-312.

Ledoux, S., Choquet, M., Flament, M. (1991). Eating disorders among adolescents in an unselected French population. *International Journal of Eating Disorders, 10*, 81-89.

Maceyko, S.J., Nagelberg, D.B. (1985). The assessment of bulimia in high school students. *Journal of School Health, 55*, 135-137.

Mumford, D.B., & Whitehouse, A.M. (1988). Increased prevalence of bulimia nervosa among Asian schoolgirls. *British Medical Journal, 297*, 718-719.

Patton, G.C., Johnson-Sabine, E., Wood, K., Mann, A.H., & Wakeling, A. (1990). Abnormal eating attitudes in London schoolgirls - a prospective epidemiological study: Outcome at twelve month follow-up. *Psychological Medicine, 20*, 383-394.

Polivy, J., Herman, P. (1983). *Breaking the Diet Habit*. New York: Basic Books.

Pope, H.G., Hudson, J.I., Yurgelun-Todd, D., & Hudson, M.S. (1984). Prevalence of anorexia nervosa and bulimia in three student populations. *International Journal of Eating Disorders, 3*, 45-51.

Raich, R.M., Rosen, J.C., Deus, J., Pérez, O., Requena, A., & Gross, J. (1992). Eating disorder symptoms among adolescents in the United States and Spain: A comparative study. *International Journal of Eating Disorders, 1*, 63-72.

Russell, G.F. (1979). Bulimia nervosa: An ominous variant of anorexia nervosa. *Psychological Medicine, 9*, 429-448.

Shaffer, D., Gould, M.S., Brasic, J., Ambrosini, P., Bird, H.R., & Aluwahlia, S. (1983). A children's global assessment scale (CGAS). *Archives of General Psychiatry, 40*, 1228-1231.

Szabo, P., & Tury, F. (1991). The prevalence of bulima nervosa in a Hungarian college and secondary school population. *Psychotherapy and Psychosomatics, 56*, 43-47.

Timmerman, M.G., Wells, L.A., & Chen, S. (1990). Bulimia Nervosa and associated alcohol abuse among secondary school students. *Journal of the American Academy of Child and Adolescent Psychiatry, 29*, 118-122.

Whitaker, A., Johnson, J., Shaffer D, Rapoport JL, Kalikow K, Walsh BT, Davies M, Braiman S, & Dolinsky A. (1990). Uncommon troubles in young people: Prevalence estimates of selected psychiatric disorders in a nonreferred adolescent poulation. *Archives of General Psychiatry, 47*, 487-496.

# Transcultural Comparisons of Adolescent Eating Disorders

*Hans-Christoph Steinhausen, Svetlana Boyadjieva, and Klaus-Jürgen Neumärker*

## 1    Introduction

There is considerable evidence that sociocultural factors play an important role in the etiology of the eating disorders (DiNicola, 1990a; DiNicola, 1990b; Garfinkel & Garner, 1982; Garner, Garfinkel, & Olmsted, 1983). The supporting evidence for the sociocultural approach is based on the following facts: (a) there is a female predominance; (b) middle and upper classes are more frequently affected (c) the incidence is increasing; (d) there is a development gradient across cultures in this Western type of illness; (e) certain types of occupation such as dancers, models, or athletes carry a greater risk; (f) developmental, family, social, and cultural factors serve as predisposing elements, and (g) life stress events function as precipitating factors.

The evidence that the eating disorders are culture-bound syndromes raises further important research questions. Transcultural studies should try to find how much different societies and cultures contribute to the clinical phenomena of the eating disorders. In principle, this could be done by using either of the three main approaches, namely (a) inter-cultural studies - e.g., by comparing European and Asian patients; (b) intracultural studies - e.g., by contrasting different ethnic groups or migrants in one host country; or (c) the study of cultural change and its effects - e.g., by studying patients in the rapidly changing East European societies with former socialistic political and economic structure. Research issues in this transcultural approach pertain to the incidence and prevalence, the clinical phenomena, the psychopathological features, the treatment facilities and strategies, and the outcome of the eating disorders. Concomitantly, the importance of sociodemographic factors, economic conditions, cultural roots and beliefs, and the distress coming from migration should be studied.

Some of these issues are currently addressed by the international collaborative study of eating disorders in adolescence (ICOSEDA) that has some rather unusual historical characteristics. Originally, the study was started in West Berlin in the 1970's as a consequence of a previous study that investigated the long-term outcome of former anorectic patients (Steinhausen & Glanville, 1983a; Steinhausen & Glanville, 1983b). Already in this study, a broad, multidimensional approach to evaluation and an adequately long follow-up period were decided upon. The study was flawed primarily by its follow-back, catch-up character and the small sample size. In the face of these methodological restrictions, a prospective outcome study was initiated in West Berlin in the late 1970's that included the entire consecutive cohort of admitted adolescent in-patients. This study also used a multidimensional approach that included self-evaluation of the patient as well as expert evaluation by the therapists and nursing staff.

As was the case in other areas of medicine, when work on the prospective Berlin study commenced in the 1980's, there was little knowledge about the frequency and possible peculiarities of the affected patients in the German Democratic Republic (GDR) and other East Block countries. The impression was that official propaganda declared eating disorders as a product of bourgeois society and, with that, persisted in obscuring the significance of the eating disorders as a clinical phenomena. At the same time, both poor access to publications from the East Block countries and little personal contact to clinics and researchers in these countries, as well as the expectation that eating disorders were indeed to some extent a product of western affluent society, prevented any serious consideration of the question of whether these disorders were observed as frequently in the GDR. The publications by Döll and Neumärker (1982) made it quite clear, however, that intensive clinical and research activity had begun in East Berlin that were based on an increasingly expanding cohort of patients.

In divided Berlin, for the times and the prevailing political situation, Steinhausen and Neumärker succeeded in realizing a quite unusual feat that demanded very careful preparation. They agreed upon a prospective long-term outcome study of patients in West and East Berlin using the same methodology, and, for the purpose of transcultural comparisons, to conduct additional field studies in both parts of the city. The unusual political circumstances of the divided city, each part of which had been cut off from the other for several decades and each having different political systems, and above all, undergoing different developments of historical life-events, were, aside from the tragedy of the outward circumstances, favorable to such a transcultural comparison. The fall of the Berlin Wall and the subsequent reunification of Germany quickly terminated these unusual circumstances. In the meantime, the data that resulted from this collaboration has undergone evaluation from various points of view. A comparison of two self-report questionnaires in field studies and in patients, the Eating Attitudes Test (Garner & Garfinkel, 1979) and the Eating Disorders Inventory (Garner, Olmsted, & Polivy, 1983) was published not long ago (Neumärker, Dudeck, Vollrath, Neumärker, & Steinhausen, 1992; Steinhausen, Neumärker, Vollrath, Dudeck, & Neumärker, 1992).

Soon after the fall of the Berlin Wall, the former East Block collapsed and gave way to fundamental societal changes in East Europe. Within this process, one of us (S. B.) noticed a progressively increasing number of adolescent eating disorders in Bulgaria, underlining the need to build up appropriate treatment programs and the desire to develop concomitant research programs for evaluation. Thus, in November 1991, contacts were formed and, soon after, the Berlin study was extended to an international collaborative study. In the meantime, data from a Zurich cohort were also incorporated into the study and data from further sites in East Europe will be integrated in the near future.

## 2   Samples and Methods

Each of the four samples compared in this chapter form a series of consecutively admitted patients that were treated in the participating centers: (a) The West Berlin cohort consisted of 60 adolescent eating-disordered patients who underwent inpatient treatment between 1979 and 1988 on two university clinic wards. (b) The East Berlin sample consists of 39 adolescent patients with eating disorders who underwent inpatient treatment between 1985 and 1989 on another university clinic ward. Two thirds of this sample originated directly from the city and one third from the surrounding areas. (c) The Zurich sample was taken from the same time period as the West Berlin sample, i.e., between 1979 and 1988, and consisted of the entire cohort of 64 consecutively admitted patients of a community-based service with mainly outpatients. (d) The Sofia sample consisted of 53 patients who were admitted between 1987 and 1993 to a university clinic ward with admissions from the whole country of Bulgaria.

All four samples complied with the ICD-10 diagnostic criteria for eating disorders. The original diagnostic criteria that had been used in the beginning of the West and East Berlin study were those of Feighner and coworkers (1972) and modified for adolescents by Steinhausen and Glanville (1984). Subsequent evaluation confirmed that these two samples were also in accordance with the more recent ICD-10 criteria. A systematic documentation of clinical data that had been developed for this study was used in all participating centers. Statistical tests included Chi-square tests and analyses of variance (ANOVA).

## 3  Results

A comparison of the quantitative clinical features of the four samples is given in Table 1. Whereas weight and height at admission were similar in the two Berlin samples, the Sofia patients weighed less and the Zurich patients were smaller. The Sofia patients had the lowest BMI and were the youngest at age at onset. The premorbid weight was lowest in the Zurich cohort, whereas the amount of absolute weight loss was greatest in the Sofia and the West Berlin sample. Menarche occured at a later age in the Zurich cohort.

Table 1.  Comparison of Quantitative Clinical Features

|  | West Berlin (N = 60) Mean SD | East Berlin (N = 39) Mean SD | Zurich (N = 64) Mean SD | Sofia (N = 53) Mean SD |
|---|---|---|---|---|
| Weight at admission (kg)[1] | 38.6   7.1 | 39.6   6.3 | 37.2   6.2 | 34.8   6.5 |
| Height (cm)[2] | 164.6   6.1 | 163.0   6.8 | 159.1   7.2 | 161.8   7.7 |
| BMI[3] | 14.2   2.3 | 14.8   1.8 | 14.6   1.7 | 13.2   1.8 |
| Premorbid weight (kg)[4] | 53.4   7.8 | 53.7   12.1 | 48.0   8.2 | 52.2   9.5 |
| Weight loss (kg)[5] | 14.8   7.4 | 14.2   8.5 | 10.8   5.6 | 17.4   5.5 |
| Age at admission (y) | 15.7   1.6 | 14.8   1.4 | 14.9   2.2 | 14.8   2.0 |
| Age at onset of the disease (y)[6] | 14.6   1.6 | 13.9   1.6 | 14.1   1.9 | 13.4   1.7 |
| Menarche (y)[7] | 12.9   1.3 | 12.4   1.3 | 13.9   2.5 | 12.9   1.8 |

[1] West Berlin/East Berlin>Sofia
[2] West Berlin>Zurich
[3] East Berlin/Zurich>Sofia
[4] West Berlin/East Berlin>Zurich
[5] Sofia/West Berlin>Zurich
[6] West Berlin>Sofia
[7] West Berlin/East Berlin/Sofia<Zurich

As Table 2 shows, anorexia nervosa was the most frequently cited diagnosis in all four cohorts, whereas bulimia nervosa was rarely observed among these adolescent patients. Although not significantly different for all parameters, the diagnostic and clinical criteria of the four cohorts, which are depicted in Table 3, are informative. They show that the clinical picture was almost identical in all four sites. Only periodic hyperactivity was consistently seen in all cases in the Sofia sample, whereas it was observed far less in the other three sites.

Table 2.  Diagnostic Classification

|  | West Berlin (N = 60) N | % | East Berlin (N = 39) N | % | Zurich (N = 64) N | % | Sofia (N = 53) N | % |
|---|---|---|---|---|---|---|---|---|
| Diagnoses |  |  |  |  |  |  |  |  |
| Anorexia nervosa | 48 | 80.0 | 31 | 79.5 | 54 | 85 | 42 | 79 |
| Anorexia and bulimia nervosa | 6 | 10.0 | 8 | 20.5 | 3 | 5 | 11 | 21 |
| Bulimia nervosa | 5 | 8.3 | 0 | 0 | 1 | 2 | 0 | 0 |
| Atypical anorexia nervosa | 1 | 1.7 | 0 | 0 | 4 | 6 | 0 | 0 |
| Atypical bulimia nervosa | 0 | 0 | 0 | 0 | 2 | 3 | 0 | 0 |

Table 3.  Comparison of Diagnostic and Clinical Criteria

|  | West Berlin (N = 60) N | % | East Berlin (N = 39) N | % | Zurich (N = 64) N | % | Sofia (N = 53) N | % |
|---|---|---|---|---|---|---|---|---|
| Disturbed attitude towards eating, food, and weight | 58 | 97 | 35 | 90 | 64 | 100 | 53 | 100 |
| Body-image disturbance | 54 | 90 | 31 | 79 | 63 | 98 | 52 | 98 |
| Amenorrhea | 43 | 72 | 29 | 74 | 40 | 65 | 37 | 70 |
| Premenarchal | 10 | 17 | 7 | 18 | 16 | 26 | 12 | 23 |
| Periodic hyperactivity[1] | 31 | 52 | 20 | 51 | 34 | 53 | 53 | 100 |
| Binge episodes | 17 | 28 | 7 | 18 | 18 | 28 | 13 | 25 |
| Vomiting | 21 | 35 | 10 | 26 | 20 | 31 | 24 | 45 |
| Laxative abuse | 12 | 20 | 5 | 13 | 11 | 17 | 12 | 23 |

[1] $p < 0.00001$

The rate of prenatal and perinatal risk factors and early-childhood eating disorders was relatively low in all four samples, and the distribution was the same, as shown in Table 4. On the other hand, premorbid obesity was more frequently observed in the Sofia and the East Berlin sample. Trigger events recorded more often for the Zurich patients included family problems, whereas criticism of obesity was most frequent in the Sofia sample. Developmental crisis typical of adolescence was most frequently noted in the Zurich sample.

Table 4. Comparison of Developmental Histories

|  | West Berlin (N = 60) N | West Berlin (N = 60) % | East Berlin (N = 39) N | East Berlin (N = 39) % | Zurich (N = 64) N | Zurich (N = 64) % | Sofia (N = 53) N | Sofia (N = 53) % |
|---|---|---|---|---|---|---|---|---|
| Pregnancy complications | 10 | 17 | 8 | 21 | 9 | 14 | 4 | 8 |
| Perinatal complications | 10 | 17 | 5 | 13 | 12 | 19 | 7 | 13 |
| Eating disorders in 1st year | 8 | 13 | 9 | 23 | 8 | 13 | 15 | 28 |
| Eating disorders in childhood | 8 | 13 | 7 | 18 | 6 | 9 | 4 | 8 |
| Premorbid obesity[1] | 9 | 15 | 15 | 38 | 8 | 13 | 18 | 34 |
| Trigger events |  |  |  |  |  |  |  |  |
| Family problems[2] | 11 | 18 | 2 | 5 | 32 | 89 | 18 | 34 |
| Criticized because of being overweight[2] | 12 | 20 | 22 | 56 | 12 | 33 | 40 | 76 |
| Developmental crisis[2] | 9 | 15 | 10 | 25 | 28 | 78 | 31 | 59 |

[1] $p=0.002$  [2] $p<0.00001$

A comparison of the family background, as given in Table 5, indicates a remarkably high rate of partnership problems in the parents of the Zurich sample. The Sofia cohort comes second with regard to this issue. Chronically ill parents were most frequently seen in the West Berlin sample, but this was also quite common in the Sofia cohort. The life-time rate of eating disorders - either anorexia nervosa or bulimia nervosa - in other family members was relatively low in all samples except the Sofia cohort.

Table 5. Comparison of Family Background

|  | West Berlin (N = 60) N | West Berlin (N = 60) % | East Berlin (N = 39) N | East Berlin (N = 39) % | Zurich (N = 64) N | Zurich (N = 64) % | Sofia (N = 53) N | Sofia (N = 53) % |
|---|---|---|---|---|---|---|---|---|
| Partnership problems[1] | 13 | 22 | 6 | 15 | 40 | 63 | 21 | 40 |
| Divorce | 9 | 15 | 3 | 8 | 6 | 9 | 2 | 4 |
| Single Parenting | 9 | 15 | 2 | 5 | 8 | 13 | 4 | 8 |
| Chronically ill parent | 23 | 38 | 5 | 13 | 3 | 5 | 12 | 23 |
| Eating-disordered family member[2] | 2 | 3 | 4 | 10 | 4 | 6 | 12 | 23 |

[1] $p<0.00001$  [2] $p=0.004$

## 4  Discussion

This transcultural study of eating disorders in adolescence was started under quite unusual historical and political conditions, i.e., the divided city of Berlin, and later extended to further sites. Whereas the Zurich data were taken from a period of wealth and remarkable socioeconomic stability, the data from Sofia stem from a time of enormous cultural change after the collapse of the socialistic societies in East Europe. Thus, the central question of the present paper is whether or not the data collected in these different sites and under differing sociocultural conditions reflect to any extent some of these varying background factors.

First, the comparison of the quantitative clinical features revealed some interesting differences among the four samples. Although the age at admission did not differ between the four groups, the Sofia patients stood out as being the youngest at the age at onset of the eating disorder; on average they had the lowest weight at admission and the lowest BMI. This may point to a relatively severe form of the eating disorder and may also reflect the fact that the Bulgarian patients were admitted for treatment rather late, considering that their younger age at onset was not matched by a younger age at admission. In Bulgaria, there were very few child and adolescent psychiatric settings in general, especially settings with years of experience in the treatment of eating disorders. Despite the official political goal of early intervention in medicine, the identification of a clinical eating problem may have been rather late because of limited information among professionals and the general population, which contrasts strikingly with the almost 'glamorizing' discussion of the eating disorders in the lay public in many western countries.

However, this argument of different identification and referral practice should not be overly stressed, because a more complex interaction of identification of the clinical problem, referral practices, and underlying etiologic factors may have been operating. The data from the four sites do not show any significant trends either for the time interval between age at onset of the disorder and admission or for the interval between menarche and age at onset of the disease. It is interesting to note in this context that, in contrast to the other samples, the Swiss patients from the canton of Zurich were rather late with regard to their menarche. However, on the average, they were the first who received professional treatment. Again, the standard of professional information in a - at this time - relatively highly developed health system, may have been responsible for admission with rather short delay.

The distribution of diagnoses showed no remarkable differences among the four samples. Above all, patients with anorexia nervosa were treated, and there were only a few cases of anorexia with bulimic features or pure bulimia nervosa. Both the distribution of the diagnoses and the distribution of the diagnostic and clinical criteria point to the universality of the expression of the eating disorders from varying cultural, sociopolitical, and economical conditions. What may be affected by these conditions is the frequency of manifestation of the eating disorders. This would effect incidence and prevalence rates, an issue that could not be studied in the present investigation.

Similar to the clinical phenomena, a comparison of the histories of the patients showed no differences as far as the early phase of development was concerned. However, among the trigger events, premorbid obesity was more common in the Sofia and the East Berlin samples. One may speculate that a more restricted supply of foods with a high amount of fat and carbohydrates in Bulgaria and the GDR may have contributed to the higher rate of premorbid obesity, which is alone a risk factor for the development of anorexia or bulimia nervosa. Consequently, the patients with premorbid obesity were more often subjected to criticism from their families and peers. Interestingly, the highest rate of family problems and developmental crises among the trigger events was observed in the sample with the least cultural squeeze, namely in the Swiss sample from Zurich.

The latter finding was also reflected by a high rate of partnership problems, which was the main distinguishing factor of the family background in the Zurich sample. The West Berlin parents stood out because of their high rate of chronic illnesses, whereas the rate of other family members with life-time diagnoses of either anorexia or bulimia nervosa was, surprisingly, highest in the Sofia sample. The diversity of the distributions of these family factors again point to a very complex interaction of sociocultural and familial factors in the etiology of the eating disorders that has to be considered in any model of the nature of these disorders.

In conclusion, these limited findings from the international collaborative study of eating disorders in adolescence have been looked at from a transcultural point of view. They were obtained at four sites under different political and sociocultural conditions. Whereas the universality of the clinical expression and phenomena of the eating disorders was strongly supported by the present study, there were some hints that differences in the medical system may contribute to the mode of treatment, including the identification of patients with adolescent eating disorders. Also, this study shows that there is still much to learn about the complex interaction of sociocultural, familial, and biological factors in the etiology of the eating disorders.

### Acknowledgment

The authors are grateful to the large number of clinical coworkers who contributed to data collection over many years in the participating countries.

### References

DiNicola, V.F. (1990a). Anorexia multiforme: Self-starvation in historical and cultural context: Part I. Self-starvation as a historical chameleon. *Transcultural Psychiatric Research Review, 27*, 165-196.

DiNicola, V. F. (1990b). Anorexia multiforme: Self-starvation in historical and cultural context: Part II. Anorexia nervosa as a culture-reactive syndrome. *Transcultural Psychiatric Research Review, 27*, 165-196.

Döll, R. & Neumärker, K.J. (1982). Bemerkungen zur Therapie der Pubertätsmagersucht. *Deutsches Gesundheitswesen, 37*, 677-680.

Feighner, J.P., Robins, E., Guze, S.B., Woodruff, R.A., Winokur, G. & Munoz, R. (1972). Diagnostic criteria for use in psychiatric research. *Archives of General Psychiatry, 26*, 57-63.

Garfinkel, P.E. & Garner, D.M. (1982). *Anorexia nervosa - a multidimensional perspective* . New York: Brunner/Mazel.

Garner, D.M. & Garfinkel, P.E. (1979). The eating attitude test: An index of the symptoms of anorexia nervosa. *Psychological Medicine, 9*, 273-279.

Garner, D.M., Garfinkel, P.E. & Olmsted, M.P. (1983). An overview of sociocultural factors in the development of anorexia nervosa. In D.V. Darby, P.E. Garfinkel, D.M. Garner & I.V. Coscina (Eds.), *Anorexia nervosa: Recent developments in research* (pp. 65-82). New York: Liss.

Garner, D.M., Olmsted, M.P. & Polivy, J. (1983). Development and validation of a multidimensional eating disorder inventory for anorexia nervosa and bulimia. *International Journal of Eating Disorders, 2*, 15-34.

Neumärker, U., Dudeck, U., Vollrath, M., Neumärker, K.J. & Steinhausen, H.-C. (1992). Eating attitudes among adolescent patients and normal school girls in East Berlin and West Berlin. A transcultural comparison. *International Journal of Eating Disorders, 12*, 281-289.

Steinhausen, H.-C. & Glanville, K. (1983a). A long-term follow-up of adolescent anorexia nervosa. *Acta Psychiatrica Scandinavica, 68*, 1-10.

Steinhausen, H.-C. & Glanville, K. (1983b). Retrospective and prospective follow-up studies in anorexia nervosa. *International Journal of Eating Disorders, 2*, 221-235.

Steinhausen, H.-C. & Glanville, K. (1984). Der langfristige Verlauf der Anorexia nervosa. *Der Nervenarzt, 55*, 236-248.

Steinhausen, H.-C., Neumärker, K.-J., Vollrath, M., Dudeck, U. & Neumärker, U. (1992). A transcultural comparison of the Eating Disorder Inventory in former East and West Berlin. *International Journal of Eating Disorders, 12*, 407-416.

# Part II

# Clinical and Psychological Issues

# Individual and Family Factors in Adolescents with Eating Symptoms and Syndromes

*Howard Steiger and Stephen Stotland*

## 1 Introduction

Although the eating disorders (EDs) Anorexia and Bulimia Nervosa (AN and BN) typically develop during adolescence and afflict at least 2-4% of school-aged girls in full-blown, clinical forms (Fairburn & Beglin, 1990; Lucas, Beard, O'Fallon, & Kurland, 1991), most reviews in the area emphasize psychological and family features seen in adult samples (e.g., Vitousek & Manke, 1994; Wonderlich, 1992). This chapter offers an update on features associated with eating syndromes in adolescents and attempts to situate findings within a multidimensional, biopsychosocial framework (Garfinkel & Garner, 1982; Johnson & Connors, 1987; Strober, 1991). In this model, EDs are regarded as being multiply determined by biological factors (e.g., heritable aspects of mood and temperament), social pressures (promoting body-consciousness or problems of self-definition), and psychological vulnerabilities (e.g., personality or "self" disturbances).

## 2 The Role of Dietary and Bodily Concerns

In a social context that equates slimness with many cultural ideals, it is not surprising to find that from 40-80% of high-school girls experience body dissatisfaction (Davies & Furnham, 1986; Eisele, Hertsgaard & Light, 1986) and that 50-70% diet (Rosen & Gross, 1987; Wardle & Beales, 1986). Such factors have an almost certain role in ED development: Studies show body dissatisfaction to predict later occurrence or exacerbation of eating problems in adolescents (e.g., Attie & Brooks-Gunn, 1989; Striegel-Moore, Silberstein, Frensch, & Rodin, 1989) and link ED onset to definable episodes of sustained, intensive dieting (e.g., Agras & Kirkley, 1986). However, it is equally apparent that "clinical ED sufferers" differ from "compulsive dieters" on diverse psychopathological indices (e.g., Garner, Olmsted, Polivy, & Garfinkel, 1984; Steiger, Leung, & Houle, 1992), and this implies that the EDs have as much to do with psychopathological processes as they do with attitudes concerning dieting or body image.

## 3  Individual Psychopathology

### 3.1  Theory

Although theories on the psychopathology of the EDs are very diverse, there is some consensus on the belief that eating syndromes express underlying "self" or "self-image" disturbances (e.g., Bruch, 1973; Garfinkel & Garner, 1982; Johnson & Connors, 1987). For decades, there has been a stereotype of the anorexic "restricter" (the classical anorexic who exercises excessive dietary control) as being a compliant, isolated, and anxious girl, who gravitates to orderliness or control. Bruch (1973) understood such features as reflecting pervasive feelings of low self-worth and ineffectiveness and developmental deficits in awareness of "self" and feeling states. Similarly, Crisp (1980) emphasized reserved, compliant children with marked conflicts around pubertal demands. He formulated Anorexia Nervosa (AN) as a phobic-avoidance response, reinforced by a literal escape from maturational changes at puberty. Strober's (1991) recently articulated "organismic-developmental" paradigm again addresses pathological adaptations to adolescence but emphasizes an incompatibility between developmental imperatives and a heritable temperament characterized by harm-avoidance, reactivity to social approval, and preference for sameness.

Thinking on bulimic syndromes (and on anorexic variants that include bulimic symptoms) emphasizes an alternative spectrum of psychopathology: self-regulatory deficits, dramatic fluctuations in self-concept and mood, and erratic efforts to regulate inner tensions (e.g., Humphrey, 1991; Johnson, 1991; Root, Fallon & Freidrich, 1986). A nicely integrative view is provided by Johnson (1991), who postulates that restrictive and bulimic ED variants, although they occur along a continuum of "narcissistic-borderline" disturbances, differ as to key aspects of defensive organization. He characterizes defenses in restricters as "paranoid, rigid, and over-determined" attempts to protect a vulnerable ego from external demands (p. 170), and those in "bingers" as "frantic, diffuse, and chaotic" compensations for inner emptiness and dysphoria (p. 171). In other words, "self" in the "restricter" is conceptualized as being structured around defense from outside influences whereas, in the "binger", there is an outwardly directed quest for self-soothing and need-fulfillment.

## 3.2 Findings

### 3.2.1 Psychiatric Syndromes

Research in adult ED sufferers indicates a striking tendency towards comorbidity with other psychiatric syndromes. For example, comorbid Mood and Anxiety Disorders are each estimated to occur in at least 25-50% of cases (Laessle, Kittl, Fichter, Wittchen, & Pirke, 1987; Strober & Katz, 1988; Toner, Garfinkel, & Garner, 1986). Available data imply that adolescent sufferers show a comparable range (if not severity) of comorbid psychopathology. For example, in a controlled study of 51 Swedish adolescents with restrictive or bulimic AN, Råstam (1992) reported 86% as having a psychiatric disturbance, 49% a DSM-III-R Mood Disorder, and 29% as having a past or present Anxiety Disorder. Similarly, Herzog, Keller, Lavori, and Bradburn (1991) documented a 56% rate of comorbid Major Depression in a sample of bulimic adolescents. Such figures are very striking when one considers that latent disturbances will often not manifest themselves by adolescence.

### 3.2.2 Personality Disturbances

Early psychometric studies using the Eysenck Personality Inventory led to a general characterization of anorexic adolescents as being "neurotic" and "introverted" (Smart, Beaumont, & George, 1976; Strober, 1980) but also implied that purging anorexics were the more disturbed and the more emotionally labile (Ben-Tovim, Marilov, & Crisp, 1979). A similar series of studies using the Minnesota Multiphasic Personality Inventory (MMPI) showed "restricter" and "binger" anorexics to display depressive and socially anxious features but indicated that the "bingers" were more impulsive, oppositional, or antisocial (Leon, Lucas, Colligan, Ferlinande, & Kamp, 1985; Casper, Hedeker, & McClough, 1992; Edwin, Andersen, & Rosell, 1988). Such observations have led to two concepts that strongly influence thinking on personality factors in the EDs – (a) that the EDs often coincide with characterological disturbances and (b) that differences exist between "restricter" and "binger/purger" patients along personality dimensions that involve "overcontrol" or "dyscontrol".

However, given that many studies fail to report or control the stage of illness at which personality is assessed, many concerns exist about the degree to which personality features observed in eating-disordered adolescents will represent stable "traits", versus "states" existing only during the active ED. Numerous investigations note that weight restoration in teenaged anorexics leads to significant normalization of scores on standardized psychometric tests (Edwin et al., 1988; Leon et al., 1985; Strober, 1980). Such findings indicate that an active ED will often produce features with a "characterological coloring" or will significantly exacerbate latent personality problems. At the same time, two types of studies support the idea that EDs are associated with stable, underlying disturbances in personality that exist independently of the ED–(a) restrospective studies that examine premorbid personality traits in ED sufferers and (b) prospective studies that assess personality traits in sufferers after recovery from the ED.

The first approach, although subject to biases inherent in restrospective designs, yields fairly consistent evidence of premorbid disturbances. Halmi (1974) reported that 21% of 71 anorexics had been timid premorbidly, 64% had been "anxious", and 61% had been "obsessive-compulsive". Casper, Eckert, Halmi, Goldberg and Davis (1980), using a structured assessment of premorbid traits in mixed "restricter" and "binger" anorexics, found both groups as showing premorbid timidity and perfectionism but more of the bingers (86% versus 57%) as having been "outgoing". Similarly, Beumont, George, and Smart (1976) concluded that premorbidly, 14 "vomiters/purgers" had been more extroverted and emotionally expressive than 17 "restricters" had been. A more recent study uses extensive interviews with patients and parents to estimate the likelihood of a premorbid DSM-III-R personality *disorder* (PD) in 51 adolescent "restricter" and "binger" anorexics (Råstam, 1992). It estimates 67% to have shown a PD prior to ED onset and 35% to have shown Obsessive-Compulsive PD (the most frequently diagnosed personality disturbance). Restricter/binger differences were not reported.

Stability of at least some components of personality disturbance is also indicated by examinations of traits in recovered or recovering patients. For example, Casper (1990) compared California Personality Inventory and Multidimensional Personality Questionnaire scores across 25 restricter anorexics (six years after weight restoration), 15 matched nonanorexic sisters, and 23 age-matched controls. The recovered anorexics showed *less* novelty seeking, flexibility, independence, social closeness, and social potency, and *more* constraint, risk avoidance, and conformity than did the controls. Similarly, both Strober (1980) and Windauer, Lennerts, Talbot, Touyz, and Beumont (1993) report that obsessional traits in weight-restored anorexics are strikingly invariant over several years. Similar findings based on adult bulimic samples suggest the existence of primary "borderline" characteristics that are exacerbated during the active ED phase (e.g., Steiger, Leung, Thibaudeau, Houle, & Ghadirian, 1993).

Direct inferences about personality processes in adolescent patients cannot be drawn using findings on Personality Disorders in adult ED sufferers, but these are at least informative about prognosis in the adolescent in whom an ED goes unresolved. We therefore summarize main themes from a large literature based on applications of formal personality-diagnostic criteria in eating-disordered adults. Relevant studies are summarized in several excellent and current reviews (see Johnson & Wonderlich, 1992; Sohlberg & Strober, 1994; Vitousek & Manke, 1994). Overall, findings support the following generalizations. Estimates of PD prevalences in mixed anorexic/bulimic samples are high but vary considerably (from roughly 30% to over 90%, with modal figures in the 50-75% range). Restrictive AN appears to show the most consistent comorbidity pattern, characterized by an affinity for Anxious-Fearful (Cluster C) PDs. Conversely, multiple comorbid diagnoses on Axis II, which can include simultaneous Dramatic-Erratic (Cluster B) and Anxious-Fearful (Cluster C) diagnoses, are often reported in "anorexic bingers". In normal-weight bulimics, Borderline and Histrionic PDs are the most frequently reported diagnoses, but Obsessive-Compulsive, Avoidant, and Dependent (Cluster C) PDs occur more often than previously thought. Taken together, results imply elusive "restricter/binger" differences that coincide partially with loadings on Anxious/Fearful versus Dramatic/Erratic personality variants. "Fit" is imperfect, however, and important within-subtype heterogenities are noted.

Several studies have directly addressed the issue of specificity of characterological features to eating syndromes. Some provide no indications of ED-specific features at all. For example, Smith and Steiner (1992) found that depressed and anorexic adolescents produce comparable scores on self-reported "ineffectiveness", "perfectionism", and "interpersonal distrust", whereas Steiner (1990) found no striking differences on a measure of maladaptive defenses across anorexic, bulimic, and depressed adolescents. However, intriguing differences are obtained in several comparisons. An early psychometric study by Strober (1980) compared 22 adolescent anorexics to 22 age-matched subjects with depressions and 22 subjects with conduct disorders, and found that compulsivity, obsessiveness, interpersonal insecurity, and minimization of affect were more characteristic of the anorexics than of other groups. In a related study, Strober (1981) differentiated anorexic patients from depressed and conduct-disordered adolescents on measures suggesting "high anxiety and social conformity", and from conduct disorders on measures reflecting "low stimulus seeking and emotional constriction". Swift, Bushnell, Hanson, and Logemann (1986) noted that a group of 30 anorexics (restricters and bingers) showed a more disturbed profile on Offer Self-Image Questionnaire scales than did a group of 30 depressed adolescents. Finally, although they involved adult samples, we note that two studies by our research group have found that anorexic and bulimic women display more elevated "self-criticism" (Steiger, Goldstein, Mongrain & Van der Feen, 1990) and "pathological narcissism" (Stotland & Steiger, 1994) than comparison groups composed of women with other psychiatric disorders. Together, results suggest that ED sufferers may be distinguished from other "psychiatric" groups, not only by ED-specific features, but by unusually heavy loadings on certain theoretically relevant dimensions (risk-avoidance, conformity, obsessiveness, self-criticism, "narcissistic" needs for approval, etc.).

### 3.2.3 Nonclinical Samples

Selection biases could cause observations in clinical samples to reflect unusually severe or chronic EDs and, hence, to misrepresent the "typical" ED sufferer, who probably never comes to clinical attention. Such concerns have generated interest in community-based studies that describe concurrent features in nonclinical subjects displaying ED-like symptoms. Investigations of this type consistently associate ED-spectrum disturbances with qualitatively and, often, quantitatively, similar psychopathological features to those seen in clinical samples: Representative studies have linked "maladaptive eating" in nonclinical, high-school samples to negative emotionality, low interoceptive awareness (Leon, Fulkerson, Perry, & Cudeck, 1993), introversion (Patton, 1988), and self-criticism (Steiger, Leung, Puentes-Neuman, & Gottheil, 1992). They have also indicated that "anorexic symptoms" in such populations coincide with perfectionism (Steiger,

Puentes-Neuman, & Leung, 1991) and elevated neuroticism (Whitaker, Davies, Shaffer, Johnson, Abrams, Walsh & Kalikow, 1989), whereas "bulimic symptoms" have been linked to low self-esteem, social anxiety (Gross & Rosen, 1988), mood lability, and "borderline" features (Steiger, Leung, & Houle, 1992). Furthermore, Steiger, Puentes-Neuman, and Leung (1991) found predictable differences on measures of perfectionism and impulsivity between schoolgirls reporting "restrictive" and "bulimic" eating patterns (Steiger et al., 1991). Such findings suggest that concurrent features in nonclinical subjects showing ED-like symptoms are strikingly similar to those seen in full-blown, clinical syndromes.

## 4 The Family

Even 19th Century theories emphasized the role of the family in the EDs–enough so that some clinicians recommended removal of the affected child from the family's influence at the start of treatment (Gull, 1874). The concept that family factors cause and maintain EDs has persisted for over a century and remains prominent in contemporary formulations.

### 4.1 Familial Transmission

Well-controlled studies using explicit criteria and blind assessments have shown clear familial aggregation (among females) for anorexia nervosa (e.g., Strober, Lampert, Morrell, et al., 1990) and less-consistently, for bulimia nervosa (Kassett, Gershon, Maxwell, et al., 1989; Hudson, Pope, Jonas, et al., 1987). Such findings suggest that the EDs may be familially transmitted syndromes. However, as the following indicates, various tenable hypotheses exist to explain such effects.

### 4.1.1 Biological Bases

Several studies show concordance for AN and BN to be substantially higher in monozygotic than in dizygotic twins (e.g., Holland, Sicotte, & Treasure, 1988; Kendler, MacLean, Neale, Kessler, Heath, & Eaves, 1991), and in turn, suggest genetic effects. However, the scope and implications of such effects need clarification. For example, Treasure and Holland (1989) reported monozygotic twins to show pronounced concordance for AN, but not for BN, and therefore proposed that AN and BN may be etiologically distinct – the former having strong family-genetic determinants, the latter more environmentally based causes. Whether or not this is the case, available twin studies are subject to various biases (related to shared environmental influences and other factors), and further evidence is needed before we can assume any specific genetic transmission effects.

Heritable effects could, alternatively, be enacted through the familial transmission of disturbances that indirectly enhance vulnerability to ED development. Given substantial clinical and neurobiological overlap with the EDs, Mood Disorders (MDs) could represent one such class of disturbance (e.g., Swift, Andrews & Barklage, 1986). Indeed, controlled studies show lifetime prevalences of Mood Disorders (MDs) to be considerably elevated in relatives of anorexics (Kassett et al., 1989; Strober et al., 1990) and bulimics (Kassett et al., 1989), although bulimic syndromes probably account for the strongest effects of this type (e.g., Piran, Kennedy, Garkinkel, & Owens, 1985). Recent findings tend, however, to rule out simple co-transmission of Eating and Mood Disorders within families – instead they show the elevated familial prevalences of MDs in families of anorexic and bulimic probands to be explained mainly by the probands who themselves show mood manifestations (Kassett et al., 1989; Strober et al., 1990). Such observations suggest independence of pathways more than they do shared causal mechanisms.

Another pathway for family-genetic effects, as postulated by Strober (1991), could relate to heritable temperamental traits that indirectly heighten susceptibility to ED development. Although feasible, findings on specific personality configurations (or "trait" dimensions) in relatives of ED sufferers have been frustratingly inconsistent; Strober, Salkin, Burroughs, and Morrell (1982) obtained expected differences on MMPI scores between parents of "restricter" and "bulimic" anorexics: The former were generally emotionally reserved, the latter displayed hostile/depressive qualities. Supporting the same "family-trait" concept, Casper (1990) noted that not only anorexics, but their nonanorexic sisters, tended toward conventionality and control. However, using standardized psychometric tests, Garfinkel, Garfinkel, Rose, et al. (1983) and Crisp, Harding, and McGuinness (1974) identified rather negligible differences between parents of anorexics and normal controls. Similarly, Steiger, Stotland, Ghadirian, and Whitehead (in press), measuring self-reported compulsivity, anxiousness, affective instability, and narcissism, found no substantial differences among the mothers, fathers, sisters, or brothers of adult "restricter", "binger", and "control" probands. Findings consistent with familial temperamental traits have, therefore, been suggestive but somewhat elusive.

## 4.1.2 Psychosocial Induction

It is intuitively appealing to assume that familial transmission in the EDs depends upon psychosocial induction effects that create a "family culture" of concerns with body image, weight, and eating. Indeed, studies in nonclinical samples, although perhaps of limited relevance to clinical EDs, imply that mothers' eating attitudes influence daughters' beliefs and behaviors around eating (e.g., Hill, Weaver, & Blundell, 1990; Pike & Rodin, 1991). However, in clinical populations, as many studies report that parents of ED sufferers have normal eating attitudes (Hall, Leibrich, Walkley, & Welch, 1986; Garfinkel et al., 1983; Steiger et al., in press) as report them to show abnormal attitudes (Hall & Brown, 1983; Wold, 1985). It, thus, appears incorrect to assume that these parents will invariably manifest eating anomalies. As for actual weight problems, a modest link between familial obesity and bulimic disorders is evident, but there is little evidence of a consistent link to restrictive syndromes (e.g., Halmi, Strauss, & Goldberg, 1978; Strober, 1981a).

## 4.2 Theories on Family Dynamics

Perhaps the most popular of family conceptualizations of the EDs are those that explain eating syndromes in terms of dynamic family interaction patterns. In theory, food-refusal has usually been conceptualized as expressing the child's struggle to achieve self-control (and to limit others' influence) in families characterized by overinvolvement or excessive emotional investment. For example, theorists construe restrictive AN as an essentially "phobic-obsessional" reaction to parents' overprotective or engulfing presence (e.g., Bruch, 1973; Johnson, 1991). A related concept, prominent in systems theories, emphasizes familial enmeshment and "boundary" problems (i.e., inadequate psychological separation among members) and emotional conflicts that result from deficits in the family's capacity to acknowledge affects (e.g., Minuchin, Rosman, & Baker, 1978; Palazolli, 1978). In both conceptualizations, Anorexia Nervosa is assumed to embody the child's struggle to establish a separate "self" definition and to mount a protest against the family's habitual mode of functioning. Less prominently, AN is linked to "oedipal" conflicts thought to motivate the child's avoidance of adult sexuality (Frazier, Faubion, Giffin, & Johnson, 1955; Sights & Richards, 1984). In support, "anorexic families" are noted as being characterized by quasi-incestuous father-daughter alliances or problematic identifications of daughters with sexually maladjusted mothers.

Family models of bulimic syndromes address an alternative spectrum of problems reflecting the child's frantic struggle to satisfy needs in a disengaged or neglectful family unit. Johnson (1991) links bulimic symptoms (and the "needy"/"impulsive" self organizations with which he believes bulimia coincides) to parental "neglect", which, in his view, spans a continuum from "nonmalevolent" forms (e.g., in families in which children are forced to function pseudomaturely, to meet parents' needs) to "malevolent" ones (occurring in blatantly abusive families). Humphrey (1991) formulates her conceptualization of bulimia in similar terms, referring to family-wide deficits in nurturance and tension regulation, and systems that ensnare members in mutually destructive, hostile projections. In both views, bulimic eating patterns are conceptualized as playing a self- and mood-regulatory function, and as being metaphors for family interactions colored by members' neediness, hostility, and criticism. Two family variants addressed by Root, Fallon, and Friedrich (1986) are compatible with those just described. One refers to "perfectionistic" families in which children receive implicit critical demands from parents, and the other refers to "chaotic and disengaged" families in which children are blatantly neglected or abused. A third variant resembles the stereotype of the anorexic family – it overprotectively locks the affected child into struggles around self-determination and control.

## 4.3 Empirical Findings on Family Dynamics

There is partial empirical support for many of the family concepts reviewed above. However, we preface our review by emphasizing that the real test of theory is in its capacity to answer the deceptively simple question: "Why an ED rather than some other disorder ?" Bearing this question in mind, doubts remain about the extent to which any dynamic family theory truly addresses ED-specific processes.

Consistent with theory, self-report studies on families of anorexic adolescents quite consistently report these families as limiting members' autonomy (Leon et al., 1985), as avoiding open criticism of members or the family unit (Heron & Leheup, 1984), or as showing unusually low levels of conflict (Monck, Graham, Richman, & Dobbs, 1990). Observational studies in adolescent samples, which are designed to elucidate dynamics of which family members themselves may not be aware, often corroborate the "enmeshed, conflict-avoiding family" concept. Crisp, Hsu, Harding, and Hartshorn (1980), in a semi-formal study, reported disturbed parent-child interactions in about half of 102 cases of AN, with "enmeshment" being the most commonly reported theme. Using coded records of parent-child interactions, Goldstein (1981) found that families of hospitalized anorexic adolescents manifested more dependency issues, requests for protection, and conflict avoidance, than did those of hospitalized non-anorexics or adolescents at-risk for schizophrenia. In a related vein, families of adolescent anorexics have been noted to display unusually low levels of Expressed Emotion (EE) (Hodes & LeGrange, 1993), which is to some extent compatible with conflict-avoidance.

Other studies loosely corroborate concepts of unusual gender-based or "oedipally-tinged" alliances in families where AN occurs. For example, Owen (1973), using a semantic differential task, found mothers of anorexics to be overly identified with their daughters. Similarly, Houben, Pierloot, and Vandereycken (1989) found that patterns featuring strong attachments to mothers and father-daughter boundary problems were more characteristic of anorexics' families than of control families.

Findings from studies on bulimic syndromes (anorexic and normal-weight) consistently point to an alternative family organization characterized by overt conflict and distress. Using various measures to obtain perceptions of family functioning from 105 DSM-III bulimics (young adults, aged 18-28) and 86 age-matched controls, Johnson and Flach (1985) noted that bulimics, relative to controls, perceived their families as being incohesive, high in conflict, and limited at expressing feelings. Degree of dysfunction in the family coincided with severity of bulimic symptoms. McNamara and Loveman (1990) obtained comparable results with the Family Assessment Device, in a comparison of 31 young-adult bulimics, 61 repeat dieters, and 59 nondieters. Bulimics rated their families as showing difficulties with affective involvement, affective responsiveness, communication, problem solving, and behavioral control. Various other self-report studies in bulimic families (see Wonderlich, 1992, for a full review) contribute to a portrait of an incohesive, disorganized, and conflictual family environment.

Observational studies bear out the impression of the bulimic's family as non-nurturant and conflict-laden, although they suggest that it may not be so much "incohesion" as a destructive sort of overinvolvement that is characteristic. Sights and Richards (1984) observed interactions in small numbers of families with college-aged bulimic or non-bulimic daughters and found the bulimics' families to be characterized by domineering and demanding mothers and greater parent-daughter stress. Similar themes are conveyed by Laura Humphrey's work (reviewed more fully in the following section), which emphasizes a fascinating observational system – the Structural Analysis of Social Behavior (SASB: Benjamin, 1974). Comparing interactions of 16 bulimic-anorexic triads (Mother-Father-Adolescent Daughter) to those of 24 normal triads, clinical families were noted to be more blameful, rejecting, and neglectful, and less nurturing and comforting (Humphrey, Apple & Kirschenbaum, 1986; Humphrey, 1987).

### 4.3.1 Restricter / Binger Differences

Many studies have explored restricter/binger differences in family functioning using validated, multiscale family assessment questionnaires (e.g., Garner, Garfinkel, & O'Shaughnessy, 1985; Kog, Vertommen, & Vandereycken, 1987; Steiger, Liquornik, Chapman, & Hussain, 1991; Thienemann & Steiner, 1993; Waller, Calam, & Slade, 1989). While inconsistencies exist (perhaps explained by differences in samples and settings), a recurring trend in reports of probands and relatives suggests that bulimic families display more overt structural and interactional problems.

A number of observational studies imply parallel restricter-binger differences: Szmukler, Eisler, Russell, and Dare (1985) rated EE in the families of 51 hospitalized patients (adolescents and adults, with mean age of 23), one-third of whom were bulimic. Results indicated higher EE (i.e., more open conflict and critical comments) in the bulimics' families. A series of observational studies by Humphrey in adolescent or young adult populations reiterates the theme that bulimic ED subtypes coincide with more openly conflictual or neglectful family-interaction styles. Using the Structural Analysis of Social Behavior to contrast experience of family process in 80 females with DSM-III Bulimia, Bulimic AN, Restrictive AN, or no ED, Humphrey (1986) identified deficits in parental nurturance and, to some extent, empathy in both bulimic subgroups. Two other reports use the SASB system to study 74 family triads, representing the same diagnostic groupings (Humphrey, 1988, 1989). Findings associated the restricter subtype with "nurturant enmeshment" in the family, and both anorexic and normal-weight "binger" subtypes with "hostile enmeshment". Rather than restricter-binger differences, however, Kog and Vandereycken (1989) reported an "anorexic-bulimic" distinction when comparing interaction patterns in families of 30 ED patients (adolescents and young adults) to those of 30 normal controls. They observed the families of anorexics (restricting and bulimic) as showing boundary problems and conflict avoidance, those of normal-weight bulimics as showing the opposite – firmer interpersonal boundaries and open disagreement. Across studies, findings converge (albeit inconsistently) to suggest two broad and opposing tendencies – one linking dietary restraint to familial enmeshment and conflict avoidance, the other linking bulimic symptoms to open conflicts and hostilities. It is equally evident, however, that a "restricter-binger" classification corresponds only imperfectly to distinct family interaction styles. For example, Kog, Vertommen, and Vandereycken's (1987) study of 55 families of patients with heterogeneous types of EDs identified important within-subtype heterogeneities. Notably, a pattern characterized by "boundary problems, rigidity, and low conflict" (that would theoretically coincide with the "restricter" pattern) was found to be as much associated with bulimic as with restrictive variants.

As an addendum to our discussion on restricter/binger differences in families, we briefly note an intriguing trend found in recent studies on the association between childhood sexual traumata and the EDs (see Vanderlinden and Vandereycken, this volume, for a review). Several studies in this area have noted sexual traumata to be more strongly linked to bulimic than to restrictive ED variants. While further data are needed to confirm this impression, the trend in question would be consistent with an overall portrait of the bulimic family as being the more blatantly disturbed or abusive.

## 4.3.2 Family Dynamics and Treatment

Treatment studies have suggested diverse types of effects linking dysfunctional family interactions to daughters' eating disorders. Crisp et al. (1974) reported that weight restoration in anorexics led to exacerbation of parental neuroticism, and suggested that this reflected a buffering role of the ED in the family dynamic. LeGrange, Eisler, Dare, and Hodes (1992) found that a high degree of Expressed Emotion at pre-treatment predicted poor response of anorexic adolescents to six-month outpatient therapies. Their result suggests a possible maintaining role of parental criticism in anorexic syndromes. Finally, Russell, Szmukler, Dare, and Eisler (1987) reported that family therapy benefitted teenaged patients in a group of 80 heterogeneous EDs, but that older patients responded better to individual supportive therapy. Their finding could imply that family dynamics have a maintaining role in the EDs, but more so in younger patients, who remain more influenced by their families.

### 4.3.3 Nonclinical Populations

Earlier, we described community-based studies that showed remarkable similarities, on individual psychopathological traits across clinical and nonclinical cases displaying ED-like symptoms. Parallel findings link nonclinical ED-spectrum disturbances to subject-reported family disturbances (e.g., Coburn & Ganong, 1989; Kagan & Squires, 1985; Scalf-McIver & Thompson, 1989; Steiger, Puentes-Neuman, & Leung, 1991). Furthermore, two studies address "restricter/binger" differences in community samples. Steiger and colleagues (1991) found that bulimic symptoms were more-consistently linked to subject-reported "family incohesion" than were restrictive ones. Using a similar self-report methodology, Smolak and Levine (1993) studied the link between separation issues and ED-spectrum disturbances in 198 nonclinical females (mean age of 20.5). They classified 19 cases as "bulimia-like", eight as "restricter-like", 11 as showing "mixed features", and 109 as showing "some ED symptoms". The restricter/binger distinctions that were obtained were intriguing: Cases with bulimic symptoms appeared "overseparated" from parents in terms of attitudinal independence, but "underseparated" in actuality, whereas "restricter-like" cases tended to be "underseparated" in both respects. We need not note the resemblance of such findings to those obtained in clinical samples.

## 5 Conclusions

Findings consistently link ED syndromes in adolescents to diverse psychopathological features and family problems. However, taken together, they support only a very unsatisfying generalization – that EDs occur in individuals with relatively diffuse "characterological/affective" problems and in families showing diffuse forms of dysfunction. Much work remains to be done to determine whether such individual and family factors act specifically in ED development or, instead, represent very nonspecific developmental and psychobiological processes that translate only indirectly into vulnerability to developing an ED. Recent studies conducted in adult samples converge on the idea that severity of deficits in family functioning may more closely predict the severity of personality disturbances in the ED sufferer, than they do the severity of his/her eating symptoms (Head & Williamson, 1990; Steiger, Liquornik, Chapman, & Hussain, 1991; Wonderlich & Swift, 1990). If this impression is correct, it may be that family disturbances are linked to generalized self-image problems in affected children, but that neither the family disturbances nor the individual problems act in any truly ED-specific fashion. Nonetheless, traits of compulsivity and dyscontrol, whether transmitted through biological or psychosocial pathways, are likely to play a role in structuring the expression of eating symptoms – i.e., in shaping the restricter's tendency to phobically avoid eating and weight gain, or the binger's tendency to give unbridled vent to impulses and then "undo". Therefore, clarification of the possible influences of individual and family processes in ED development remains relevant to the goal of developing an integrated causal formulation.

If EDs are indeed as multiply determined as biopsychosocial etiological theory would have it (e.g., Garfinkel & Garner, 1982; Johnson & Connors, 1987; Strober, 1991), pathways to them will likely be immensely complex and heterogeneous, and singularly psychological or family-based models will, at best, provide partial explanations. Following from this line of thinking, we propose that what may be of greatest interest about the EDs is, in fact, their tendency to have relatively nonspecific individual and family causes. The study of the EDs may (paradoxically) inform us more about the way in which many forms of psychopathology represent a "collision" between social pressures and psychological vulnerabilities than it does about the development of eating problems per se. In other words, in understanding the pathogenesis of the EDs, we may be learning about psychobiological processes that render affected individuals excessively permeable to contextual (social) influences and values. In Western social contexts, such vulnerabilities may often become manifest in the form of extreme susceptibility, especially in adolescent females, to social ideals of thinness. However, the same basic vulnerabilities may (in other contexts and life stages) account for diverse maladaptive investments (e.g., "workaholism", religious asceticism), that may equally reflect the adverse impacts of social ideals upon diffuse "self" deficits.

## References

Agras, W., & Kirkley, B. (1986). Bulimia: Theories of etiology. In K. Brownell & J. Foreyt (Eds.), *Handbook of eating disorders*. New York: Basic Books.
Attie, I., & Brooks-Gunn, J. (1989). Development of eating problems in adolescent girls: A longitudinal study. *Developmental Psychology, 25*, 70-79.
Beumont, P., George, G., & Smart, D. (1976). "Dieters" and "vomiters and purgers" in anorexia nervosa. *Psychological Medicine, 6*, 617-621.
Benjamin, L.S. (1974). Structural analysis of social behavior. *Psychological Review, 81*, 392-425.
Ben-Tovim, D., Marilov, V., & Crisp, A. (1979). Personality and mental state (PSE) within anorexia nervosa. *Journal of Psychosomatic Research, 23*, 321-325.

Bruch, H. (1973). *Eating disorders: Obesity, anorexia nervosa and the person within.* New York: Basic Books.

Casper, R. (1990). Personality features of women with good outcome from restricting anorexia nervosa. *Psychosomatic Medicine, 52,* 156-170.

Casper, R., Eckert, E., Halmi, K., Goldberg, S., & Davis, J. (1980). Bulimia: Its incidence and clinical importance in patients with anorexia nervosa. *Archives of General Psychiatry, 37,* 1030-1035.

Casper, R., Hedeker, D., & McClough, J. (1992). Personality dimensions in eating disorders and their relevance for subtyping. *Journal of the American Academy of Child and Adolescent Psychiatry, 31,* 830-840.

Coburn, J. & Ganong, L. (1989). Bulimic and non-bulimic college femles' perceptions of family adaptability and family cohesion. *Journal of Advanced Nursing, 14,* 27-33.

Crisp, A.H. (1980). *Anorexia nervosa: Let me be.* London: Academic Press.

Crisp, A.H., Harding, B. & McGuinness, B. (1974). Anorexia nervosa. Psychoneurotic characteristics of parents: Relationship to prognosis. *Journal of Psychosomatic Research, 18,* 167-173.

Crisp, A.H., Hsu, L., Harding, B. & Hartshorn, J. (1980). Clinical features of anorexia nervosa: A study of a consecutive series of 102 female patients. *Journal of Psychosomatic Research, 24,* 179-191.

Davies, E., & Furnham, A. (1986). Body satisfaction in adolescent girls. *British Journal of Medical Psychology, 59,* 279-287.

Edwin, D., Andersen, A., & Rosell, F. (1988). Outcome prediction by MMPI in subtypes of anorexia nervosa. *Psychosomatics, 29,* 273-282.

Eisele, J., Hertsgaard, D., & Light, H. (1986). Factors related to eating disorders in adolescent girls. *Adolescence, 82,* 283-290.

Fairburn, C., & Beglin, S. (1990). Studies of the epidemiology of bulimia nervosa. *American Journal of Psychiatry, 147,* 401-408.

Frazier, S.H., Faubion, M.H., Giffin, M.E. & Johnson, A.M. (1955). A specific factor in symptom choice. *Staff Meetings of the Mayo Clinic, 30,* 227-243.

Garfinkel, P., & Garner, D. (1982). *Anorexia nervosa: A multidimensional perspective.* New York: Brunner/Mazel.

Garfinkel, P.E., Garner, D., Rose, J., Darby, P., Brandes, J.S., O'Hanlon, J., & Walsh, N. (1983). A comparison of characteristics in the families of patients with anorexia nervosa and normal controls. *Psychological Medicine, 13,* 821-828.

Garner, D.M., Garfinkel, P.E. & O'Shaughnessy, M. (1985). The validity of the distinction between bulimia with and without anorexia nervosa. *American Journal of Psychiatry, 142,* 581-587.

Garner, D., Olmsted, M., Polivy, J., & Garfinkel, P. (1984). Comparison between weight preoccupied women and anorexia nervosa. *Psychosomatic Medicine, 46,* 255-266.

Goldstein, H.J. (1981). Family factors associated with schizophrenia and anorexia nervosa. *Journal of Youth and Adolescence, 10,* 385-405.

Gross, J., & Rosen, J. (1988). Bulimia in adolescents: Prevalence and psychosocial correlates. *International Journal of Eating Disorders, 7,* 51-61.

Gull, W.W. (1874). Anorexia nervosa (apepsia/hysterica, anorexia hysterica). In M.R. Kaufman & M. Helman (Eds.), *Evolution of psychosomatic concepts: Anorexia nervosa.* New York: International Press.

Hall, A. & Brown, L.B. (1983). A comparison of the attitudes of young anorexia nervosa patients and non-patients with those of their mothers. *British Journal of Medical Psychology, 56,* 39-48.

Hall, A., Leibrich, J., Walkley, F. & Welch, G. (1986). Investigation of "weight pathology" of 58 mothers of anorexia nervosa patients and 204 mothers of schoolgirls. *Psychological Medicine, 16,* 71-76.

Halmi, K.A., (1974). Anorexia nervosa: Demographic and clinical features in 94 cases. *Psychosomatic Medicine, 36,* 18-26.

Halmi, K.A., Strauss, A. & Goldberg, S.C. (1978). An investigation of weights in the parents of anorexia nervosa patients. *Journal of Nervous and Mental Disease, 166,* 358-361.

Head, S.B. & Williamson, D.A. (1990). Association of family environment and personality disturbance in bulimia nervosa. *International Journal of Eating Disorders, 9,* 667-674.

Heron, J.M. & Leheup, R.F. (1984). Happy families? *British Journal of Psychiatry, 148,* 136-138.

Herzog, D.B., Keller, M.B., Lavori, P.W., & Bradburn, I.S. (1991). Bulimia nervosa in adolescence. *Developmental and Behavioral Pediatrics, 12,* 191-195.

Hill, A.J., Weaver, C. & Blundell, J.E. (1990). Dieting concerns of 10-year-old girls and their mothers. *British Journal of Clinical Psychology, 29,* 346-348.
Hodes, M. & LeGrange, D. (1993). Expressed emotion in the investigation of eating disorders: A review. *International Journal of Eating Disorders, 13,* 279-288.
Holland, A.J., Sicotte, N. & Treasure, J. (1988). Anorexia nervosa: Evidence for a genetic basis. *Journal of Psychosomatic Research, 32,* 561-571.
Houben, M.E., Pierloot, R. & Vandereycken, W. (1989). The preception of interpersonal relationships in families of anorexia nervosa patients compared with normals. In: Vendereycken, W., Kog, E. & Vanderlinden, J. (Eds*.). The family approach to eating disorders.* New York: PMA Publishing, pp. 147-160.
Hudson, J.I., Pope H.G., Jr., Jonas, J.M. et al. (1987). A controlled family history study of bulimia. *Psychological Medicine, 17,* 883-890.
Humphrey, L.L. (1986). Structural analysis of parent-child relationships in eating disorders. *Journal of Abnormal Psychology, 93,* 395-402.
Humphrey, L.L. (1987). A comparison of bulimic-anorexic and non-distressed families using structural analysis of social behavior. *Journal of the Amercian Academy of Child and Adolescent Psychiatry, 26,* 248-255.
Humphrey, L.L. (1988). Relationships within subtypes of anorexic, bulimic and normal families. *Journal of the American Academy of Child and Adolescent Psychiatry, 27,* 544-551.
Humphrey, L.L. (1989). Observed family interactions among subtypes of eating disorders using structural analysis of social behavior. *Journal of Consulting and Clinical psychology, 57,* 206-213.
Humphrey, L.L. (1991). Object relations and the family system: An integrative approach to understanding and treating eating disorders. In Johnson, C. (Ed.), *Psychodynamic Treatment of Anorexia Nervosa and Bulimia.* New York: Guilford Press.
Humphrey, L.L., Apple, R.F. & Kirschenbaum, D.S. (1986). Differentiating bulimic-anorexic from normal families using interpersonal and behavioral observational systems. *Journal of Consulting and Clinical psychology, 54,* 190-195.
Johnson, C. (1991). Treatment of eating-disordered patients with borderline and false-self/narcissistic disorders. In Johnson, C. (Ed.). *Psychodynamic Treatment of Anorexia Nervosa and Bulimia.* New York: Guilford Press.
Johnson, C., & Connors, M. (1987). *The etiology and treatment of bulimia nervosa.* New York: Basic Books.
Johnson, C. & Flach, A. (1985). Family characteristics of 105 patients with bulimia. *American Journal of Psychiatry, 142,* 1321-1324.
Johnson, C., & Wonderlich, S. (1992). Personality characteristics as a risk factor in the development of eating disorders. In J.H. Crowther, D.L. Tennenbaum, S.E. Hobfell, & M.A.P. Stephens, (Eds.), *The etiology of bulimia nervosa: The individual and family context.* Hemishpere Publishing: Ohio.
Kagan, D.M. & Squires, R.L. (1985). Family cohesion, Family adaptability and eating behaviors among college students. *International Journal of Eating Disorders, 4,* 267-279.
Kassett, J.A., Gershon, E.S., Maxwell, M.E., et al. (1989). Psychiatric disorders in the first-degree relatives of probands with bulimia nervosa. *American Journal of Psychiatry, 146,* 1468-1471.
Kendler, K.S., MacLean, C., Neale, M., Kessler, R., Heath, A. & Eaves, L. (1991). The genetic epidemiology of bulimia nervosa. *Amercian Journal of Psychiatry, 148,* 1627-1637.
Kog, E. & Vandereycken, W. (1989). Family interaction in eating disorder patients and normal controls. *International Journal of Eating Disorders, 8,* 11-23.
Kog, E., Vertommen, H. & Vandereycken, W. (1987). Minuchin's psychosomatic family model revised: A concept validation study using a multitrait-multimethod apporach. *Family Process, 26,* 235-253.
Laessle, R., Kittl, S., Fichter, M., Wittchen, H., & Pirke, K. (1987). Major affective disorder in anorexia nervosa and bulimia: A descriptive diagnostic study. *British Journal of Psychiatry, 151,* 785-789.
LeGrange, D., Eisler, I., Dare, C. & Russell, G.F.M. (1992). Evaluation of family treatments in adolescent anorexia nervosa: A pilot study. *International Journal of Eating Disorders, 12,* 347-357.
Leon, G., Fulkerson, J.A., Perry, C.I., & Cudeck, R. (1993). Personality and behavioral vulnerabilities associated with risk status for eating disorders in adolescent girls. *Journal of Abnormal Psychology, 102,* 438-444.

Leon, G., Lucas, A., Colligan, R., Ferlinande, R., & Kamp, J. (1985). Sexual, body-image, and personality attitudes in anorexia nervosa. *Journal of Abnormal Child Psychology, 13*, 245-258.

Lucas, A.R., Beard, C.M., O'Fallon, W.M., & Kurland, L.T. (1991). 50-year trends in the incidence of anorexia nervosa in Rochester, Minn.: A population-based study. *American Journal of Psychiatry, 148*, 917-922.

McNamara, H. & Loveman, C. (1990). Differences in family functioning among bulimics, repeat dieters and nondieters. *Journal of Clinical Psychology, 46*, 518-523.

Minuchin, S., Rosman, B.L., & Baker, L. (1978). *Psychosomatic families: Anorexia nervosa in context.* Cambridge, Ma: Harvard University Press.

Monck, E., Graham, P., Richman, N. & Dobbs, R. (1990). Eating and weight-control problems in a community population of adolescent girls aged 15-20 years. In H. Remschmidt & M.H. Schmidt (Eds.), *Anorexia nervosa* (pp. 1-12). Toronto: Hogrefe and Huber Publishers.

Owen, S.E.H. (1973). The projective identification of the parents of patients suffering from anorexia nervosa. *Australian and New Zealand Journal of Psychiatry, 7*, 285-290.

Palazolli, M. (1978). *Self-starvation: From individual to family therapy in the treatment of anorexia nervosa.* New York: Jason Aronson.

Patton, G. (1988). The spectrum of eating disorder in adolescence. *Journal of Psychosomatic Research, 32*, 579-584.

Pike, K.M. & Rodin, J. (1991). Mothers, daughters, and disordered eating. *Journal of Abnormal Psychology, 100*, 198-204.

Piran, N., Kennedy, S., Garfinkel, P.E. & Owens, M. (1985). Affective disturbance in eating disorders. *Journal of Nervous and Mental Disease, 173*, 395-400.

Råstam, M. (1992). Anorexia nervosa in 51 Swedish adolescents: Premorbid problems and comorbidity. *Journal of the American Academy of Child and Adolescent Psychiatry, 31*, 819-829.

Root, M.P., Fallon, P. & Friedrich, W.N. (1986). *Bulimia: A systems approach to treatment.* New York: W.W. Norton.

Rosen, J., & Gross, J. (1987). Prevalence of weight reducing and weight gaining in adolescent girls and boys. *Health Psychology, 6*, 131-147.

Russell, G.F.M., Szmukler, G.I., Dare, C. & Eisler, I. (1987). An evaluation of family therapy in anorexia and bulimia nervosa. *Archives of General Psychiatry, 44*, 1047-1056.

Scalf-McIver, L. & Thompson, J.K. (1989). Family correlates of bulimic characteristics in college females. *Journal of Clinical Psychology, 45*, 467-472.

Sights, J.R. & Richards, H.C. (1984). Parents of bulimic women. *International Journal of Eating Disorders, 3*, 3-13.

Smart, D., Beumont, P., & George, G. (1976). Some personality characteristics of patients with anorexia nervosa. *British Journal of Psychiatry, 128*, 57-60.

Smith, C., & Steiner, H. (1992). Psychopathology in anorexia nervosa and depression. *Journal of the American Academy of Child and Adolescent Psychiatry, 31*, 841-843.

Smolak, L. & Levine, M.P. (1993). Separation-individuation difficulties and the distinction between bulimia nervosa and anorexia nervosa in college women. *International Journal of Eating Disorders, 14*, 33-41.

Sohlberg, S., & Strober, M. (1994). Personality in anorexia nervosa: An update and a theoretical integration. *Acta Psychiatrica Scandinavica, 89* (supp 378), 1-15.

Steiger, H., Goldstein, C., Mongrain, M., & Van der Feen, J. (1990). Description of eating-disordered, psychiatric and normal women on cognitive and psychodynamic measures. *International Journal of Eating Disorders, 9*, 129-140.

Steiger, H., Leung, F., & Houle, L. (1992). Relationships among borderline features, body-dissatisfaction and bulimic symptoms in nonclinical females. *Addictive Behaviors, 17*, 397-406.

Steiger, H., Leung, F., Puentes-Neuman, G., & Gottheil, N. (1992). Psychosocial profiles of adolescent girls with varying degrees of eating and mood disturbances. *International Journal of Eating Disorders, 11*, 121-131.

Steiger, H., Leung, F., Thibeaudeau, J., Houle, L. & Ghadirian,A.M. (1993). Comorbid features in bulimics before and after therapy: Are they explained by Axis II diagnoses, secondary effects of bulimia, or both ? *Comprehensive Psychiatry, 34*, 45-53.

Steiger, H., Liquornik, K., Chapman, J. & Hussain, N. (1991). Personality and family disturbances in eating-disorder patients: Comparison of "restricters" and "bingers" to normal controls. *International Journal of Eating Disorders, 10*, 501-512.

Steiger, H., Puentes-Neuman, G. & Leung, F. (1991). Personality and family features of adolescent girls with eating symptoms: Evidence for restricter/binger differences in a nonclinical population. *Addictive Behaviors, 16*, 303-314.

Steiger, H., Stotland, S., Ghadirian, A.M. & Whitehead, V. (in press). Controlled study of eating concerns and psychopathological traits in relatives of eating-disordered probands: Do familial traits exist ? *International Journal of Eating Disorders*.

Steiner, H. (1990). Defense styles in eating disorders. *International Journal of Eating Disorders, 9*, 141-151.

Stotland, S., & Steiger, H. (1994). Narcissistic personality pathology and eating disorders. Paper presented at the *Sixth International Conference on Eating Disorders*, New York, April 30, 1994.

Striegel-Moore, R., Silberstein, L., Frensch, P., and Rodin, J. (1989). A prospective study of disordered eating among college students. *International Journal of Eating Disorders, 8*, 599-509.

Strober, M. (1980). Personality and symptomatological features in young nonchronic anorexia nervosa patients. *Journal of Psychosomatic Research, 24*, 353-359.

Strober, M. (1981). A comparative analysis of personality organization in juvenile anorexia nervosa. Journal of Youth and Adolescence, 10, 285-295.

Strober, M. (1981a). The significance of bulimia in juvenile anorexia nervosa: An exploration of possible etiologic factors. *International Journal of Eating Disorders, 1*, 28-43.

Strober, M. (1991). Disorders of the self in anorexia nervosa: An organismic-developmental paradigm. In C. Johnson (Ed.), *Psychodynamic treatment for eating disorders*. New York:

Strober, M., & Katz, J. (1988). Depression in the eating disorders: A review and analysis of descriptive, family, and biological findings. In D. Garner & P. Garfinkel (Eds.), *Diagnostic issues in anorexia nervosa and bulimia nervosa*. New York: Brunner/Mazel.

Strober, M., Lampert, C., Morrell, W., et al. (1990). A controlled family study of anorexia nervosa: Evidence of familial aggregation and lack of shared transmission with affective disorders. *International Journal of Eating Disorders, 9*, 239-253.

Strober, M., Salkin, B., Burroughs, M. & Morrell, W. (1982). Validity of the bulimic-restricter distinction in anorexia nervosa: Parental personality characteristics and family morbidity. *Journal of Nervous and Mental Disease, 170*, 345-351.

Swift, W.J., Andrews, D., & Barklage, N.E. (1986). The relationship between affective disorder and eating disorders: A review of the literature. *American Journalo of Psychiatry, 143*, 290-299.

Swift, W., Bushnell, N., Hanson, P., & Logemann, T. (1986). Self-concept in adolescent anorexics. *Journal of the American Academy of Child Psychiatry, 25*, 826-835.

Szmukler, G.I., Eisler, I., Russell, G.F.M. & Dare, C. (1985). Anorexia nervosa, parental "expressed emotion" and dropping out of treatment. *British Journal of Psychitry, 151*, 174-178.

Thienemann, M. & Steiner, H. (1998). Family environment of eating disordered and depressed adolescents. *International Journal of Eating Disorders, 14*, 43-48.

Toner, B., Garfinkel, P., & Garner, D. (1986). Long-term follow-up of anorexia nervosa. *Psychosomatic Medicine, 48*, 520-529.

Treasure, J. & Holland, A.J. (1989). Genetic vulnerability to eating disorders: Evidence from twin and family studies. In: Remschmidt, H., Schmidt, M.H. (eds). *Child and Youth Psychiatry: European Perspectives*. New York: Hogrefe and Huber.

Vitousek, K., & Manke, F. (1994). Personality variables and disorders in anorexia nervosa and bulimia nervosa. *Journal of Abnormal Psychology, 103*, 137-147.

Waller, G., Calam, R. & Slade, P. (1989). Eating disorders and family interaction. *British Journal of Clinical Psychology, 28*, 285-286.

Wardle, J., & Beales, S. (1986). Restraint, body image and food attitudes in children from 12-18 years. Appetite, 7, 209-217.

Whitaker, A., Davies, M., Shaffer, D., Johnson, J., Abrams, S., Walsh, B. & Kalikow, K. (1989). The struggle to be thin: A survey of anorexic and bulimic symptoms in a non-referred adolescent population. *Psychological Medicine, 19*,143-163.

Windauer, U., Lennerts, W., Talbot, P., Touyz, S., & Beumont, P. (1993). How well are "cured" anorexia nervosa patients? An investigation of 16 weight-recovered anorexic patients. *British Journal of Psychiatry, 163*, 195-200.

Wold, P.N. (1985). Family attitudes toward weight in bulimia and affective disorders-a pilot study. *The Psychiatric Journal of the University of Ottawa, 10*, 162-164.

Wonderlich, S.A. (1992). Relationship of family and personality factors in bulimia. In Crowther, J.H., Tennenbaum, D.L., Hobfell, S.E. & Stephens, M.A.P. (Eds.). *The etiology of bulimia nervosa: The individual and family context.* Hemishpere Publishing: Ohio.

Wonderlich, S.A. & Swift, W.J. (1990). Borderline versus other personality disorders in the eating disorders. *International Journal of Eating Disorders, 9,* 629-638.

# Social Avoidance, Social Negativism, and Disorders of Empathy in a Subgroup of Young Individuals with Anorexia Nervosa

*Maria Råstam, Christopher Gillberg, and I. Carina Gillberg*

## 1 Introduction

Anorexia nervosa is a common disorder, often with adolescent onset. It affects more than 1% of females and 0.1% of males under age 18 years (Råstam et al., 1989; Rathner and Messner, 1993). Premorbid constitutional and personality factors may play an important role in the pathogenesis of the disorder or at least in the expression of the symptoms associated with the eating disorder (Dally, 1969; Gartner et al.,1989; Casper, 1990; Råstam, 1992). Co-morbidity patterns of anorexia nervosa, particularly the relation to other eating disorders, affective disorders, and anxiety disorders have currently been explored (Toner et al., 1988; Halmi et al., 1991). It now seems clear that anorexia nervosa sometimes develops into bulimia nervosa. A very high rate of comorbid depression in anorexia nervosa has also been repeatedly demonstrated (Cantwell et al., 1977; Hendren, 1983).

Operationalized criteria (American Psychiatric Association, 1980; Loranger et al., 1987) and structured instruments for diagnosing personality disorders (American Psychiatric Association, 1987; Spitzer et al., 1992) have only appeared in the last ten to fifteen years. Cluster C DSM-III-R personality disorders (i.e., avoidant, dependent, obsessive-compulsive, and passive-aggressive, all of which involve a restriction of the social interaction repertoire) were found to be exceptionally common in a study by Halmi et al. (1991). Avoidant personality disorder was more common in clinically referred anorexia nervosa cases than in a control group in the study by Casper (1990). Råstam (1992) reported that obsessive compulsive personality disorder (OCPD) occurred in 35% of the cases of anorexia nervosa drawn from the general population compared with 4% of non-anorexia nervosa comparison cases matched for age, sex and school. Diagnoses were made by a rater blind to eating disorder status on the basis of case notes prepared from structured interviews covering personality variables and personality disorders. C. Gillberg and Råstam (1992) further suggested that a subgroup of cases with anorexia nervosa might have underlying autistic-like conditions with severe restrictions of social interaction, communication and imagination, behaviour and interest patterns.

## 2 Methods

### 2.1 Subjects

Twenty-three female subjects (including one patient ascertained as meeting DSM-III-R criteria for anorexia nervosa who refused participation in the post-screening neuropsychiatric part of the study) and two male subjects constituted the total population of individuals born in Göteborg in 1970 who developed DSM-III-R-defined anorexia nervosa before the age of 18 years. The details of the epidemiological study have already been published (Råstam et al., 1989; Råstam, 1992; Råstam and C. Gillberg, 1991). In the first report, reference is made to 20 subjects diagnosed under age 16 years. The population was later followed up to age 18 years and five further subjects had onset at age 16 or 17 years. The findings correspond to a population prevalence of anorexia nervosa of 1.08% for females and 0.09% for males, in those 17 years and younger and a population-corrected female:male ratio of 11.6:1.0. The Göteborg study of anorexia nervosa is the only clear population study that comprises a reasonable number of subjects in the field. Because every single teenager was examined without clothing, had his/her growth chart scrutinized in detail, was followed up for more than a year by the same school nurse and because 99.7% (N=4280) of the entire population completed an anorexia nervosa screening questionnaire, we believe that we have not missed any anorexia nervosa cases in this population.

The population group (22 female and 2 male subjects plus the female subject who refused in-depth study) was pooled with another population screening sample of subjects with anorexia nervosa (26 females and 1 male) who were reported to the research team by school health nurses, doctors, pediatricians, and child psychiatrists during the first two years of follow-up of the original population group. This sample was less comprehensive than the original one, but it was not a clinically referred group. In fact, more than one third of this group had not been treated for the eating disorder. We have estimated that the latter sample comprises about 60% of all anorexia nervosa cases in their birth cohort.

All 51 subjects in this study met DSM-III-R criteria for the disorder. Forty-eight of these met or had met such criteria already at the time of the first diagnostic study, but three were classified as partial syndrome of anorexia nervosa at that time. However, these three subjects later met full DSM-III-R criteria.

Thus, the study group consisted of (a) *anorexia nervosa-total-1* (comprising the 17 female subjects (excluding the one who refused participation in the neuropsychiatric study) and 2 male subjects in the first population group who had onset of anorexia nervosa before age 16 years), (b) *anorexia nervosa-total-2* (comprising the 5 female subjects belonging to the first population group who had onset of anorexia nervosa at age 16 or 17 years) and, (c) *anorexia nervosa-screen* (comprising the 26 female subjects and 1 male subject with adolescent onset anorexia nervosa in this subgroup, who were reported during the follow-up of groups (a) and (b). In this subgroup, however, more cases were reported to be in contact with treatment facilities. This is not surprising given that, as a direct consequence of the research project as such, both interest in treatment and intensive efforts at referring for treatment increased during the follow-up of the original population group. The collapsed (anorexia nervosa - total-1 and total-2 groups in this paper will be pooled with the *anorexia nervosa-screen group* to produce the *anorexia nervosa-group*.

The three anorexia nervosa subgroups have been compared with regard to several hundred background measures (relating to aspects of development, personality, physical illness, family situation, family interaction, etc.) and found to be similar in virtually all aspects other than treatment received. The anorexia nervosa-total-1 group was referred to as the anorexia nervosa-P group and the collapsed anorexia nervosa-total 2 and anorexia nervosa-screen group as the anorexia nervosa-M group in a previous publication (Råstam et al., 1992) that analyzed the premorbid personality disorder pattern in the present samples. The anorexia nervosa-group will be compared throughout with 51 sex and age-matched healthy subjects from the same school and recruited by the school nurse at the time of the original diagnostic study. This group will be referred to as the *COMP-group*. There was no drop out from the follow-up study and all 102 individuals assigned for study were seen personally and examined in accordance with the procedure described below.

The mean age of reported anorexia nervosa onset was 14.3 years (95% confidence interval 13.9-14.7). The mean age at first examination was 16.1 (95% confidence interval 15.7-16.5) years in the anorexia nervosa-total group, 16.0 years (95% confidence interval 15.5-16.5) in the anorexia nervosa-screen group and 16.0 years (95% confidence interval 15.5-16.5) in the COMP group. The mean age at follow-up examination was 21.0 years (95% confidence interval 20.5-21.4) in the anorexia nervosa group and 20.8 years (95% confidence interval 20.3-21.3) in the COMP group. The anorexia nervosa-total and anorexia nervosa-screen groups were of almost identical age at follow-up. The average time that had elapsed from reported onset of anorexia nervosa to the time of the follow-up study was 6.7 years (95% confidence interval 6.3-7.0). The average time that had elapsed from the first examination to the time of the follow-up study was 4.9 years (95% confidence interval 4.7-5.2) in the anorexia nervosa group and 4.6 years (95% confidence interval 4.3-4.9) in the COMP group. The anorexia nervosa-total group had been followed up for a slightly longer period of time than had the anorexia nervosa-screen group. Some of the characteristics of the anorexia nervosa and COMP groups at age 16 and 21 years are shown in Table 1.

## 2.2 Methods Used

At the time the clinical subjects were diagnosed with anorexia nervosa, the subjects of both the anorexia nervosa and COMP group had a mean age of 16 years. The subjects were seen by a psychiatrist (MR) who interviewed them and their mothers in depth concerning family history, family situation, early development, temperament, personality, physical and mental symptoms, and the extent to which the family and child had sought assistance or treatment for anorexia nervosa and other problems or disabilities. MR also performed a limited neurodevelopmental examination.

After this assessment, MR prepared deidentified case-notes covering physical, mental, and behavioural development and problems up to the age of about 10, i.e., one or several years before the development of anorexia nervosa. These case-notes from the anorexia nervosa and comparison group were then put in random order and submitted to CG, who was blind to the children's diagnoses, for scrutiny. CG used the DSM-III-R and made diagnoses of premorbid Axis I diagnoses in accordance with this. He also used criteria by I.C. Gillberg and C. Gillberg (1989) for diagnosing Asperger syndrome.

Table 1. Weight and Height SD at Age 16 and Age 21 Years in Anorexia Nervosa and COMP Groups

|  | AN (N=51) Age 16 yrs | AN (N=51) Age 21 yrs | COMP (N=51) Age 16 yrs | COMP (N=51) Age 21 yrs |
|---|---|---|---|---|
| **Weight** | | | | |
| Mean | 49.4** | 58.9 | 56.2 | 60.4 |
| S.D. | 8.8 | 11.8 | 6.6 | 7.9 |
| Confidence limits | 47.0-51.8 | 55.6-62.2 | 54.4-58.0 | 58.2-62.6 |
| **Height** | | | | |
| Mean | 164.3 | 166.2* | 166.7 | 169.1 |
| S.D. | 5.8 | 6.4 | 6.9 | 6.8 |
| Confidence limits | 162.7-165.9 | 164.4-168.0 | 164.8-168.8 | 167.2-171.0 |
| Extremely under-weight (n) | 15*** | 4* | 0 | 0 |
| Extremely over-weight (n) | 1 | 3* | 0 | 0 |
| Extremely short (n) | 0 | 6* | 0 | 0 |

AN=Anorexia Nervosa; COMP=Comparison; *** $p<.001$ AN and COMP compared; ** $p<.01$ AN and COMP compared; * $p<.05$ AN and COMP compared

The individuals with anorexia nervosa and those in the COMP group were later followed up at a mean age of 21 years by another clinician (psychiatrist), who is also a psychologist (ICG), blind to the original group status. Only a few (N=4) of the anorexia nervosa cases were noticeably underweight at that time, and it was not possible for the clinician (ICG) to determine which original diagnostic group they had belonged to. Furthermore, each individual was specifically instructed by the receptionist nurse not to mention anything about whether or not she/he had suffered from an eating disorder. The clinician (ICG) performed the Structured Clinical Interview-II (SCID-II, Spitzer et al., 1992) in order to elicit information to make appropriate personality disorder diagnoses. She also made an overall judgement as to each individual's capacity for empathizing with the perspectives, thoughts, and feelings of others (see below). She administered the Dewey social awareness test (Dewey, 1991) and performed neurodevelopmental and neurological tests. She also administered the Wechsler Adult Intelligence Scale (WAIS-R, Wechsler, 1992) and requested some information relating to overall functioning.

In addition, all individuals were examined again by the psychiatrist who had performed the diagnostic study (MR). She used the SCID-I (Spitzer et al., 1992) to elicit information for establishing appropriate Axis I diagnoses according to the DSM-III-R. She also interviewed the young adults, using the revised version of the Morgan-Russell anorexia nervosa outcome scales (Morgan & Hayward, 1988). In addition, she made a rating of emphatic skills as reflected during interview, corresponding to the rating made by the clinician (ICG) (see below). Finally, she weighed all the individuals in the study. Height was reported by the individuals themselves at interview.

At the end of the interviews, DSM-III-R diagnoses were made independently by the two psychiatrists (Axis I by MR and Axis II by ICG). Paranoid, schizoid and schizotypal personality disorder (Cluster A personality disorders) were classified as a group of personality disorders considered as reflecting *social negativism*. Avoidant, dependent, and obsessive-compulsive personality disorders (OCPD) (i.e., three of the four Cluster C personality disorders) were considered as reflecting *social withdrawal*. ICG also checked a list of 20 symptoms and diagnostic criteria for *Asperger syndrome* as outlined in I.C. Gillberg and C. Gillberg (1989) and elaborated in C. Gillberg (1991). These criteria have been shown to have good interrater-reliability (Ehlers and C. Gillberg, 1993). After the completion of the study, the diagnostic criteria for Asperger syndrome of the ICD-10 were also checked. ICG also checked a list of the 16 symptoms and diagnostic criteria for the DSM-III-R. When 6-7 of the required 8 (out of 16 possible) necessary criteria for *autistic disorder* were met, a diagnosis of *other autistic-like condition* was made. *Autism spectrum disorder (ASD)* was the blanket-term used when either Asperger syndrome criteria or criteria for other autistic-like conditions were met.

After the data collection was finished and the diagnoses according to Axis I and Axis II had been made, the two psychiatrists met to make a conjoint diagnosis of "empathy disorder" on the basis of all information and observation data obtained by both of them in connection with the interviews. The psychiatrist who had been blind to original group status (ICG) remained blind throughout this procedure.

Empathy deficits were rated on a 5-point scale: 0=no problems, 0.5=possibly mild problems, 1.0=mild problems, 1.5=possibly severe problems, 2.0=severe problems. A diagnosis of *empathy disorder* was made for individuals who (a) were given a score of 2.0 and, (b) who had professed during the interview that they had a problem understanding other people's perspectives, thoughts, and feelings and, (c) who felt socially inept themselves or related in a non-reciprocal fashion with the examiner. Inter-rater reliability for empathy disorder, as diagnosed above is good if psychiatrists have worked together for at least two months and have been using this concept in their diagnostic work-up of patients. In a preliminary study, which included 20 individuals in the 20-50 year-old age range, five of whom had Asperger syndrome and the remaining 15 being a sample from the normal population, three psychiatrists showed complete agreement in 60% of the assessments. A difference across all three raters of 0.5 on a 5-point scale (as described earlier) in 15%, and a difference across all three raters of 1.0 in 25% were seen. At least two of the three psychiatrists agreed completely in 90% of the assessments (C. Gillberg, 1991).

Some of the outcome data are published in separate reports. Thus, for instance, the Morgan-Russell scale data are presented in one paper (I.C. Gillberg et al., 1994a), and the Axis I and Axis II diagnoses and psychological achievement aspects (I.C. Gillberg et al., 1994b, Råstam et al., 1994). The present study deals with personality disorders that involve social withdrawal, social negativism, ASD, and empathy disorders at age 21 years.

## 3 Results

### 3.1 Overall Outcome

IQ was above 72 in all 102 individuals. However, two anorexia nervosa and two comparison subjects, had IQs in the 73-84 range. Fifty-three percent of the anorexia nervosa group were not recovered from anorexia nervosa according to their own opinion. However, of these, almost three quarters considered themselves improved. Interestingly, a girl who considered herself recovered was diagnosed as suffering from empathy disorder and OCPD. Four girls were extremely underweight at follow-up (Table 1). Three girls still fulfilled criteria for anorexia nervosa according to DSM-III-R.

## 3.2 Empathy Disorders, ASD and Personality Disorders Considered as Reflecting Social Negativism and/or Social Withdrawal

Fifteen subjects (29%) in the anorexia nervosa group had an empathy disorder (compared with 4% in the COMP group, p<0.01) as shown in Table 2. Several of these anorexia nervosa empathy disorder subjects met criteria for ASD: Asperger syndrome (5 female subjects, 1 male subject), or autistic-like conditions (4 female subjects). A male subject with Asperger syndrome and a female subject with an autistic-like condition were diagnosed as suffering from OCPD. Another female subject with Asperger syndrome was also diagnosed with OCPD and paranoid and narcissistic personality disorder. A female subject with an autistic-like condition also received the diagnoses of paranoid and schizotypal personality disorder. A further female subject with an autistic like condition also received the diagnoses of paranoid and narcissistic personality disorder. The remaining 4 female subjects with Asperger syndrome and the one with an autistic-like condition were not given SCID Axis II diagnoses.

Table 2. ASD, Personality Disorders Involving Severe Problems of Reciprocal Social Interaction (Cluster C) and Empathy Disorders

| Type of problem | AN (N=51) N | AN (N=51) % | COMP (N=51) N | COMP (N=51) % | p-level |
|---|---|---|---|---|---|
| Autism spectrum disorders | | | | | |
| Asperger syndrome | 6 | 12[*] | 0 | | <.05 |
| Other autisticlike conditions | 4 | 8 | 0 | | <.001 |
| Any autism spectrum disorder | 10 | 20 | 0 | | <.0001 |
| Any cluster C personality or autism spectrum disorder | 25 | 49 | 5 | 10 | <.0001 |
| Empathy disorder | 15 | 29 | 2 | 4 | <.001 |

AN=Anorexia Nervosa; COMP=Comparison; [*] Including 2 cases meeting 5 of the 6 criteria for Asperger syndrome according to the elaborated criteria set out in C. Gillberg (1991); meeting full ICD-10 (WHO, 1993) criteria for Asperger syndrome in all cases (except that it is usually impossible to ascertain that the language development accorded exactly with that described in the ICD-10).

Four of the 15 individuals with empathy disorder in the anorexia nervosa group received no other diagnosis (Axis I or Axis II). However, two of the four were in the bottom five with regard to outcome according to Morgan Russell average scores. Forty-nine percent (N=25) of the anorexia nervosa group had either a personality disorder involving social negativism or social avoidance diagnosis, a diagnosis of ASD, or a diagnosis of empathy disorder compared with 10% of the individuals in the COMP group (p<.0001).

### 3.2.1 Obsessive Compulsive Symptoms and ASD in Anorexia Nervosa: Change Over Time

Almost exactly as many individuals in each of the anorexia nervosa and comparison groups showed either OCD, OCPD, ASD, or any combination of these at follow-up as they had in the original study at age 16 years (Table 3). More than three quarters who showed OCD, OCPD, or ASD at either of the two ages did so at both ages. Twenty-seven percent of the anorexia nervosa and 4% of the COMP group showed OCPD or ASD or both at both ages (p<.01). Both OCPD and ASD were diagnosed by raters blind to anorexia nervosa/COMP group status at both ages.

Of the six individuals diagnosed with Asperger syndrome at age 21 years, only the male subject had already been diagnosed with this condition at the time of the original study. Two of the five female subjects with Asperger syndrome at follow-up had been diagnosed as suffering from an autistic-like condition in the diagnostic study at age 16 years. Two further female subjects with autistic-like conditions at the time of the first study again received this diagnosis at age 21 years. The three "new" subjects with Asperger syndrome at follow-up had received diagnoses of OCPD (N=2) and "identity disorder" (N=1) at age 16 years. The two "new" subjects with autistic-like conditions had been diagnosed in the diagnostic study at age 16 years as suffering from OCPD and Tourette respectively. (It merits mention here that all diagnoses pertaining to ASD and personality disorders were made by two independent clinicians, and that both of these were blind with regard to original group status and the diagnostic assessments made by previous investigators.)

Table 3. The Development of Obsessive Compulsive Problems and ASD from Age 16 to 21 Years

| Problem | AN (N=51) N | % | COMP (N=51) N | % | p-level |
|---|---|---|---|---|---|
| Any OCD/OCPD/AS/ALC at age 16 | 30 | 59 | 5 | 10 | <.0001 |
| Any OCD/OCPD/AS/ALC at age 21 | 30 | 59 | 6 | 12 | <.0001 |
| OCD/OCPD/AS/ALC at both ages | 23 | 45 | 5 | 10 | <.001 |
| OCPD/AS/ALC at both ages | 14 | 27 | 2 | 4 | <.01 |

AN=Anorexia Nervosa; COMP=Comparison

## 4 Discussion

Empathy disorder (including Asperger syndrome and other autistic-like conditions) was present in 29% of the anorexia nervosa group and in only 4% of the comparison group. Empathy disorder is not a widely used diagnostic concept, but it has recently been suggested that it is associated with (or indeed underlies) a number of psychiatric disorders such as some instances of obsessive compulsive disorder, OCPD, some cases of Tourette syndrome, Asperger syndrome, and autism (C. Gillberg, 1992). The diagnosis can be made with a good degree of reliability. The presence of empathy disorder in the individual with anorexia nervosa predicted poor outcome better than the presence of the eating disorder per se (I.C. Gillberg et al., 1994a).

Six of the 51 individuals (12%) with anorexia nervosa (and none of those in the comparison group) met full diagnostic criteria for Asperger syndrome, as outlined in the ICD-10. Four met full criteria for Asperger syndrome as outlined by I.C. Gillberg and C. Gillberg (1989). One reason that this association has not been reported by other groups may be that the diagnosis of Asperger syndrome is not well-known in psychiatry. Children with Asperger syndrome often have attention and motor control problems (Asperger, 1944). In a recent population-based follow-up study of 6 through 16 year-old children with DAMP (deficits in attention, motor control and perception) (Hellgren et al., 1994), one individual out of 39 with DAMP and none out of 45 in the comparison group developed anorexia nervosa. DAMP, in some cases, appears to be related to ASD (C. Gillberg, 1983).

Not only were Asperger syndrome and other autistic-like conditions more frequently observed in the anorexia nervosa group but personality disorders that are considered as reflecting social negativism and social withdrawal were also more common in the anorexia nervosa than in the COMP group. The high rate of social interaction problems, communication failure, and ritualistic/obsessive compulsive phenomena in the anorexia nervosa group suggests a link with autism spectrum disorder, even in some cases that do not meet full criteria for ASD.

C. Gillberg and Råstam (1992) hypothesized that in *some* cases, anorexia nervosa may be regarded as one of the ritualistic phenomena expressed by an individual with a life-long (albeit relatively mild) autistic-like condition. Supportive of a connection between anorexia nervosa and ASD is the finding of anorexia nervosa in the extended families of some children afflicted with autism (C. Gillberg, 1992), and the occurrence of Asperger syndrome in a parent of some adolescents with anorexia nervosa (C. Gillberg & Råstam, 1992). We are aware that some clinicians (and researchers) might protest that they have never seen autistic-like problems in anorexia nervosa. We would not contradict this, but would like to point out that, that which is not sought will not be found. Most clinicians (and researchers) appear to agree that alexithymia (the inability to talk about or verbalize feelings) is common in eating disorders (Schmidt et al, 1993). We would like to posit that sometimes the alexithymia manifested by individuals with anorexia nervosa may be a reflection of an underlying empathy disorder that results not only in an inability to talk about affective states but in an impairment in the ability to conceive of and talk about mental states in general. Such an impairment has been shown to be important in autism and ASD (Steffenburg, 1991). It is noteworthy that, just as in the studies of alexithymia, there was no correlation between degree of weight loss and the presence of empathy disorders or personality disorders coded on Axis II, meaning that the emaciated state of the individuals did not contribute to the personality style. Also, at age 21 years, most of the individuals with anorexia nervosa were in good physical health and well-nourished and yet they retained the same type of empathy disorder or personality type or personality disorder that is considered as reflecting social negativism or social withdrawal.

It is also of some interest that dysdiadochokinesis, a prevalent finding in Asperger syndrome (C. Gillberg, 1991), was also a common feature of anorexia nervosa, both at age 16 and 21 years, and particularly, in cases with empathy disorders (I.C. Gillberg et al., 1994). The persistence over many years of both social communication disorders and dysdiadochokinesis in anorexia nervosa suggests the presence of an underlying neurodevelopmental disorder in some cases.

## References

American Psychiatric Association. (1980). *Diagnostic and Statistical Manual of Mental Disorders*. Washington, D.C.: APA.
American Psychiatric Association. (1987). *Diagnostic and Statistical Manual of Mental Disorders* (Third Edition - Revised ed.). Washington, D.C.: APA.
Asperger, H. (1944). Die autistischen Psychopathen im Kindesalter. *Archiv für Psychiatrie und Nervenkrankheiten, 117*, 76-136.
Cantwell, D.P., Sturzenberger, S., Burroughs, J., Salkin, B., & Green, J.K. (1977). Anorexia nervosa: an affective disorder? *Archives of General Psychiatry, 37*, 1087-1093.
Casper, R.C. (1990). Personality features of women with good outcome from restricting anorexia nervosa. *Psychosomatic Medicine, 52*, 156-170.
Dally, P. (1969). Anorexia Nervosa. London: William Heineman Medical Books.
Dewey, M. (1991). Living with Asperger's syndrome. In U. Frith (Ed.), *Autism and Asperger syndrome* (pp. 184-206). Cambridge: Cambridge University Press.
Ehlers, S., & Gillberg, C. (1993). The epidemiology of Asperger syndrome. A total population study. *Journal of Child Psychology and Psychiatry, 34*, 1327-1350.
Frith, U. (Ed.). (1991). *Autism and Asperger Syndrome*. Cambridge: Cambridge University Press.
Gartner, A.F., Marcus, R.N., Halmi, K., & Loranger, A.W. (1989). DSM-III-R personality disorders in patients with eating disorders. *American Journal of Psychiatry, 146*, 1585-1591.
Gillberg, C. (1983). Perceptual, motor and attentional deficits in Swedish primary school children. Some child psychiatric aspects. In *Journal of Child Psychology and Psychiatry, 24*, 377-403.
Gillberg, C. (1991). Clinical and neurobiological aspects of Asperger syndrome in six family studies. In U. Frith (Ed.), *Autism and Asperger Syndrome* (pp. 122-146). Cambridge: Cambridge University Press.
Gillberg, C. (1992). The Emanuel Miller Memorial Lecture 1991: Autism and autistic-like conditions: subclasses among disorders of empathy. *Journal of Child Psychology and Psychiatry, 33*, 813-842.
Gillberg, C., & Råstam, M. (1992). Do some cases of anorexia nervosa reflect underlying autistic-like conditions? *Behavioural Neurology, 5*, 27-32.
Gillberg, I.C., & Gillberg, C. (1989). Asperger syndrome - some epidemiological considerations: a research note. *Journal of Child Psychology and Psychiatry, 30*, 631-638.
Gillberg, I.C., Råstam, M., & Gillberg, C. (1994a). Anorexia nervosa outcome: Six year controlled longitudinal study of 51 cases including a population cohort. *Journal of the American Academy of Child and Adolescent Psychiatry, 33*, 729-739.
Gillberg, I.C., Råstam, M., & Gillberg, C. (1994b). Anorexia nervosa 6 years after onset. Part I. Personality disorders. *Comperhensive Psychiatry, 36*, In Press
Halmi, K.A., Eckert, E., Marchi, P., Sampugnaro, V., Apple, R., & Cohen, J. (1991). Comorbidity of psychiatric diagnoses in anorexia nervosa. *Archives of General Psychiatry, 48*, 712-718.
Hellgren, L., Gillberg, I.C., Bågenholm, A., & Gillberg, C. (1994). Children with Deficits in Attention, Motor control and Perception (DAMP) almost grown up: psychiatric and personality disorders at age 16 years. *Journal of Child Psychology and Psychiatry*, In press.
Hendren, R.L. (1983). Depression in anorexia nervosa. Journal of the American Academy of Child Psychiatry, 22, 59-62.
Loranger, A.W., Lehman Susman, V., Oldham, J.M., & Russakoff, L.M. (1987). The personality disorder examination: a preliminary report. *Journal of Personality Disorders, 1*, 1-13.
Morgan, H.G., & Hayward, A.E. (1988). Clinical assessment of anorexia nervosa. The Morgan-Russell outcome assessment schedule. *British Journal of Psychiatry, 152*, 367-371.
Rathner, G., & Messner, K. (1993). Detection of eating disorders in a small rural town: an epidemiological study. *Psychological Medicine, 23*, 175-184.
Råstam, M. (1992). Anorexia nervosa in 51 Swedish adolescents. Premorbid problems and comorbidity. *Journal of the American Academy of Child and Adolescent Psychiatry, 31*, 819-829.

Råstam, M., & Gillberg, C. (1991). The family background in anorexia nervosa: a population-based study. *Journal of the American Academy of Child and Adolescent Psychiatry, 30,* 283-289.
Råstam, M., Gillberg, C., & Garton, M. (1989). Anorexia nervosa in a Swedish urban region. A population-based study. *British Journal of Psychiatry, 155,* 642-646.
Råstam, M., Gillberg, C., & Gillberg, I.C. (1994). Anorexia nervosa 6 years after onset. Part II.Comorbid psychiatric problems. *Comperhensive Psychiatry, 36,* In Press
Schmidt, U., Jiwany, A., & Treasure, J. (1993). A controlled study of alexithymia in eating disorders. *Comprehensive Psychiatry, 34,* 54-58.
Spitzer, R.L., Williams, J.B., Gibbon, M., & First, M.B. (1992). The Structured Clinical Interview for DSM-III-R (SCID). I: History, rationale, and description. *Archives of General Psychiatry, 49,* 624-629.
Steffenburg, S. (1991). Neuropsychiatric assessment of children with autism: a population-based study. *Developmental Medicine and Child Neurology, 33,* 495-511.
Toner, B.B., Garfinkel, P.E., & Garner, D.M. (1988). Affective and anxiety disorders in the long-term follow-up of anorexia nervosa. *International Journal of Psychiatry in Medicine, 18,* 357-364.
Wechsler, D. (1992). *Wechsler Adult Intelligence Scale Revised.* Stockholm: Psykologiförlaget (Swedish version).
World Health Organization. (1993). *The ICD-10 Classification of Mental and Behavioural Disorders. Diagnostic criteria for research.* Geneva: Author.

# Risk Factors For The Development of Early Onset Bulimia Nervosa

*Ulrike Schmidt, Jane Tiller, Matthew Hodes, and Janet Treasure*

## 1 Introduction

Dieting is a well-known risk factor for the development of bulimia nervosa (Patton et al., 1990). A significant proportion of preadolescent girls between the ages of 7 and 12 years are weight conscious and diet (Davies & Furnham, 1986; Maloney et al., 1989; Wardle & Marsland, 1990; Collins, 1991; Hill et al., 1992; Childress, et al., 1993). Prospective data from the food diaries of a group of 9-year olds confirm that those who claim to diet actually do so (Hill & Robinson, 1991). Those with a higher body weight (Wardle & Beales, 1986; Hill et al., 1989; Hill et al., 1992) and those perceiving themselves as overweight (Wadden et al., 1989; Hill et al., 1992; Hill et al., 1993) are more likely to diet. Other factors associated with dieting in preadolescence and early adolescence include the onset of menarche and dating (Gralen et al., 1990), as during pubertal development girls are frequently distressed about their increase in body fat (Brooks-Gunn & Warren, 1988). Maternal and peer influences are also important (Hill et al., 1990). In one study, over two-thirds of the girls reported that their mother had dieted at some time and 45% reported that they had a friend who dieted (Maloney et al., 1989). In another study (Attie & Brooks-Gunn, 1989), a relationship between the girls' pubertal development and mothers' menstrual status and dieting was found. Early maturing girls whose mothers were premenopausal dieted less than early maturers whose mothers were menopausal. This was thought to be linked to the greater body fat of the menopausal mothers who, therefore, dieted more.

There is some evidence that dieting in preadolescent girls is a relatively new phenomenon (Hill, 1993), which may be the result of increased socio-cultural pressures to be slim in the context of a secular trend for pubertal development to occur at an increasingly lower age (Tanner, 1989). The preoccupation with weight in increasingly younger children has been thought to lead to an increase in eating disorders in this group (Lask & Bryant-Waugh, 1992).

In bulimia nervosa, although the typical age of onset is thought to be around age 18 (Mitchell et al., 1987), some reports of cases with an early onset are now beginning to appear. One series described eleven cases with an onset of bulimia nervosa between the ages of 13 and 16 (Remschmidt & Herpertz-Dahlmann, 1990). In a cohort of patients presenting to a tertiary referral centre 25 % had started to binge before the age 16 (Blake-Woodside & Garfinkel, 1992). Premenarchal bulimia nervosa is, however, still a rarity. Only three subjects of a cohort of 323 patients with bulimia nervosa described a pre-menarchal onset (Kent et al., 1992). None of them had a pre-pubertal onset.

Dieting alone is unlikely to be a sufficient precondition for the development of eating disorders. Bulimia nervosa is generally thought to be a multifactorial disorder and, apart from dieting, other risk factors include: (a) a family history of affective disorder, alcoholism, and obesity (Kassett et al., 1989); (b) deficits in childhood care with high levels of discord, neglect, and physical and sexual abuse (for review see Schmidt et al., 1993a); (c) distressing life events and difficulties (Schmidt, Hodes, & Treasure, 1992); and (d) acculturation stress (Mumford & Whitehouse, 1988). The aim of the present study was to determine whether early and typical onset cases of bulimia nervosa differed in terms of the familial and individual risk factors that they have been exposed to. The study is an extension of previous work in which we compared 23 cases with early onset bulimia nervosa with a matched group of 23 typical onset cases using a retrospective case-control design (Schmidt, Treasure, Tiller, & Blanchard, 1992). Whilst there was no difference in eating symptomatology between the two groups, deliberate self-harm was more frequent in the early onset group and there was a trend for more depression amongst their relatives. Inadequate parental control, which was often associated with lack of parental warmth, occurred more often in the early onset group, but other indicators of intrafamilial disturbance did not differ in the two groups. There was also a trend for the early onset group to be exposed to more cultural stress as a result of family migration. Given the tentative nature of some of the findings from our earlier study, we wanted to see whether they would stand up to scrutiny in a sample of larger size with increased power.

## 2 Subjects

Forty cases of early onset bulimia nervosa (EO) were identified from recent consecutive referrals to the Eating Disorder Clinic (32 cases) and to the Department of Child and Adolescent Psychiatry (8 cases) at the Maudsley Hospital between 1988 and 1992. All patients were female. In order to qualify for an early onset, subjects had to fulfil DSM-III-R criteria for bulimia nervosa at the age of 15 or below. As in the previous study, this cut-off point was chosen because all the subjects in this group would have been expected to live in the parental home (or equivalent) and be in full-time education. All patients had been personally assessed by the authors.

The comparison group consisted of female patients with a typical age of onset (TO), who were identified from referrals to the Maudsley Hospital Eating Disorder Clinic and who had been seen over the same period of time as the index group. A typical onset was defined as an onset of DSM-III-R bulimia nervosa between the ages of 17 and 21. Patients with an onset after the age of 21 were not included in the TO group. Each case of early onset bulimia nervosa was matched with the subsequently referred case of typical onset bulimia nervosa from the same social class.

## 3 Method

At the time of patients' initial assessment, a standard Maudsley Hospital history was taken (Department of Psychiatry and Child Psychiatry, Institute of Psychiatry and Maudsley Hospital, 1987). The Childhood Parental Care Interview, developed by Harris et al. (1986), was administered to sixty-eight of the 72 patients seen in the adult department. This is a retrospective semistructured interview, which assesses childhood care up to the age of 17. Information is gathered on family structure and the quality of childhood care. The patient is encouraged to give concrete examples of parental behaviour. The interviewer makes ratings of intrafamilial discord, violence, parental indifference, and parental disciplinary practices. High parental indifference and low parental control were combined into a composite rating of 'lack of care', which has been found to be a predictor of adult psychiatric problems (Harris et al., 1986; Bifulco et al., 1987). Family disturbance that had arisen as a result of the eating disorder was not included. Childhood sexual abuse was also enquired about and defined as: sexual activity involving contact by a perpetrator five or more years older than the victim who was herself 16 years or younger (after Browne & Finkelhor, 1986). Ratings were made on a consensus basis by a team of raters blind to the diagnosis and age of onset of the patient. The use of this interview in eating disorder patients has been described elsewhere (Schmidt et al., 1993b). Five of the eight cases seen in the children's department were assessed with a semistructured family interview (Kinston & Loader, 1984). These and the remaining cases (three presenting to the children's department and four presenting to the adult department) were re-rated using the criteria of the childhood care interview to ensure a uniform assessment procedure. Cultural stress was rated as present if the patient was a first or second generation immigrant.

A family history of mental disorder or eating disorder was rated as present if a first degree relative had been treated by a general practitioner or a mental health professional. A family history of obesity was rated as present if the patient described their parents or siblings as markedly overweight. (Wherever possible, we attempted to get estimates of weight and height for first degree relatives). A personal history of being overweight was rated as present if the patient had had a body mass index of $> 25$ kg/m$^2$ before the onset of bulimia nervosa. Socio-economic status was based on paternal occupation and was classified according to the Hollingshead two-factor index of social position (Guy, 1976).

Data were analyzed using SPSS/PC+ (Norusis, 1988). Odds ratios with 95% confidence intervals were used for categorical data (Gardner et al., 1989) and $t$-tests for normally distributed data.

## 4  Results

### 4.1  Sociodemographic Background

At the time of referral, patients in the EO group had a mean age of 20.1 (±4.5) years and patients in the TO group a mean age of 23.9 (±3.8) years. The duration of bulimia nervosa at presentation was comparable in the two groups with 6.4 (±5.1) years in the EO group and 5.1 (±3.8) years in the TO group. The body mass index at presentation was 22.9 (±4.0) kg/m$^2$ in the EO and 21.6 (±2.2) kg/m$^2$ in the TO group. This difference is not significant. One third of patients in both groups were of working class background.

## 4.2 Clinical Features

As expected, the groups differed in their mean age at the onset of dieting - EO: 13.1 (±2.0) years vs. TO: 18.1 (±1.1) years - and their mean age at onset of bingeing - EO: 13.7 (±1.6) years vs. TO: 18.8 (±1.0) years. Mean age at menarche was identical in both groups - EO: 12.7 (± 1.3) years vs. TO: 12.7 (± 1.6) years. Only six patients had a premenarchal onset of their eating disorder.

A comparison of the clinical features between the two groups is shown in Table 1. The proportion of patients in both groups who induced vomiting, abused laxatives or appetite suppressants, or had a history of anorexia nervosa was almost identical. In contrast, a history of obesity was nearly twice as common in the early onset group as in the typical onset group, although this finding did not quite reach significance.

Table 1. Clinical Features and Concurrent Psychopathology

|  | Early Onset N | % | Typical Onset N | % | Odds Ratio (95% CI) |
|---|---|---|---|---|---|
| Self-induced vomiting | 33/40 | 83% | 35/40 | 88% | 0.7 (0.2-2.3) |
| Laxatives | 19/40 | 48% | 23/40 | 58% | 0.7 (0.3-1.6) |
| Appetite suppressants | 6/40 | 15% | 9/40 | 23% | 0.6 (0.2-1.9) |
| History of anorexia nervosa | 10/40 | 25% | 10/40 | 25% | 1.0 (0.4-2.8) |
| History of obesity | 14/38[a] | 37% | 8/40 | 20% | 2.3 (0.8-6.5) |
| Deliberate self-harm DSH | 21/39[b] | 54% | 12/40 | 30% | 2.7 (1.1-6.7) |
| Substance abuse | 13/40 | 33% | 11/40 | 28% | 1.3 (0.5-3.3) |
| Stealing | 12/37[c] | 32% | 11/40 | 28% | 1.3 (0.5-3.4) |

[a] no information available in two patients;
[b] no information available in one patient;
[c] no information available in three patients.

## 4.3 Concurrent Psychopathology

The early onset group had a significantly higher rate of deliberate self-harm (DSH) than the typical onset group (Table 1). Deliberate self-harm usually occurred after onset. The increased level of DSH in the early onset group was not a result of a longer duration of illness. Other maladaptive behaviours such as drug and alcohol abuse and stealing were not different in the two groups.

## 4.4 Family Factors

These are shown in Table 2. In contrast to our previous study, the two groups did not differ with regard to a family history of depression. In our previous study, we had included first and second degree relatives whereas, in the current study, we limited ourselves to first degree relatives because the information on second degree relatives was thought to be too unreliable.

The family structure did not differ between groups. Forty to 45% of patients came from broken homes. Levels of family disturbance were high and almost identical in both groups, with the exception of inadequate parental care, which occurred significantly more often in the EO group. The two groups did not differ with regard to the frequency of cultural stress.

## 5 Discussion

The clinical features of the early onset cases closely resembled those of the typical onset cases. There was no suggestion that those with an earlier onset are milder cases than those with a typical onset.

Most of the findings from our previous study held up in the larger sample with the exception of two of the more tentative findings: In the enlarged sample we did no longer find that a family history of depression was more common in the early onset group, nor did we find more cultural stress in this group than in the patients with a typical onset.

A new trend emerged in our enlarged sample: Nearly twice as many early onset cases compared to typical onset cases were overweight before onset. This trend fits in with other research suggesting that higher actual body weight is associated with early onset of dieting (Wardle & Beales, 1986; Hill et al., 1989; Hill et al., 1992) and predisposes for the development of bulimia nervosa (Garner & Fairburn, 1988).

Table 2. Family Factors

|  | Early Onset N | % | Typical Onset N | % | Odds Ratio (95% CI) |
|---|---|---|---|---|---|
| *Family history of:* | | | | | |
| Depression | 15/39[a] | 39% | 11/37[b] | 30% | 1.5 (0.6-3.8) |
| Substance abuse | 7/39 | 18% | 10/37 | 27% | 0.6 (0.2-1.8) |
| Eating disorders | 5/39 | 13% | 2/35[c] | 6% | 2.4 (0.4-13.4) |
| Obesity | 13/39 | 33% | 11/35 | 31% | 1.1 (0.4-2.9) |
| *Family structure* | | | | | |
| Multiple family arrangements | 16/40 | 40% | 18/40 | 45% | 0.8 (0.3-2.0) |
| Adopted | 1/40 | 3% | 3/40 | 8% | 0.3 (0.03-3.2) |
| Institutional care or boarding school | 5/40 | 13% | 3/40 | 8% | 1.8 (0.4-7.9) |
| *Family disturbance* | | | | | |
| Discord | 26/40 | 65% | 26/40 | 65% | 1.0 (0.4-2.5) |
| Violence | 10/40 | 25% | 9/40 | 23% | 1.2 (0.4-3.2) |
| Lack of care | 20/40 | 50% | 11/40 | 28% | 2.6 (1.04-6.7) |
| Childhood sexual abuse | 6/40 | 15% | 10/38[d] | 26% | 0.5 (0.2-1.5) |
| *Cultural stress* | 13/40 | 33% | 11/40 | 28% | 1.3 (0.5-3.3) |

[a] no information on one patient available because she was adopted;
[b] no information on three patients available because they were adopted;
[c] no information available on five patients (three adopted, in two additional cases patients had not been asked);
[d] in two patients no information was available.

Children's attitude to overweight is extremely negative (Richardson et al., 1961; Staffieri, 1967; Hill & Silver, 1993) and girls are less accepting of overweight same-sex peers than are males (DeJong & Kleck, 1986). Overweight children may be teased and excluded from peer groups and athletic activities (Hill, 1993). Whilst overweight 9 year olds have low body esteem but, in terms of global self-esteem, are no different than their peers (Mendelson & White, 1985; Hill et al., 1993) by the age of 13 those with low body esteem also have global low self-esteem. We did not systematically ask our patients whether they had been teased about their weight by their peers or families and, therefore, do not know whether teasing or critical comments about weight and appearance were part of the behavioural chain leading to the youngsters' decision to start a diet.

Parental lack of care was nearly twice as common in the early onset group as in the typical onset group. What is the link between parental lack of care and the early development of bulimia nervosa? From a psychodynamic point of view, it has been argued that overeating may represent an attempt to avoid feelings of emptiness and low mood associated with maternal unavailability (Johnson & Connors, 1987). At a more practical level, parents who are emotionally and physically unavailable to their teenage daughter may not provide her with regular meals. Once rigid dieting or an eating disorder have started, these parents may fail to notice, or if they do notice it, may fail to act appropriately.

None of these considerations explain why these young girls developed bulimia nervosa rather than depression, drug problems, or some other breakdown in personal functioning (Wonderlich, 1992). Parental neglect and inappropriate control are also common in the histories of patients with depression, alcohol problems, or personality disorders (e.g., Crook, et al., 1981; Parker, 1983; Harris et al., 1986; Bifulco et al., 1987; Andrews et al., 1990; Zweig & Paris, 1991). An interesting intergenerational study of London working-class women and their adolescent and young adult daughters sheds some light on this point (Andrews et al., 1990). Both mothers and daughters were asked about the childhood care they had received. In both generations, parental neglect and abuse had a negative effect on later mental health. Whereas the most common psychiatric disorder in the generation of the mothers was depression, in the daughters bulimia and depression were equally common. This supports Russell's hypothesis that bulimia nervosa is a contemporary Western expression of neurosis (Russell, 1986) arising in a culture that equates slimness with youth, health, and beauty. Individuals from a neglectful family environment with a damaged view of themselves and poor ability to cope may be particularly vulnerable for subjecting themselves to a relentless pursuit of slimness - resulting in bulimia - in an attempt to deal with emotional upset, take control of their lives and solve their problems.

Deliberate self harm occurred in 50% of the early onset group, i.e., considerably more commonly than in the typical onset patients. Usually it occurred after the onset of the eating disorder. It is well-known that deliberate self-harm often is an impulsive act that occurs at a time of crisis in order to communicate distress to others that are close to them. In the majority of early onset cases, self-harm was associated with severe family problems. This is in line with studies of adolescent suicide attempters (De Wilde et al., 1992), which found them to differ from both depressed adolescents who had never made a suicide attempt and non-depressed adolescents. The suicide attempters had experienced more family difficulties that began in childhood and had not stabilized in adolescence. The deliberate self-harm in our young onset group may, thus, have been a desperate attempt to signal to others within or outside the family that all was not well.

Another possibility is that depression associated with an eating disorder was a contributing factor in facilitating deliberate self-harm. Unfortunately, we did not assess life-time depression in our sample, so we are unable to address this point.

Those young onset patients who do show some outward disturbance, e.g., deliberate self-harm, may be more readily identified and referred for treatment, whereas the older patients who are more independent can more easily refer themselves. Thus, it is possible that our clinic population of young onset cases is not representative of young onset cases at large and that the increased incidence of deliberate self-harm is simply an artifact of being referred.

Given its retrospective nature and the varying initial assessment procedure, the study is limited. However, by limiting ourselves to cases that had been assessed in depth using semistructured interviews and that were all known to the authors personally, we hope to have minimized potential sources of bias. In the long term, it would be desirable to conduct a prospective study of premenarchal or prepubertal onset cases of bulimia nervosa.

## Acknowledgement

We would like to thank Professor G.F.M. Russell and Dr. C. Dare for giving permission to include their patients in this study. Ulrike Schmidt and Jane Tiller were supported by Solvay Duphar. Matthew Hodes was supported by an M.R.C. grant during part of the study.

## References

Andrews, B., Brown, G.W., & Creasey, L. (1990). Intergenerational links between psychiatric disorder in mothers and daughters: the role of parenting experiences. *Journal of Child Psychology and Psychiatry 31*, 1115-1129.

Attie, I., & Brooks-Gunn, J. (1989). The development of eating problems in adolescent girls: A longitudinal study. *Developmental Psychology 25*, 70-79.

Bifulco, A.T., Brown, G.W., & Harris, T.O. (1987). Childhood loss of parents, lack of adequate parental care and adult depression: a replication. *Journal of Affective Disorders 12*, 115-128.

Blake-Woodside, D.B., & Garfinkel, P.E. (1992). Age of Onset in Eating Disorders. *International Journal of Eating Disorders 12*, 31-36.

Brooks-Gunn, J., & Warren, M. (1988). The psychological significance of secondary sexual characteristics in nine-to-eleven-year old girls. *Child Development 59*, 1061-1069.

Browne, A., & Finkelhor, D. (1986). Impact of child sexual abuse: a review of the research. *Psychological Bulletin 99*, 66-77.

Childress, A.C., Brewerton, T.D., Hodges, E.L., Jarrell, M.P. (1993). The kids' eating disorder survey (KEDS): a study of middle school students. *The Journal of the American Academy of Child and Adolescent Psychiatry 32*, 843-850.

Collins, M.E. (1991). Body figure perceptions and preferences among preadolescent children. *International Journal of Eating Disorders 10*, 199-208.

Crook, T., Raskin, A., & Eliot, J. (1981). Parent-child relationships and adult depression. *Child Development 52*, 950-957.

Davies, E., & Furnham, A. (1986). The dieting and body shape concerns of adolescent females. *Journal of Child Psychology and Psychiatry 27*, 417-428.

DeJong, W., & Kleck, R.E. (1986). The social psychological effects of overweight. In: C.P. Herman, M.P. Zanna, & Higgins, E.T. (eds.) Physical Appearance, Stigma and Social Behaviour. The Ontario Symposium 3, 65-87. Hillsdale, NJ, Erlbaum.

Department of Psychiatry and Child Psychiatry, Institute of Psychiatry and Maudsley Hospital (1987). Psychiatric Examination. 2nd edition. Oxford Medical Publications.

De Wilde, E.J., Kienhorst, I.C.W.M., Diekstra, R.F.W., & Wolters, W.H.G. (1992). The relationship between adolescent suicidal behavior and life events in childhood and adolescence. *American Journal of Psychiatry 149*, 45-51.

Gardner, S.B., Winter, P.D., & Gardner, M.J. (1991). Confidence Interval Analysis. Microcomputer Manual and Disc. Version 1.1. British Medical Journal.

Garner, D.M., & Fairburn, C.G. (1988). Relationship between anorexia nervosa and bulimia nervosa: Diagnostic implications. In: Garner, D.M., & Garfinkel, P.E. (eds.). Diagnostic Issues in Anorexia Nervosa and Bulimia Nervosa. New York: Brunner/Mazel.

Gralen, S.J., Levine, M.P., Smolak, L., & Murnen, S.K. (1990). Dieting and disordered eating during early and middle adolescence: do the influences remain the same? *International Journal of Eating Disorders 9*, 501-512.

Guy, W. (1976). ECDEU assessment manual for psychopharmacology. Rockville, MD: US Department of Health, Education and Welfare, 516-520.

Harris, T.O., Brown, G.W., & Bifulco, A. (1986). Loss of parent in childhood and adult psychiatric disorder: the role of lack of adequate parenting. *Psychological Medicine 16*, 641-659.

Hill, A.J. (1993). Preadolescent dieting: implications for eating disorders. *International Review of Psychiatry 5*, 87-100.

Hill, A.J., Jones, E., & Stack, J. (1993). A weight on children's minds: body shape dissatisfactions at 9-years old. *Submitted to International Journal of Obesity*.

Hill, A.J., Oliver, S., & Rogers, P.J. (1992). Eating in the adult world: the rise of dieting in childhood and adolescence. *British Journal of Clinical Psychology 31*, 95-105.

Hill, A.J., & Robinson, A. (1991). Dieting concerns have a functional effect on the behaviour of nine-year old girls. *British Journal of Clinical Psychology 30*, 265-267.

Hill, A.J., Rogers, P.J., & Blundell, J.E. (1989). Dietary restraint in young adolescent girls: a functional analysis. *British Journal of Clinical Psychology 28*, 165-176.

Hill, A.J., & Silver, E. (1993). Fat, friendless and unhealthy: 9-year old children's perception of body shape stereotypes (in preparation).

Hill, A.J., Weaver, C., & Blundell, J.E. (1990). Dieting concerns of 10-year old girls and their mothers. *British Journal of Clinical Psychology 29*, 346-348.

Johnson, C., & Connors, M.E. (1987). The Etiology and Treatment of Bulimia Nervosa. New York Basic Books.

Kassett, J.A., Gershon, E.S., Maxwell, M.E., Guroff, J.J., Kazuba, D.M., Smith, A.L., Brandt, H.A., & Jimerson, D.C. (1989). Psychiatric disorders in the first-degree relatives of probands with bulimia nervosa. *American Journal of Psychiatry 146*, 1468-1471.

Kent, A., Lacey, J.H., & McCluskey, S.E. (1992). Pre-menarchal bulimia nervosa. *Journal of Psychosomatic Research 36*, 205-210.

Kinston, W., & Loader, P. (1984). Eliciting whole family interaction with a standardized clinical interview. *Journal of Family Therapy 6*, 347-363.

Lask, B., & Bryant-Waugh, R. (1992). Early-onset anorexia nervosa and related eating disorders. *Journal of Child Psychology and Psychiatry 33*, 281-300.

Maloney, M.J., McGuire, L., Daniels, S.R., & Specker, B. (1989). Dieting behaviour and eating attitudes in children. *Pediatrics 84*, 482-489.

Mendelson, B.K., & White, D.R. (1985). Development of self-body-esteem in overweight youngsters. *Developmental Psychology 21*, 90-96.

Mitchell, J.E., Hatsukami, D., Pyle, R.L., Eckert, E.D., & Soll, E. (1987). Late onset bulimia. *Comprehensive Psychiatry 28*, 323-328.

Mumford, D.B., & Whitehouse, A.M. (1988). Increased prevalence of bulimia nervosa among Asian schoolgirls. *British Medical Journal 297*, ii, 718.

Norusis, M.J. (1988). SPSS/PC+ V2. Chicago: SPSS.

Parker, G. (1983). Parental 'affectionless control' as an antecedent to adult depression. *Archives of General Psychiatry 40*, 956-960.

Patton, G.C., Johnson-Sabine, E., Wood, K., Mann, A.H., & Wakeling, A. (1990). Abnormal eating attitudes in London schoolgirls - a prospective epidemiological study: outcome at twelve month follow-up. *Psychological Medicine 20*, 383-394.

Remschmidt, H., & Herpertz-Dahlmann, B. (1990). Bulimia in children and adolescents. In: Fichter, M. (ed.). Bulimia Nervosa. Basic Research, Diagnosis and Therapy. pp. 84-98. John Wiley and Sons, Chichester.

Richardson, S.A., Hastorf, A.H., Goodman, N., & Dornbusch, S.M. (1961), Cultural uniformity in reaction to physical disabilities. *American Sociological Review 26*, 241-247.

Russell, G.,F. M. (1986). The changing nature of anorexia nervosa: an introduction to the conference. In: Szmukler, G.I., Slade, P.D., Harris, P., Benton, D., & Russell, G.F.M. (Eds.). Anorexia Nervosa and Bulimic Disorders. Oxford, Pergamon Press.

Schmidt, U., Hodes, M., & Treasure, J. (1992). Early onset bulimia nervosa: who is at risk? A retrospective case-control study. *Psychological Medicine, 22*, 623-628.

Schmidt, U., Treasure, J., Tiller, J., & Blanchard, M. (1992). Life events and difficulties in eating disorders. *Neuroendocrinology Letters 14*, 256.

Schmidt, U., Tiller, J., & Treasure, J. (1993a). Psychosocial factors in bulimia nervosa. *International Review of Psychiatry 5*, 51-59.

Schmidt, U., Tiller, J., & Treasure, J. (1993b). Setting the scene for eating disorders: Childhood care, classification and course of illness. *Psychological Medicine 23*, 663-672.

Staffieri, J.R. (1967). A study of social stereotype of body image in children. *Journal of Personality and Social Psychology 7*, 101-104.

Tanner, J.M. (1989). Foetus into Man: Physical Growth from Conception to Maturity, 2nd ed. Ware: Castlemead Publications.

Wadden, T.A., Foster, G.D., Stunkard, A.J., & Linowitz, J.R. (1989). Dissatisfaction with weight and figure in obese girls: discontent but not depression. *International Journal of Obesity 13*, 89-97.

Wardle, J., & Beales, S. (1986). Restraint, body image and food attitudes in children from 12 to 18 years. *Appetite 7*, 209-217.

Wardle, J., & Marsland, L. (1990). Adolescent concerns about weight and eating: a social-developmental perspective. *Journal of Psychosomatic Research 34*, 377-391.

Wonderlich, S. (1992). Relationship of family and personality factors in bulimia. In: Crowther, J.H., Tennenbaum, D.L., Hobfoll, S.E., & Stevens, M.A.P. (eds.). The Etiology of Bulimia Nervosa: The Individual and Family Context. Washington, DC, Hemisphere Publishing.

Zweig-Frank, H., & Paris, J. (1991). Parents' emotional neglect and overprotection according to the recollections of patients with borderline personality disorder. *American Journal of Psychiatry 148*, 648-651.

# Precursors and Risk Factors of Juvenile Eating Disorders

*Hans Steiner, Mary Sanders, and Erika Ryst*

## 1    Introduction

A large number of recent cross-sectional studies report that disordered eating in the general adolescent population is very high. Somewhere between 40% and 60% of high school girls in the U.S. diet to lose weight (Maloney & Ruedisueli, 1993; Lucas, Beard, O'Fallon; & Kurland, 1991; Field, Wolf, Herzog, Cheung, & Colditz, 1993). According to Joel Killen et al. (1986) about 13% induce vomiting or use diet pills, laxatives or diuretics. About 30% to 40% of junior high girls also admit to concerns about weight (Childress, Brewerton, Hodges; & Jarrell, 1993; Richards, Regina, & Larson, 1990). These numbers are very similar in the school-age range (Field, Wolf, Herzog, Cheung, & Colditz, 1993; Maloney, Mcguire, Daniels, & Specker, 1989). These findings have raised some concerns. However, direct examination as to what dieting in fact refers to in this age range reveals that actual food intake varies very little between self-reported dieters and non-dieters. Stating that one is dieting seems to reflect a concern with weight and body shape, not necessarily a syndromal eating disorder. Furthermore, of this large number of girls who worry about their weight, only a small fraction develop actual eating disorders. Studies have shown a possible link between dieting and subsequent anorexia (e.g., Patton, 1992) but it seems that actual food restriction or repeated and syndromal purgation represents one of the last stations on the road to eating pathology. Other factors must be operating in concert with altered handling of food to produce disorders as defined in the DSM-IV, which, when identified properly, could lead to prevention of the onset of the disorders and open new avenues for treatment.

The task of identifying risk factors involved in eating disorders is important for both theoretical and practical reasons. Theoretically, the field of eating disorders offers certain opportunities in studying the genesis of psychopathology. Like few other psychopathological syndromes, eating disorders usually appear during a very precise window of developmental time. This characteristic makes it easier to define whether or not predicted risk groups in a longitudinal study actually develop the disorder.

In addition, the psychosomatic nature of eating disorders means that they probably evolve as an interplay of biological and psychosocial factors. This offers a chance to observe the relative impact of environment and constitution in the creation of psychopathology. Because the risks also appear to accumulate slowly over a period of preadolescent years, the study of risk factors also allows an investigation of the additive effect of risks across time.

On a practical level, discovering risk factors for eating disorders can save human suffering and money. Anorexia and bulimia are two chronic illnesses that require costly long-term intervention and have relatively high morbidity and mortality rates. These costs can be avoided by intervening in ways suggested by the risk factors found operating at different stages of development. Causal models informed by this study can, in turn, point toward new interventions which, when successful, will further refine the etiological model of the disorder.

## 2  The Status of Research in the Field

Until now, few investigators have attempted the kind of large-scale prospective studies necessary to identify the definitive etiology of eating disorders. Part of the problem has to do with the enormous costs involved. Due to the rare and mostly gender-specific nature of eating disorder pathology, large population samples are necessary for such a study. Any testing of competitive risk models for example, environmental versus biological further increases the size of the subject sample and concomitant costs. These enormous costs demand suitable prior groundwork to make the endeavor viable.

Fortunately, cross-sectional- and time-lagged-design research can provide us with such a foundation. As a quick and productive way of identifying possible leads, these research methods have proven invaluable in preparing for the more definitive, longitudinal studies. Certain problems are of course inherent in interpreting this cross-sectional and even time-lagged data. One of the greatest difficulties in research that compares normals with disordered adolescents is that it can become tautological. That is, so-called "risk factors" can be confused with manifestations of the disorder. In order to truly identify risk pre-dating the disorder, we must study subjects before they become disordered.

Previously, in the 1970s, the strategy in tackling risk factor assessment was to study the characteristics of rehabilitated eating disorder patients. Researchers employing this method assumed that any psychological or biological traits remaining after recovery existed prior to the illness onset. These characteristics then became the "risk factors" believed to be associated with eating disorders (Vigersky, 1977). The major flaw of this approach was that malnutrition for long periods of time produces changes that may have little to do with premorbid make-up. This was systematically studied by Keys and his group in their assessment of starving normal males in a camp for conscientious objectors (Keys, Brozek, Henschel, Mickelsen, & Taylor, 1950). Their findings are convincing: Many changes - both psychological and biological - are brought about by prolonged starvation, some of which are quite reminiscent of "pathognomonic symptoms" of eating disorders. Furthermore, it is not known how much time needs to elapse before someone recovering from an eating disorder can return to baseline. Some of Keys' subjects had problems for months after nutritional rehabilitation. As a result of this strategy, researchers came up with many "false positives" – abnormalities at all levels of functioning that supposedly indicated premorbid illness characteristics for eating disorders which, when studied over a longer period of time, actually returned to normal (Laue, Gold, Richmond, & Chrousos 1991; Kaye, Gwirtsman, George, Jimerson, Ebert, & Lake, 1990; Kaye, Ebert, Raleigh, & Lake, 1984).

The current strategy of looking for risk factors in very young subjects with illness of relatively short duration offers a better chance of identifying true precursors to the disorder. Problems with this methodology also exist, however. Because we do not know at which age risk factors surface, we run the risk of studying an age that is too early or too late, thus running into the problem of identifying both false negatives and false positives. Developmental issues also cloud interpretation of this kind of research, as we don't know if psychopathology looks the same at different ages. For example, the drive for thinness and dieting in a fourteen- year-old could manifest quite differently in a child of eight, as the current epidemiological studies tell us: At age eight speaking of dieting results in no or small changes in caloric intake; in mid-adolescence, however, such statements seem to be tied to some form of purgation. Normative cognitive distortions at younger ages may also mimic the abnormal body image distortions found in eating disorder patients of older age. Still, we believe the benefits of using this method outweigh its uncertainties. In combination with the study of persistent problems after weight rehabilitation and at prolonged follow-up we believe it can lead us to a clearer picture as to where to look for relevant disturbances long before eating becomes manifestly disordered.

## 3  The Model

Taking the data that we have from cross-sectional research, we can build a model for risk to test prospectively. This current model may be over-inclusive in scope, given our current uncertainty about the integral features of anorexia nervosa and bulimia. However, starting with such an extensive model gives us an appropriate range with which to work.

The basic framework of the model we propose is one of multifactorial etiology and cumulative risk. As we conceptualize it, many antecedents to eating disorder build slowly over the course of years, until the stress of adolescence causes disorder to manifest. It is of course possible that only a few factors may eventually emerge as the most powerful determinants. But until we know this for sure, the safest course is to investigate the interaction of many factors potentially adding to risk.

Our theory is that these multiple factors are all important but not sufficient conditions for the generation of eating disorders. Each one in isolation may present no particular threat. However, with each additional factor a child's risk grows greater, until some precipitant event – such as facing new unexpected demands in adolescence – catalyzes the transformation of risk into disorder.

What form the disorder takes may depend on specific risks. We think that the precursors to bulimia and anorexia are related and in some cases overlap. However the total risk profiles for the two disorders are not identical. Some clues for the relevant risks come from relationships between associated pathology (see Figure 1), such as affective disorders, anxiety disorders, and disturbed habits. Anorexia and bulimia carry a differential risk for psychiatric comorbidities, which in turn provide clues as to their different risks and etiologies (see Figures 2 and 3).

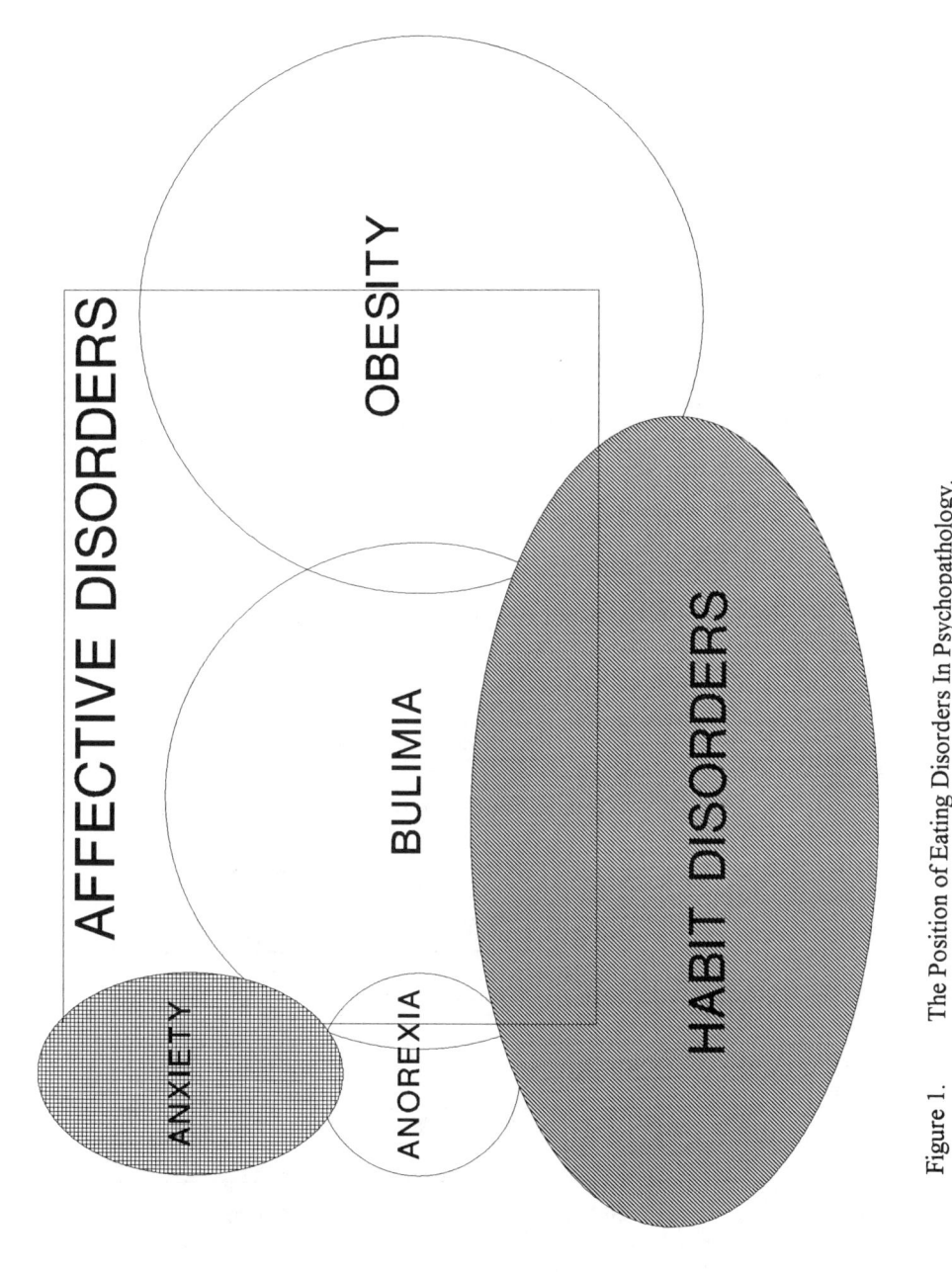

Figure 1. The Position of Eating Disorders In Psychopathology.

```
                    ┌─────────────────────────────┐
                    │ Cultural and Familial Press │
                    └─────────────────────────────┘
                  ┌─────────────────────────────────┐
                  │  Lack of Preparation for Exit   │
                  └─────────────────────────────────┘
            ┌──────────────────────────────────────────────┐
            │ Weak Self Concept, Inadequate Peer Relationships │
            └──────────────────────────────────────────────┘
               ┌────────────────────────────────────────┐
               │ Anxious Attachment, Separation Problems │
               └────────────────────────────────────────┘
         ┌──────────────────────────────────────────────────┐
         │ Insecure Parenting, Emphasis on Appearance and Fitness │
         └──────────────────────────────────────────────────┘
       ┌────────────────────────────────────────────────┐
       │ Fussy Eating, Altered Hunger / Satiety Regulations │
       └────────────────────────────────────────────────┘
    ┌──────────────────────────────────────────────────────┐
    │ Fat Distribution, Shy Temperament, Body Mass Index, Gender │
    └──────────────────────────────────────────────────────┘
    ─────────────────────────────────────────────────────────►
    Birth                    Time                   Puberty
```

Figure 2.   The Stacking of Risk Factors for Anorexia Nervosa.

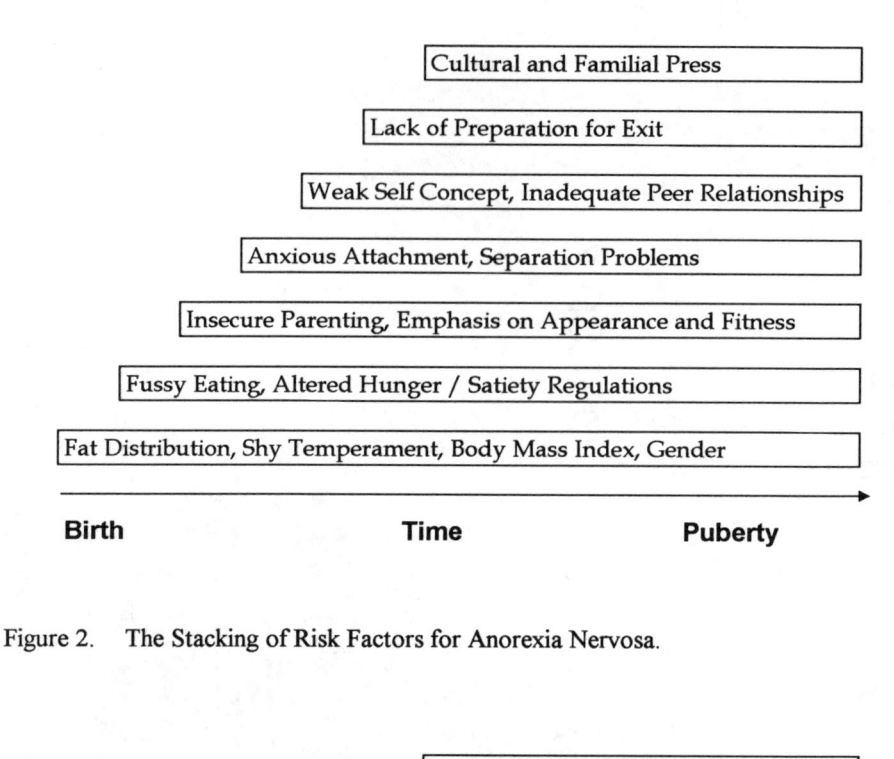

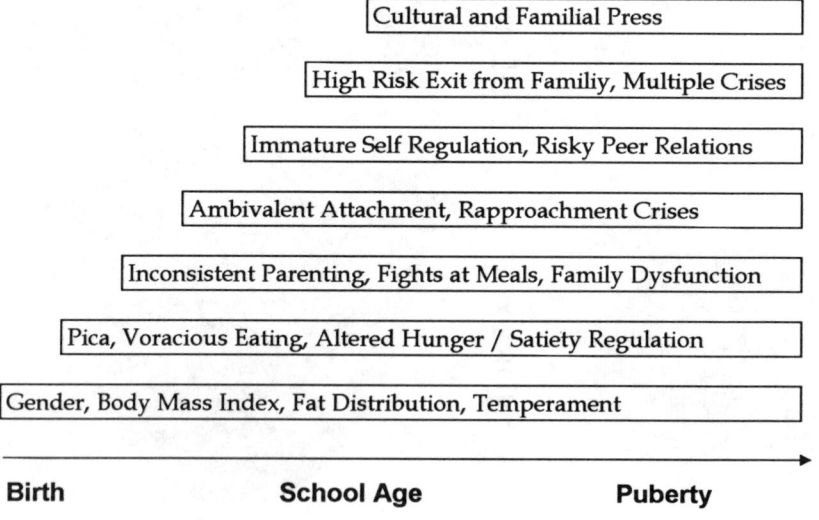

```
                    ┌─────────────────────────────┐
                    │ Cultural and Familial Press │
                    └─────────────────────────────┘
                ┌───────────────────────────────────────┐
                │ High Risk Exit from Familiy, Multiple Crises │
                └───────────────────────────────────────┘
               ┌────────────────────────────────────────┐
               │ Immature Self Regulation, Risky Peer Relations │
               └────────────────────────────────────────┘
              ┌─────────────────────────────────────────┐
              │ Ambivalent Attachment, Rapprochement Crises │
              └─────────────────────────────────────────┘
          ┌──────────────────────────────────────────────────┐
          │ Inconsistent Parenting, Fights at Meals, Family Dysfunction │
          └──────────────────────────────────────────────────┘
         ┌──────────────────────────────────────────────────────┐
         │ Pica, Voracious Eating, Altered Hunger / Satiety Regulation │
         └──────────────────────────────────────────────────────┘
    ┌──────────────────────────────────────────────────┐
    │ Gender, Body Mass Index, Fat Distribution, Temperament │
    └──────────────────────────────────────────────────┘
    ─────────────────────────────────────────────────────────►
    Birth              School Age                 Puberty
```

Figure 3.   The Stacking of Risk Factors for Bulimia.

Our model also postulates a developmental dimension to the eating disorders: As a child passes through time and acquires more and more risks in addition to the ones it inherently possesses at birth, these factors get organized and congealed into more encompassing traits that are increasingly manifested in behavior and mentation. Such an increasing pervasiveness of certain tendencies is then said to reflect a characteristic self organization. When given the final precipitating factors, these traits transform into manifest syndromes by virtue of becoming excessive and all encompassing.

Another important principle in generating risk models for the disorders must be that they are non-circular in the definition of risk and syndrome. In order to be able to provide a non-tautological interpretation of what risks may be involved, we have constructed models depicting a progression of possible factors that are not included in the current DSM-IV definition of the syndromes. Such a step, we believe, is a necessary one if we are to further our understanding of the genesis of the eating disorders. Research that argues that pre-syndromal disordered eating is a risk factor for the eating disorders is a necessary stepping stone, but it is much less helpful in leading us to better understand the etiology of the disorders and to truly new and helpful prevention and treatment.

Some of the elements in Figure 2 and Figure 3 are putative only and have little empirical support; others have substantial research backing. Our model attempts to address in a plausible way how biological, psychological, and social domains interact to produce an ultimate outcome of disorder. The specific nature and role of risks in each of these domains will be examined in the following discussion.

## 4  Biological Factors

As eating disorders represent classic psychosomatic syndromes, all of them show a variety of biological deficits as the illnesses unfold. The syndrome itself is defined in part by dysfunction of the Hypothalamic-Pituitary-Gonadal axis. There is little doubt that biological factors play an important role in both the ongoing illness and recovery and that disturbances are pervasive in many organ systems (Palla & Litt, 1990). It also seems very likely that some of these biological accompaniments represent risk factors that are premorbidly present. Whether some of them (or any of them) are genetically induced, however, remains an open question until answered by appropriate extensive prospective studies (Strober, 1990). In the study of biological risk factors for eating disorders, one common method has been to study familial aggregations of the syndromes (Hudson, Pope, Jonas, Yorgelun-Todd, & Frankenburg, 1987). Using this approach, shared characteristics of afflicted family members can be extrapolated to possible biological substrates. Mono- and dizygotic twins serve as particularly important sources of this kind of information. Studies have indeed shown that there is a familial aggregation of eating problems such that one's risk to suffer an eating disorder is much greater when a member of the immediate family suffers one as well. Numerous studies have been done in an attempt to determine risk factors within families for the onset of eating disorders. Evidence of a high prevalence of eating disorders with siblings: 3 to 10% (Morgan & Russell, 1975); parents: 27% of mothers and 16% of fathers (Kalucy, Crisp, & Harding, 1977); and first-degree relatives: 29% (Crisp, Hsu, Harding, & Harshorn, 1980) raises the question of genetic versus environmental transmission of risk factors (Strober , 1990). Unfortunately, most studies to date have only cursorily assessed the issue of shared or non-shared psychosocial environments (Kendler, McLean, Neal, Kessler, Heath, & Eaves, 1991 and Rutherford, McGuffin, Katz, & Murray, 1993). There is no detailed study as to how developmental environments were alike and different, and it is highly unlikely that such differences can be properly assessed by ten or even twenty retrospective questions about clothes, friends, and classrooms. As long as such studies limit themselves to such questions, it is unlikely that we will receive definitive answers about the differential association rates of eating problems, even using mono- and dizygotic twins as comparison groups. Familial aggregation confounds possible biological causes with psychosocial influences. Studies of twins reared in different families could control for psychosocial environments, but such projects are exceedingly difficult to do given the numbers involved, and they still would also require some controlled assessment of the two different psychosocial environments in which the children are raised. Still, it is reasonable to think at this point that the increased frequency of eating disorders in certain families may be due to factors that are biological in nature and causally related to the disorders.

We will now discuss some promising leads as to which mediating variables might be relevant in the risk for development of eating disorders. We will concentrate on those variables that are not a part of the syndromal definitions and that appear to have some empirical support or at least theoretical relevance.

## 4.1 Gender, Fat Distribution, and Body Mass Index

At the most elementary level of analysis, these three factors pose a significant risk for young individuals: being of female gender, having a pear shaped fat distribution and a body mass index high in fat. Repeated analyses have shown a preponderance of women who have eating disorders, which indicates a significant risk for the female gender. The biological dimension of gender may not be the major operator here; however – we suggest that at least in part this is so considering that during the course of many decades it has been primarily women who have been afflicted with eating disorders. Role expectations have changed dramatically over the past 4-5 decades, while the occurrence of eating disorders in women has remained relatively stable, suggesting that it is the biology of being a woman that confers a risk for the development of eating disorders rather than societal expectations in terms of gender related roles.

Excessive fat distribution in the buttocks and thighs has been associated with much higher occurrences of eating disorders (Radke-Sharpe, Whitney-Saltiel, & Rodin, 1990). In a recent study of 77 women it was shown that waist and hip measurements correlated significantly with body dissatisfaction and disordered eating. These body characteristics are most likely genetic or metabolic in origin (Hammer, 1993). A high Body Mass Index (an index of body composition and a proxy measure for obesity) also appears to confer significant risk for eating disorders, especially bulimia. Evidence that the heritability estimate for Body Mass Index is about 64% suggests that it, too, is most likely genetically determined (Rutherford, Mc Guffin, Katz, & Murray, 1993).

## 4.2 Puberty

Another general biological factor to be considered in the genesis of these disorders is puberty. Killen and his group (Killen, Hayward, Litt, Hammer, Wilson, Miner, Taylor, Varady, & Shisslak, 1992) have found evidence that girls who manifested relatively early maturity also showed more bulimic symptoms. In this sample of 971 high schoolers, the odds ratio for the association between bulimic symptoms and Tanner stages of sexual maturity was 1.8, controlling for age. Findings like this make sense given the hormonally induced, rapid, and uncontrollable weight gain that occurs during puberty. Such weight gain in girls, which involves relatively more adipose tissue than in boys, seems to be accompanied by sharp increases in concern and dissatisfaction about body appearance.

All the above factors are rather general and must have relatively weak influences, as most women, most people with high thigh and buttock fat distribution, and most pubertal girls are not bulimic or anorexic. The biological factors specific to eating disorders are of greater concern to researchers than such general, non-specific factors.

### 4.3 Metabolic Abnormalities Related to Hunger and Satiety

It is attractive to think that individuals prone to eating disorders have altered pathways of responding to food. Such pathways would plausibly explain why such an individual would gravitate towards restriction or overeating in times of personal crisis. There are some leads in the current research that appear promising and deserve discussion.

For example, there is evidence that disturbances in the metabolic functions that are more specifically tied to hunger, satiety regulation, mood regulation, and impulse control may accompany eating disorders and persist after weight rehabilitation. Of interest is the finding that in adult patients, caloric requirements for weight rehabilitation and maintenance differ for bulimic, anorexic, and normal populations (Weltzin, Fernstrom, Hansen, McConaha, & Kaye, 1991; Gwirtsman, Kaye, Obarzanek, George, Jimerson, & Ebert 1989; Kaye, Gwirtsman, Obarzanek, George, Jimerson, & Ebert, 1986). We have been able to replicate some of these findings in a sample of adolescent eating disorders where we found that adolescents with restrictive anorexia required the most calories to maintain their daily weight, while bulimic patients required the least. Such differences persisted for many months following weight rehabilitation, indicating that there are possible premorbid characteristics (Brantner-Innthaler, Nasserbakht, Shih, & Steiner 1994). Such differences could help explain why it is so difficult for patients with anorexia and bulimia to regain control over their eating and weight once they are confronted with the deleterious consequences of their dietary malpractices and are trying to the best of their abilities to become either binge/purge abstinent or regain up to normal weight.

On the hormonal level, alterations of brain-gut peptides occur in eating disorder patients and possibly antedate the development of syndromes. Such disturbances would explain the altered eating patterns found in this population starting from a very early age (Marchi & Cohen, 1990). One specific hormonal deficiency associated with bulimia appears to be in the cholecystokinin system (Geracioti et al, 1992), although there are some contradictory findings (Phillipp, Pirke, Kellner, & Krieg, 1991). These findings could relate to the absence of satiety induction in bulimic patients.

Our own group studied Histidyl-Diketo-Piperazine (Cyclo-His-Pro) in normal, anorexic, and bulimic adolescents (Steiner, Wilber, Prasad, Rogers, & Rosenkrantz, 1989). This hormone is involved, among other things, in the induction of satiety. Results suggested that as anorexic patients gain weight, this correlates positively with levels of CHP, possibly indicating the induction of premature satiety. Bulimic patients seem to experience the opposite effect, as weight correlated negatively with the hormone. This could indicate insufficient release of CHP after eating, which in turn affords them inadequate satiety in response to adequate caloric intake. It is also clear, though, from a simple study of the neuroanatomical and neurophysiological facts about these particular systems, that it is highly unlikely that any single hormone or defect will be found responsible for problems in this area, as the system is exceedingly complex, relies on many hormones and neurotransmitters that act in concert and provide "failsafe wiring." The latter, of course, makes eminent sense given the importance of the functions involved for our survival (Vande Wiele, 1980; Johnson & Larson, 1982; Krieger & Hughes, 1980).

Sometimes, a disturbance in relevant hormones caused by other diseases can cause a secondary eating disorder (Striegel-Moore, Nicholson, & Tamberlane, 1992; Peveler, Fairburn, Boller, & Dunger, 1992). This seems to be the case with people suffering from diabetes mellitus, many of whom develop eating disorders after the onset of their primary illness. As many as twenty percent of these patients have been found to suffer such problems, a figure that by far exceeds that expected by chance alone. Such an association raises questions about abnormalities in the insulin-glucagon systems, which might predispose individuals to the disorders.

## 4.4 Biological Determinants of Mood

Evidence supports the idea that negative mood initiates binge and purge cycles in bulimics (Davis, Freeman, & Garner, 1988; Johnson & Larson, 1982) and possibly relates to dietary restriction in anorexic patients. Such cycles and patterns may be acquired very early in life or predetermined by hard-wired differences between individuals. Such an association is particularly interesting, as the neuroanatomy and neurotransmitters of mood and food regulation are closely linked in the hypothalamus (Jimerson, Lesem, Kaye, Hegg, & Brewerton, 1990).

To the extent that mood and anxiety states reflect biological substrates under genetic as well as environmental control, such states should be considered in the assessment of biological risks for eating disorders. Anxiety and related syndromes long post-date anorexia nervosa (Smith, Feldman, Nasserbakht, & Steiner, 1993), whereas mood disturbances, especially depressions, predominate in both anorexia and bulimia before and during the illnesses. We have more information on this link for bulimia than for anorexia. Some data suggests that depression and bulimia are related but not directly passed on together in a genetic pattern; however, they do show some shared heritability (Kendler, McLean, Neale, Kessler, Heath, & Eaves, 1993). The specific nature of this relationship is not clear (Strober & Katz, 1988).

Most of these studies are concurrent only; however, they have treatment implications and could point to some risk associated with a tendency for rapid depletion of serotonin or norepinephrine in response to challenges in life for bulimics and the obverse tendency for anorexics who might be suffering from an excess of serotonergic activity in this particular area.

## 4.5 Native Temperamental Characteristics

As one considers biological risk factors in these disorders, one is led to consider temperament. Temperament has been shown to be stable over time and to be at least under partial genetic control (Strober, 1991). Clinicians have repeatedly commented on the relatively unvaried presence of certain traits in eating disorders, and it is tempting to think that such traits might be present at birth.

We have found an association between certain temperamental characteristics and diagnostic status in a study of 37 anorexic, 28 bulimic, and 36 depressed girls who were compared to 315 normal adolescents. The groups were assessed by a self-reported, standardized inventory, measuring nine traits (Shaw, Lee, & Steiner, 1994). We have shown that parental and adolescent reporting of such characteristics is remarkably consistent (Luby & Steiner, 1993). In the study of eating disorders, the groups differed significantly on four of nine temperamental dimensions. All three pathological groups were significantly more dysphoric than normals, but differed temperamentally in other ways. Specifically, anorexic girls were more depressed, more rhythmic in their eating and sleep, and more avoidant of novel stimuli in comparison to normals. In contrast, bulimic girls were less task-oriented and less rhythmic in eating than normals, but had similar scores for approaching novel stimuli. Depressed patients, while showing no difference in daily rhythms compared to normals, did demonstrate more avoidance in their approach to novel stimuli. Such temperamental differences are interesting, as they may relate to the personality characteristics that under certain conditions, could become deficient traits. If not corrected, these factors add further weight to the growing pyramid of risk.

## 5 Psychological Factors

The possible psychological risks for eating disorders span several different domains. Personality traits – especially the regulation of mood and affect, cognitive styles, and attachment – are three different areas that have undergone scrutiny. In the realm of personality, most experts agree on a general risk profile for Anorexia that includes anxiety, obsessiveness, perfectionism and over-compliance, and another profile for Bulimia that includes emotional lability, depressed mood, and counter-phobic independence. Adolescents with eating disorders have difficulty with certain cognitive tasks such as conceptualizing realistic images of their bodies and forming appropriate attitudes about the mastery of their bodies. In the area of attachment, researchers have explored issues of separation and individuation, as well as the anorexic adolescent's fear of growing up and becoming independent.

### 5.1 Affect and Mood Regulation

Within the literature on personality traits associated with eating disorders, none has received so much attention recently as the area of affective tone and mood regulation, which accompanies eating disorders to a very high degree and even antedates the onset of symptoms in a large percentage of patients. Disordered eating and mood are almost inextricably linked in some patients. Many studies have reported correlations between depressed mood and disordered eating (e.g., Steiger, Leung, & Houle, 1992 ; Strober & Katz, 1988) whereas depression as a precursor to eating disorders is one possible interpretation of the evidence, several others also exist.

For example, it is possible that the disordered eating itself causes depression. Malnutrition has been shown to induce hormonal changes, that could lead to emotional change. The studies by Keys are still the standard for this line of investigation. (Keys, Brozek, Henschel, Mickelsen, & Taylor, 1950). However, a more recent comparison of anorexic and cystic fibrosis patients by means of contemporary standardized instruments demonstrated that malnutrition does not invariably cause depression in non-anorexic subjects (Steiner, Rahimzadeh, & Lewiston, 1989). Anorexic adolescents in this study reported significantly more depressive affect than cystic fibrosis patients matched for sex, SES, age, menstrual status, body mass, and pubertal development. This information argues well for the theory of premorbid depression. In the same data base, we also were able to establish that malnutrition – in this case induced by malabsorption – did not lead to cognitive distortions of body image, drive for thinness or other thought patterns characteristic of anorexia, thereby highlighting the possible importance of these elements in the genesis of the syndrome.

Those who argue against depression as a risk factor describe its role in anorexia as primarily comorbid. They view depression as a *state* accompanying the illness, rather than a premorbid *trait*. Maria Råstam's finding of similar rates of prior depressive disorders in individuals with anorexia and normal subjects supports this notion. (Råstam, 1992)

We have no doubt that depressive disorder overlaps considerably with anorexia and bulimia. What we wish to suggest is that a propensity toward depression – a nonsyndromal trait – may precede the onset of anorexia. Such a depressive predisposition would not surface in a study like Råstam's, which only measured clinical manifestations of disorder. Yet it might help explain why anorexic patients with less initial depression are less at risk for chronic eating problems (Smith, Feldman, Nasserbakht, & Steiner, 1993).

It may be that factors like low self-esteem and depression put an adolescent at risk for psychopathology in general rather than eating disorders in specific. Other variables associated with risk may also fall into this category. For example, Gloria Leon and her associates identified interoceptive awareness as a strong predictor of risk for eating disorders (Leon, Fulkerson, Perry, & Cudeck, 1992; Leon, Perry, Mangelsdorf, & Tell, 1989). Yet other researchers found this same factor – as well as ineffectiveness and interpersonal distrust – equally represented among eating disorder and depressed patients (Smith & Steiner, 1992).

If depressed mood, low-self-esteem, ineffectiveness, interpersonal distrust, and lack of interoceptive awareness act only as general risk factors for eating disorders, then more specific traits must also be added to the risk profile. Consistent descriptions of such traits have been provided by a consensus of researchers working from different theoretical orientations.

## 5.2 Personality Traits

The two personality trait descriptions for anorexia and bulimia paint a picture of two quite different adolescents. In general, the anorexic teenager is anxious to please, driven to achieve, perfectionistic, self-restrained, shy, inhibited, and sometimes picky or obsessive (Casper, Yates, Beutler, & Arzimendi, 1992; Råstam, 1992; Strober, 1980; Fahy, Osacar, & Marks, 1993). Contrastingly, the bulimic girl is impulsive, less careful about her impression on others, and she may show borderline characteristics (Steiger, Leung, & Houle, 1992). Measuring such traits in a ego-psychological framework, anorexics appear as heavily emphasizing mature defenses, perhaps age-inappropriately so, whereas bulimics tend to appear immature in their defense profile (Steiner, 1990).

The link between each of these descriptions and eating disorder behavior makes intuitive sense. For example, the potential anorexic's concern for what others think may make her more vulnerable to the social pressure of being thin. Her desire to avoid conflict may also be served by turning her attention away from interpersonal problems and onto the more manageable arena of her body. The fact that she is self-disciplined and perfectionistic gives her the tools to maintain an obsessively strict diet and exercise regimen. All these factors taken together stack the cards in anorexia's favor.

The trait that favors bulimia is an inability to self-regulate. In social situations, this may mean less restraint and less inhibition. When it comes to food, the self-control deficit can result in difficulty controlling urges to overeat. Such binges may be precipitated by the distrust and interpersonal difficulties.

## 5.3 Cognitive Processing

How a young woman thinks, certain ways of assimilating incoming information, may facilitate the development of an eating disorder. Several interesting recent studies have explored this topic.

One approach by Alfred Heilbrun and Alison Flodin involves the study of food cues and perceptual distortions (Heilbrun & Flodin, 1989). Their investigation examined whether women at risk for eating disorders would rate models as fatter in the presence of food cues. They found that food cues did indeed cause women who scored high on anorexic characteristics (such as drive for thinness) to perceive body shapes as bigger, but only if they were really stressed. For this group, it seemed, stressful conditions elicited a cognitive strategy that is highly useful in the attempt to lose weight. The interaction of stress with other characteristics also highlights how cumulative risks work together in the evolution of eating disorder.

Another cognitive strategy used by anorexia-prone women under stress is a "disattention" similar to repression (Heilbrun & Worobow, 1990). When applied to internal hunger sensations, the disattention allows anorexia-prone women under stress to ignore their need to eat. The end result is a lack of interoceptive awareness, which is a factor that has been implicated in eating disorders (Leon, Fulkerson, Perry, & Cudeck, 1992). The cognitive strategies to avoid weight gain developed by women with eating problems probably take years to acquire. Interpersonal processes which begin at an early age most likely predate such risks. Research into separation-individuation problems puts us right at the bottom of the risk pyramid. This is an area that has the potential to clarify many of the mysterious origins of problems with eating, yet it clearly has received only very little systematic attention. No doubt, it is the difficulty of measuring states, traits, and interactions at this stage of development that poses formidable obstacles.

## 5.4 Attachment Status

Learning to separate 'self' from 'other' and retaining a permanent image of an attachment figure, no matter what the situation, is one of the most pervasive achievements of development. This is an area with which individuals with anorexia and bulimia appear to have trouble. In fact, dependency conflicts and a difficulty differentiating one's own needs from those of others have been shown to be strongly predictive of Eating Disorder Measures (Friedlander & Siegel, 1990). Girls with eating disorders do not seem to have a clear sense of who they are, which suggests early deficiencies in the developmental process of identity formation.

Attachment theory sets up early mother-infant interactions as an important foundation for this process. Of these interactions, none is more primary than that of feeding and mealtimes. Infants with difficult temperaments who are fussy eaters can exhibit behaviors that are reinforced in turn by mothers unsure of how to respond to their demands. Mother and infant in this way both fuel a continuing negative interaction that reaches far into the future and that specifically involves food and meals as vehicles for interpersonal processes. The persistence of the behavior evinces itself in feeding problems that last from three months of age until at least four years (Dahl & Sundelin, 1992).

The consequences of these feeding problems has been looked at from both the angles of infant temperament and mother response style. One study has found that picky eating and childhood digestive problems predict adolescent anorexia. Similarly, pica predicts bulimia (Marchi & Cohen, 1989). Whereas infant eating behavior may influence later development of anorexia, so it seems does early mother feeding practices. In a retrospective study, mothers of anorexic teenagers recalled more schedule feeding and earlier introduction of solids than comparison control mothers (Steiner, Smith, Rosenkrantz, & Litt, 1990). The combination of these two factors – early infant temperament and maternal response – could set up an early chain of events ultimately leading to eating disorder.

## 6 Familial Risk Factors

Families might be involved in several ways in the generation of risk for eating disorders in their children. The literature to date has been very focussed on interactions between members, mostly under the influence of Minuchin's interesting ideas; however, other areas appear to us as deserving of our attention (Minuchin, Rosman, & Baker, 1978; McNamara & Lovemann, 1990; Gowers, Kadambari, & Crisp, 1985; Råstam & Gilberg, 1991; Gordon, Beresin, & Herzog, 1989; Yager, 1982). The handling of food, fitness, bodily functioning, appearance, indepence, competition, competence, preparation for exit from the family, and the clustering of psychiatric syndromes that might contribute specifically to risk by influencing these areas of family functioning all need to be explored.

## 6.1 Family Interactions

Theorists have promoted the idea that family patterns and relationships contribute to the onset of eating disorders (Minuchin, Rosman, & Baker, 1978; Strober & Yager, 1985) and that certain family patterns are characteristic of "eating disorder families". The idea is attractive to clinicians who report certain invariant patterns occurring in families with patients with eating disorders and who see improvement of their patients after such patterns have been changed. From a theoretical point of view, the role of the family in shaping a child's expectations regarding role, beauty, body, food, love and attachment is most important. The family can be seen as a transducer of cultural values that will shape the child's expectations and realistic appraisal of her own abilities and desires.

However, empirical studies that have attempted to determine distinguishing family interactions have indicated differing results. Currently, the strongest series of studies, examining directly the interactions between family members of eating disorder patients after the onset of the disorders (Humphrey, 1988), employed a structural analysis in which family members rated themselves and their relationships with family members. The teenage daughters diagnosed with bulimia and anorexia with bulimia both indicated greater neglect and rejection as well as less nurturance in their families relative to a control population. The girls diagnosed with anorexia denied parent-child problems, but did report severe marital distress. Each family was videotaped (Humphrey, 1989) and their interactions were coded. The parents of the girls diagnosed with anorexia communicated a combination of nurturance and neglect of their daughter's needs to express feelings, and the daughters were found to appear ambivalent about disclosing their feelings. However, the parents of the girls diagnosed with bulimia appeared to be enmeshed in a hostile pattern and also to undermine their daughter's self assertion and attempts to "separate".

Another study (Grigg, Friesen, & Shappy, 1989) utilized the same structural analysis to assess reported transactional patterns of families with girls diagnosed with anorexia and compared them with those of a control population. Findings showed that families tended to fall in cluster groups. Of the seven distinct family clusters, the families with girls diagnosed with anorexia fell predominantly into three groups, whereas the control population fell predominantly into a separate cluster. These findings indicate that interaction patterns may differentiate control families from families experiencing anorexia but that there does not appear to be a single "anorexigenic family system." The major limitation of these findings is that the communication patterns are observed after the child has been ill for some time. It is thus not possible to distinguish whether these patterns antedate the illness, or whether they are indeed a driving force of the illness.

Futhermore, comparing the self reports of children with another type of chronic illness and their families to those of patients with anorexia and bulimia shows no distinguishing features. Thienemann and Steiner (1993) gave a self report measure to assess the family environment of families of teenage daughters diagnosed with either anorexia, anorexia with bulimia, bulimia, or depression in comparison to a control population. They found that the report of a negative family environment was associated with the level of reported depression independent of diagnosis. This argues against a specific familial environment for eating disorders, or raises once again issues regarding the overlap between eating disorders and depression.. The obvious limitation here is that self report may simply be too blunt an instrument to answer the question satisfactorily.

The results of these empirical studies indicate that families experiencing significant eating issues tend to indicate some negative aspects in regards to their relationships. However, as the Thienemann and Steiner (1993) study indicates, these reports may be more indicative of other mediating variables such as depression. All of these studies are retrospective or concurrent, so they may be more indicative of an "effect" of the problem(s) rather than be contributory to the problem. The family's response to the stress of the problem may contribute to reported negative experiences rather than reflect premorbid risk factors or enduring family characteristics.

Another research strategy to address familial risk factors would be to examine the longitudinal effect of the course of illness on the family to see which specific changes lead to improvement in the patient. While not decisive evidence, positive findings would lend some more weight to certain factors if it can be shown that they are linked to improvement. In an attempt to determine if the family's response to the problems changes or evolves over time, Galante, Sanders, & Steiner (1994) gave several self report measures to families of teenage daughters diagnosed with anorexia, bulimia, or with both disorders at different phases of their experience with the problem. They found that independent of diagnosis, families perceive themselves as more cohesive and more adaptable in the beginning of their experience with the problem as compared to later in their experience. Therefore, rather than appearing to have premorbid risk characteristics, a family may perceive and present themselves differently depending on the duration of their struggle with the problem.

Another possible risk factor relates to the fact that sometimes an eating disorder appears to provide a protective function in the family by diverting attention from parental neuroticism or marital dysfunction. Crisp, Harding, & McGuiness (1974) found that parents' neuroticism increased as their child improved. They suggest that symptoms in children may have an organizing, settling effect on parents, keeping certain family structures and hierarchies intact.

## 6.2 Familial Attitudes Towards Food, Health, Fitness and Appearance

There are a few studies that have looked in detail at familial expectations for these patients, father's and mother's ideals of beauty and body, preoccupation with dieting and appearance, and connotation of food and nourishment (Pike & Rodin, 1991; Hall & Brown, 1983; Hill, Weaver, & Blundell, 1990). Hill, in a series of studies, showed that parents of prepubertal girls who are showing excessive concern about appearance, weight, and dieting, reflect those same concerns in their own lives. For the study of risk research, these are all very important areas to explore crossectionally. Because of the powerful reinforcement value of food, almost any message is easily paired with it during the daily rituals of eating and replenishment. Interactions around these issues are intense and carry lots of weight (so to speak). All these are areas deserving of our attention in addition to the fine-grained assessments of interactions in these families.

## 6.3 Premorbid Parental Characteristics

Investigation into possible premorbid parental characteristics indicates a variety of parental physical illness (Kalucy, Crisp, & Harding 1977; Strober, Morrell, Burroughs, Salkin, & Jacobs, 1985; Strober, Salkin, Burroughs, & Morrell, 1982) and psychiatric illness (Cantwell, Sturzenberger, Borroughs, Salkin, & Green, 1977) associated with the onset of eating issues in children. In addition, associations have been reported for various parent-child interaction patterns (Morgan & Russell, 1975).

## 6.4 Abuse in the Family

A special issue, which has recently received much attention, is the role of abuse – especially sexual victimization – in the genesis of eating disorders (Palmer, Oppenheimer, Dignon, Chaloner, & Howells, 1990; Rorty, Yager, & Rossotto, 1994). The high prevalence of eating disturbances and sexual abuse in women raises the question of whether a history of sexual abuse may predispose women to eating disorders. However, research conducted in an attempt to clarify this relationship has indicated diverse findings with some studies indicating no relationship between eating issues and abuse (Finn, Hartmann, Leon, & Lawson, 1986) and others reporting significantly high rates of sexual abuse associated with eating disorders (Hall, Tice, Beresford, Wooley, & Hall, 1989) and especially associated with bulimia (Root & Fallon, 1988; Waller, 1992). Rorty, Yager, & Rossotto (1994) found higher rates of physical, psychological, and multiple abuse rather than sexual abuse associated with a diagnosis of bulimia.

Comparison of studies is difficult due to methodological differences such as differing diagnostic criteria used to assess eating issues as well as differing definitions of abuse which could include an array of traumatic experiences of various length and severity. Connors & Morse (1993) report that the studies they reviewed indicated that around 30% of women with diagnosed eating disorders also reported a history of sexual abuse and that this was similar to the percentage reported for the general female population (Finkelhor, 1984; Russell, 1986) and is a lower percentage than has been reported by other diagnostic groups, such as somatization disorder (Morrison, 1989) and borderline patients (Herman, Perry, & van der Kolk, 1989).

Pitts and Waller (1993) found that the mediating variables of self esteem and severity of self-denigratory beliefs following abuse were linked to severity of eating problems rather than the abuse per se. The above findings suggest that sexual abuse may not be necessary or sufficient in contributing to the onset of eating issues in general. In cases of incestuous abuse, the abuse may be a significant contributing factor and evidence of the dysfunction of a particular family. In cases of both incestuous and extrafamilial abuse, the patient may experience a link between the abuse and eating issues.

## 7 Cultural Factors

Recent research indicates that the incidence of anorexia nervosa and bulimia has been on the increase in Western societies over the past fifteen years (Lucas, Beard, O'Fallon, & Kurland, 1991; Theander, 1970; Duddle, 1973; Cooper & Fairburn, 1982; Halmi, Jones, & Schwartz, 1981; Chiodo & Latimer, 1983). The rise seemingly cannot be attributed just to greater diagnostic sophistication and improved case finding.

By contrast, the incidence of eating disorders in non-Western cultures such as Latin America (Carlos, 1972), West India (Neki, 1973), Africa (German, 1973; Nwaefuna, 1981; Buchan & Gregory, 1984), Sudan (El Sarag, 1968), Egypt (Okasha, Karmel, Sadek, Lotaif, & Bishry, 1977), India (Prince, 1985), Malaysia (Buhrich, 1981), and Singapore (Ong, Tsoi, & Cheah, 1982) has been described as rare to absent. Some of these cultures even value plumpness as an attractive and desirable characteristic (Rudofsky, 1972; El Sarag, 1968; Buhrich, 1981; Orbach, 1978, Powers, 1980).

### 7.1 Exposure to Western Culture

Yet eating disorders do appear in non-Western countries that are influenced by Western values. For example, several researchers have found that women from non-Western cultures indicated greater body consciousness after exposure to a Western industrialized society (Worsley, 1981; Furnham & Alibhai, 1983, Fichter et al, 1983; Nasser, 1986). Some have also suggested that the non-Western individuals who do develop anorexia nervosa have strong Western affiliations and high social status (Norris, 1979).

Given this wide body of evidence, there can be little doubt that living within a Western culture puts adolescents at significant risk for eating disorders. This leads us to the obvious question: What is it about our culture that engenders such risk?

One answer concerns pervasive Western value judgments about health and body image. The post-World War II emphasis on reducing "fat", which was supported by insurance campaigns, worked to convince the North American population that animal fat was dangerous. Within this cultural context, weight loss began to be seen as "healthy", while being "fat" meant that you were not trying hard enough to take care of yourself (DeJong, 1980). Furthermore, being overweight opposed the American ideal that if you "just try hard enough" you can obtain your goals (Seid, 1994). Increasingly, North America became a "healthist" culture, emphasizing healthy behavior as a moral duty and illness as an individual moral failing. Within this climate the thin person became an example of mind-over-body mastery as well as virtuous self-denial (Crawford 1984).

These generally unrealistic attitudes toward health affect women in especially damaging ways. This is because the reality of the cultural ideal is an "unrealistic" body type for most of the female population. At this point in time the "ideal" female body type represents approximately 5 to 10% of American women (Garner & Garfinkel, 1980). What this means is that 90 - 95% of American women are invited to feel they are "too fat," or, as viewed through the cultural lens, "less of a person". Yet the biological standards are both "unrealistic" and "unhealthy" for the majority of the female population, in the sense that if women were to attempt to meet them, they would, in fact, become anorexic.

As puberty changes girls' bodies in a direction away from these standards, it puts them particularly at risk. Evidence supporting this idea shows that postmenarcheal girls have more risk for eating disorders than premenarchial girls of common age . Other studies indicate that early maturity also puts girls at greater risk (Killen, Hayward, Litt, Hammer, Wilson, Miner, Taylor, Varady, & Shisslak, 1992). Because these early maturers tend to be heavier, fatter, and slightly shorter, it is not unreasonable to suggest that their bodies' deviation from social norms plays a role in their distress.

Whereas these fundamental underlying values make living in Western culture a general risk for eating disorders, several more specific social factors have also been implicated as risks.

## 7.2 Gender Roles

Given that prevalence of eating issues is so much higher for women than men, the influence of gender role differences has been investigated as a risk factor. Thornton (1991) found that women who endorsed either stereotypic female (not aggressive) attributes or stereotypic male (aggressive) attributes *and* the "superwoman" ideal of success were more prone to eating disorders than less "stereotyped" participants. As a gender class in a society that stresses perfection, women may be more concerned with body image. Therefore, those who strive for "perfection" or "superwomen" status may be more at risk for eating issues (Steiner-Adair, 1986).

It is plausible to view eating disorder prevalence in women as being due to the changing of women's roles, whereas men may have yet to experience such gender transition in our culture. Likewise, men may be subject to sociocultural conflict in regards to gender but they may be less concerned with eating or body image.

## 7.3 Class

Individuals from higher SES appear to be at higher risk for development of eating disorders (Anderson & Hay, 1985) and subthreshold eating disorders (Dwyer & Mayer, 1970). In contrast, obesity correlates with lower economic status (Hsu, 1989). These relationships may represent the fact that today's fasting began among financially comfortable and well-educated females, as well as those marked for success. However, there is some indication that eating disorders are becoming more evenly distributed according to social class (Pumariega, Edwards, & Mitchell, 1984; Pumariega, 1986; Pate, Pumariega, Hester, & Garner, 1992).

## 7.4 Ethnicity

Caucasian females tend to be more likely to see themselves as overweight and attempt to diet as compared to their black counterparts (Heunemann, Shapiro, Hampton, & Mitchell, 1966; Hooper & Garner, 1986). However, also emerging is the greater incidence of eating disorder diagnoses in ethnic groups in which such diagnoses were previously absent, such as blacks (Robinson & Andersen, 1985; Hsu, 1987; Lawlor & Rand, 1985; Lacey & Dolan, 1988), hispanics (Pumeriega, 1986), Asians (Lacey & Dolan, 1988; Bryant-Waugh & Lask, 1991; Mumford & Whitehouse, 1988), Native Americans (Rosen, Shafer, Dummer, Cross, Deumann,

& Malmberg, 1988) and Vietnamese refugees (Kope & Sack, 1987). Reports may underestimate the prevalence of of eating disorder diagnoses in ethnic minority groups due to their incapability or tendency not to seek treatment.

## 7.5 Competitive Sub-Populations

Even the study of subgroups within Western culture might shed some light on the contribution cultural factors make in the genesis of these syndromes. If we examine groups that have to perform under the excessive influence of Western ideals of beauty and grace, we should find an increase in the eating problems. Indeed, dancing, gymnastics, and modelling (McKenna, 1989) all show increased risk.. An increased incidence of eating issues is found in dancers and models after they enter the profession compared to other competitive "nonappearance" related professions (Crago, Yates, Beutler, & Arizmendi, 1985; Garner & Garfinkel, 1980). It is as if in these cases, individuals are exposed to an especially concentrated form of expectations. The alternative interpretation – that such professions tend to attract individuals who are prone to eating disorders – also must be considered and, although it has never received appropriate study and attention, is equally plausible.

## 8 Conclusions

We have attempted to outline relevant factors from four major domains - biological, psychological, familial and cultural - which may be considered as being premorbidly present risk factors for eating disorders. In an effort to push current thinking beyond a narrow definition of the disorders, we have tried to avoid the tautological definitions of risk that are sometimes found inearly risk research. In general, we have found that within each domain there are at least some studies that address issues satisfactorily, but it is exceedingly uncommon to find studies that address any other domains or factors simultaneously or that integrate multiple domains into a more cohesive picture. It appears that we will need to concentrate on the building of more complex models and to support them with appropriate studies if we are to go successfully beyond the current state of knowledge and are to be truly effective in prevention and treatment.

## References

Anderson, A., & Hay, A. (1985). Racial and socio-economic influences in anorexia nervosa and bulimia. *International Journal of Eating Disorders, 4*, 479-487.

Bryant-Waugh, R., & Lask, B. (1991). Anorexia nervosa in a group of Asian children living in Berlin. *British Journal of Psychiatry, 158*, 229-233.

Brantner-Inthaler, S., Nasserbakht, A., Shih, G., & Steiner, H. (1994). *Differences in caloric utilisation in eating disordered adolescsents.* Submitted for publication.

Buchan, T., & Gregory, L. (1984). Anorexia nervosa in a black Zimbabwean. *British Journal of Psychiatry, 145*, 326-330.

Buhrich, N. (1981). Frequency of presentation of anorexia nervosa in Malaysia. *Australian and New Zealand Journal of Psychiatry, 15*, 153-155.

Cantwell, D.P., Sturzenberger, S., Borroughs, J., Salkin, B., & Green, J.K. (1977). Anorexia nervosa - an affective disorder? *Archives of General Psychiatry, 34*, 1087-1093.

Carlos, A. (1972). Psychiatry in Latin America. *British Journal of Psychiatry, 121*, 121-136.

Casper, R., Hedecker, D., & McClough, J. (1992). Personality dimensions in eating disorders and their relevance for subtyping. *Journal of the American Academy of Child and Adolescent Psychiatry, 31*(5), 830-840.

Childress, A., Brewerton, T., Hodges, E., & Jarrelll, M. (1993). The kids eating disorder survey (KEDS): A study of middle school students. *Journal of the American Academy of Child and Adolescent Psychiatry, 32*(4), 843-850.

Chiodo, S., & Latimer, P. (1983). Vomiting as a learned weight-control technique in bulimia. *Journal of Behavior Therapy and Experimental Psychiatry, 14*, 131-135.

Connors, M., & Morse, W. (1993). Sexual abuse and eating disorders: A review. *International Journal of Eating Disorders, 13*(1), 1-11.

Cooper, P.& Fairburn, C. (1982). Binge eating and self-induced vomiting in the community. A preliminary study. *British Journal of Psychiatry, 15*, 1955-2025.

Crago, M., Yates, A., Beutler, L.E., & Arizmendi, T.A. (1985). Height weight ratios among female athletes: Are collegiate athletics the precursors to anorexic syndrome? *International Journal of Eating Disorders, 4*, 79-82.

Crawford, R. (1984) A cultural account of "health": Control, release, and the social body. In J. B. McKinlay (Ed.), *Issues in the political economy of health care* (pp. 60-103). New York: Tavistock Publications.

Crisp, A.H., Harding, B., & McGuinness, B. (1974). Anorexia nervosa, psychoneurotic characteristics of parents: Relationship to prognosis. *Journal of Psychosomatic Research, 18*, 167-173.

Crisp, A. H., Hsu, L. K. G., Harding, B., & Hartshorn, J. (1980). Clinical features of anorexia nervosa. *Psychosomatics, 24*, 179-191.

Dahl, M., & Sundelin, C. (1992). Feeding problems in an affluent society. Follow-up at four years of age in children with early refusal to eat. *Acta Pediatrica, 81*, 575-579.

Davis, R., Freeman, R.J., & Garner, D.M. (1988). A naturalistic investigation of eating behavior in bulimia nervosa. *Journal of Consulting and Clinical Psychology, 56*(2), 273-279.

DeJong, W. (1980). The stigma of obesity: The consequences of naive assumptions concerning the causes of physical deviance. *Journal of Personality and Social Psychology, 21*, 75-87.

Devlin, M.J., Walsh, B.T., Kral, J.G., Heymsfield, S.B., Pi-Sunyer, F.X., & Dantzic, S. (1990). Metabolic abnormalities in bulimia nervosa. *Archives of Genereal Psychiatry, 47*, 144-148.

Duddle, M. (1973). An increase in anorexia nervosa in a university population. *British Journal of Psychiatry, 123*, 711-712.

Dwyer, J., & Mayer, J. (1970). Potential dieters: Who are they? *Journal of the American Diabetic Association, 5*, 510-514.

El Sarag, M. (1968). Psychiatry in Northern Sudan: A study in comparative psychiatry. *British Journal of Psychiatry, 114*, 946-948.

Fahy, T., Osacar, A., & Marks, I. (1993). History of eating disorders in female patients with obsessive-compulsive disorder. *International Journal of Eating Disorders, 14*(4), 439-443.

Fichter, M. Weyerer, S. Sourdi, L., & Sourdi, Z. (1983). Anorexia nervosa. In A. Liss (Ed.), *Recent developments in research,* (pp. 95-105). New York: Springer.

Field, A.F., Wolf, A.M., Herzog, D. B., Cheung, L., & Colditz, G.A. (1993). The relationship of caloric intake to frequency of dieting among preadolescent and adolescent girls. *Journal of the American Academy of Child and Adolescent Psychiatry, 32*, 1246-1252.

Finkelhor, D., (1984). *Child sexual abuse: New theory and research.* New York: Free Press.

Finn, S. E., Hartman, M., Leon, G., & Lawson. L. (1986). Eating disorders and sexual abuse: Lack of confirmation for a clinical hypothesis. *International Journal of Eating Disorders, 5*, 1051-1060.

Friedlander, M.L., & Siegel, S.M., (1990). Separation-individuation difficulties and cognitive-behavioral indicators of eating disorders among college women. *Journal of Counseling Psychology, 37*(1), 74-78.

Furnham, A.C., & Alibhai, N. (1983). Cross-cultural differences in the perception of female body shape. *Psychological Medicine, 13*, 829-837.

Galante, D., Sanders, M., & Steiner, H. (1994). *Characteristics of families of daughters with anorexia or bulimia: A study of treatment phases*. Unpublished manuscript.

Garner, D.M. (1980). Cultural expectations of thinness in women. *Psychological Reports, 47*, 483-491.

Garner, D.M., & Garfinkel, P. E. (1980). Socio-cultural factors in the development of anorexia nervosa. *Psychological Medicine, 10*, 647-56.

Geracioti, T.D., Liddle, R.A., Altemus, M., Demitrack, M.A., & Gold, P.W. (1992). Regulation of appetite and Cholecystokinin secretion in anorexia nervosa. *American Journal of Psychiatry, 149* (7), 958-961.

German, G. (1972). Aspects of clinical psychiatry in sub-Saharan Africa. *British Journal of Psychiatry, 121*, 461-479.

Gordon, C., Beresin, E., & Herzog, D. (1989). The parents relationship and the child's illness in anorexia nervosa. *Journal of the American Academy of Psychoanalysis, 17*(1), 29-42.

Gowers, S., Kadambari, S.R., & Crisp, A.H. (1985). Family structure and birth order of patients with anorexia nervosa. *Journal of Psychiatric Research, 19*(2,3), 247-251.

Grigg, D., Friesen, J., & Shappy, M. (1989). Family patterns associated with anorexia nervosa. *Journal of Marital and Family Therapy, 15*(1), 29-42.

Gwirtsman, H.E., Kaye, W.H., Obarzanek, E., George, D.T., Jimerson, D.C., & Ebert, M.H. (1989). Decreased caloric intake in normal-weight patients with bulimia: Comparison with female volunteers. *American Journal of Clinical Nutrition, 49*, 86-92.

Hall, A., & Brown L.B. (1983). A comparison of the attitudes of young anorexia nervosa patients and nonpatients with those of their mothers. *British Journal of Medical Psychology, 56*, 39-48.

Hall, R.C.W., Tice, L., Beresford, T. P., Wooley, B., & Hall, A. K. (1989). Sexual abuse in patients with anorexia nervosa and bulimia. *Psychosomatics, 30*, 73-79.

Halmi, K., Goldberg, S., & Casper, R. (1979). Pretreatment predictors of outcome in anorexia nervosa. *British Journal of. Psychiatry, 134*, 71-78.

Hammer, L.D. (1993). Child and adolescent obesity. In R. Behrman (Ed.), *Nelson textbook of pediatrics* (pp. 1-11). New York: W. B. Saunders Co.

Heilbrun, A.B. jr., & Flodin, A. (1989). Food cues and peceptual distortion of the female body: Implications for food avoidance in the early dynamics of anorexia nervosa. *Journal of Clinical Psychology, 45*(6), 843-851.

Heilbrun, A.B. jr & Worobow, A.L. (1990). Attention and disordered eating behavior: II. Disattention to turbulent inner sensations as a risk factor in the development of anorexia nervosa. *Psychological Reports, 66*, 467-478.

Herman, J. Perry, C., & van der Kolk, B. (1989). Childhood trauma in borderline personality disorder. *American Journal of Psychiatry, 146*, 490-495.

Heunemann, R., Shapiro, L., Hampton, M., & Mitchell, B. (1966). A longitudal study of gross body compositions and body conformation and their association with food and activity in a teenage population. *American Journal of Clinical Nutrition, 18*, 325-338.

Hill, A., Weaver, C., & Blundell, J. (1990). Dieting concerns of 10-year-old girls and their mothers. *British Journal of Clinical Psychology, 29*, 346-348.

Hooper, M.S.H., & Garner, D.M. (1986). Application of the eating disorders inventory to a sample of black, white and mixed race school girls in Zimbabwe. *International Journal of Eating Disorders, 5*(1), 161- 165.

Hsu, L.K. (1987). Are the eating disorders becoming more common in blacks? *International Journal of Eating Disorders, 6*, 113-124.

Hsu, L.G. (1989). The gender gap in eating disorders: Why are the eating disorders more common among women? *Clinical Psychology Review, 9*(3), 393-407.

Hudson, J., Pope, H., Jonas, J., Yurgelun-Todd, D., & Frankenburg, F. (1987). A controlled family history study of bulimia. *Psychological Medicine, 17*, 883-890.

Humphrey, L. L. (1988). Relationships within subtypes of anorexic, bulimic, and normal families. *Journal of the American Academy of Child and Adolescent Psychiatry, 27*(5), 544-551.

Humphrey, L. L. (1989). Observed family interactions among subtypes of eating disorders using structural analysis of social behavior. *Journal of Consulting and Clinical Psychology, 57* (2), 206-214.

Jimerson, D.C., Lesem, M.D., Kaye, W.H., Hegg, A.P., & Brewerton, T.D. (1990). Eating disorders and depression: Is there a serotonin connection? *Biological Psychiatry, 28* (5), 443-454.

Johnson, R., & Larson, C. (1982). Bulimia: An analysis of moods and behavior. *Psychomatic Medicine, 44,* 341-351.

Kalucy, R.S., Crisp, A.H., & Harding, B. (1977). A study of 56 families with anorexia nervosa. *British Journal of Medical Psychology, 50,* 381-395.

Kaye, W.H., Ebert, M.H., Raleigh, M., & Lake, C.R. (1984). Abnormalities in CNS monoamine metabolism in anorexia nervosa. *Archives of General Psychiatry, 41,* 350-355.

Kaye, W.H., Gwirtsman, H.E., George, D.T., Jimerson, D.C., Ebert, M.H., & Lake, C.R. (1990). Disturbances in noradrenergic systems in normal weight bulimia: Relationship to diet and menses. *Biology Psychiatry, 27* (1), 4-21.

Kaye, W.H., Gwirtsman, H.E., Obarzanek, E., George, T., Jimerson, D.C., & Ebert, M.H. (1986). Caloric intake necessary for weight maintainance in anorexia nervosa: Nonbulimics require greater intake than bulimics. *American Journal of Clinical Nutrition, 44,* 435-443.

Kendler, K., Maclean, C., Neale, M., Kessler, R., Heath, A., & Eaves, L. (1991). The genetic epidemiology of bulimia nervosa. *American Journal of Psychiatry, 148,* 1627-1637.

Keys, A., Brozek, J., Henschel, A., Mickelsen, O., & Taylor, H.L. (1950). *The biology of human starvation* (Vol. 1). Minneapolis: University of Minnesota Press.

Killen, J.D., Hayward, C., Litt, I., Hammer, L.D., Wilson, D.M., Miner, B., Taylor, B, Varady, A, & Shisslak, C. (1992). Is puberty a risk factor for eating disorders? *American Journal of Diseases of Children, 146,* 323-325.

Killen, J.D., Taylor, C.B., Telch, M.J., Saylor, K.E., Maron, D.J., & Robinson, T.N. (1986). Self-induced vomiting and laxative and diuretic use among teenagers: Precursors of the binge-purge syndrome? *Journal of the American Medical Association, 255*(11), 1447-1449.

Kope, T., & Sack, W. (1987). Anorexia nervosa in South East Asian refugees: A report of 3 cases. *Journal of the American Academy of Child and Adolescent Psychiatry, 26,* 795-797.

Krieger, D., & Hughes, J. eds. (1980). *Neuroendrocrinology.* Sunderland, Mass: Sinauer Associated.

Lacey, H., & Dolan, B. (1988). Bulimia in British blacks and Asians. *British Journal of Psychiatry, 152,* 73-79.

Laue, L., Gold,P.W., Richmond, A., & Chrousos, G.P.(1991). The hypothalamic-pituitary-adrenal axis in anorexia nervosa and bulimia nervosa: Pathophysiologic implications. *Advances in Pediatrics, 38,* 287-316.

Lawlor, B., & Rand, C. (1985). Bulimia nervosa in a black woman. *American Journal of Psychiatry, 142,* 12.

Leon, G.R., Fulkerson, J.A., Perry, C.L., & Cudeck, R. (1992). Personality and behavioral vulnerabilities associated with risk status for eating disorders in adolescent girls. *Journal of Abnormal Psychology, 102*(3), 438-444.

Leon, G.R., Perry, C.L., Mangelsdorf, C., & Tell, G.J. (1989). Adolescent nutritional and psychological patterns and risk for the development of an eating disorder. *Journal of Youth and Adolescence, 18*(3), 273- 282.

Levine, M., Smolak, L., Moodey, A., Shuman, M., & Hessen, L. (1994). Normative developmental challenges and dieting and eating disturbances in middle school girls. *International Journal of Eating Disorders, 15*(1), 11-20.

Luby, J., & Steiner, H. (1993). Concordance between Parent/Child Temperamental Assessment in a clinical adolescent population. *Child Psychiatry & Human Development, 23*(4), 297-305.

Lucas, A. R., Beard, M., O'Fallon, W. M., & Kurland, L. T. (1991). 50-year trends in the incidence of anorexia nervosa in Rochester, Minn.: A population-based study. *American Journal of Psychiatry, 148*(7), 917-922.

Maloney, J.J., & Ruedisueli, G., (1993). The epidemiology of eating problems in nonreferred children and adolescents. *Child and Adolescent Psychiatric Clinics of North America, 2*(1), 1-13.

Maloney, M.J., McGuire, J., Daniels, S.R., & Specker, B. (1989). Dieting behavior and eating attitudes in children. *Pediatrics, 84*(3), 482-489.

Marchi, M., & Cohen, P. (1989). Early childhood eating behaviors and adolescent eating disorders. *Journal of the American Academy of Child and Adolescent Psychiatry, 29* (1), 112-117.

McKenna, M. (1989). Assessment of the eating disordered patient. *Psychiatric Annals, 19,* 467-472.

McNamara, K.& Loveman, C. (1990). Differences in family functioning among bulimics, repeat dieters, and nondieters. *Journal of Clinical Psychology, 46*(4), 518-523.
Minuchin, S., Rosman, B.L., & Baker, L. (1978). *Psychosomatic families*. Cambridge, Mass.: Harvard.
Morgan, H.G., & Russell, G. (1975). Value of family background and clinical features as predictors of long-term outcome in anorexia nervosa: Four-year follow-up study of 41 patients. *Psychological Medicine, 5*, 355-371.
Morrison, J. (1989). Childhood sexual histories in women with somatization disorder. *American Journal of Psychiatry, 146*, 239-241.
Mumford, D., & Whitehouse, A. (1988). Increased prevalence of bulimia nervosa among Asian schoolgirls. *British Medical Journal, 297*, 718.
Nasser, M. (1986). Comparative study of the prevalence of abnormal eating attitudes among Arab female students in both London and Cairo universities. *Psychological Medicine, 16*, 621-625
Neki, J. (1973). Psychiatry in South East Asia. *British Journal of Psychiatry, 123*, 257-269.
Norris, D. (1979). Clinical diagnostic criteria for primary anorexia nervosa. *South African Medical Journal, 56*, 987-993.
Nwaefuna, A. (1981). Anorexia nervosa in a developing country. *British Journal of Psychiatry, 138*, 270-271.
Okasha, A., Karmel, M., Sadek, A., Lotaif, F., & Bishry, Z. (1977). Psychiatric morbidity among university students in Egypt. *British Journal of Psychiatry, 131*, 149-154.
Ong, Y. Tsoi, W., & Cheah, J. (1982). A clinical and psychosocial study of seven cases of anorexia nervosa in Singapore. *Singapore Medical Journal 23*, 255-261.
Orbach, S. (1978). *Fat is a feminist issue*. London: Paddington Press.
Palla, B & Litt, I.F. (1988). Medical complications of eating disorders in adolescence. *Pediatrics, 81*, 613-623.
Palmer, R., Oppenheimer, R., Dignon, A., Chaloner, D., & Howells, K. (1990). Childhood sexual experiences with adults reported by women with eating disorders: An extended series. *British Journal of Psychiatry, 156*, 699-703.
Pate, J., Pumariega, A., Hester, C., & Garner, D. (1992). Cross-cultural patterns in eating disorders: A review. *Journal of the American Academy of Child and Adolescent Psychiatry, 31*, 802-809.
Patton, G. (1992). Eating disorders: Antecedents, evolution and course. *Annals of Medicine, 24*, 281-285.
Peveler, R., Fairburn, C., Boller, I., & Dunger, D. (1992). Eating disorders in adolescents with IDDM. A controlled study. *Diabetes Care, 15*(10), 1356-1360.
Phillipp, E., Pirke, K.M., Kellner, M.B.., & Krieg, J.C. (1991). Disturbed cholecystokinin secretion in patients with eating disorders. *Life Sciences, 48*(25), 2443-2450.
Pike, K. M., & Rodin, J. (1991). Mothers, daughters, and disordered eating. *Journal of Abnormal Psychology, 100* (2), 198-204.
Pitts, C., & Waller, G. (1993). Self-denigratory beliefs following sexual abuse: Association with thesymptomatology of bulimic disorders. *International Journal of Eating Disorders, 13*(4), 407-410.
Powers, P. (1980). *Obesity: the regulation of weight*. Baltimore: William.
Prince, R. (1985). The concept of culture-bound syndromes: Anorexia nervosa and brain-fag. *Social Sciences in Medicine, 21*(2), 193-203.
Pumariega, A.J., Edwards, P., & Mitchell, C.B. (1984). Anorexia nervosa in black adolescents. *Journal of the American Academy of Child and Adolescent Psychiatry, 23*, 111-114.
Pumariega, A.J. (1986). Acculturation and eating attitudes in adolescent girls: A comparitive and correlational study. *Journal of the American Academy of Child and Adolescent Psychiatry, 25*(2), 276-279.
Radke-Sharpe, N., Whitney-Saltiel, D., & Rodin, J. (1990) Fat distribution as a risk factor for weight and eating concerns. *International Journal of Eating Disorders, 9*(1), 27-36.
Råstam, M., & Gillberg, C. (1991). The family background in anorexia nervosa: A population-based study. *Journal of the American Academy of Child and Adolescent Psychiatry, 30*(2), 283-289.
Råstam, R. (1992). Anorexia nervosa in 51 Swedish adolescents: Premorbid problems and and comorbidity. *Journal of the American Academy of Child and Adolescent Psychiatry, 31*(5), 819-829.
Richards, M., Regina, C., & Larson, R. (1990). Weight and eating concerns among pre- and young adolescent boys and girls. *Journal of Adolescent Health Care, 11*, 203-209.
Robinson, P., & Anderson, A. (1985). Anorexia nervosa in American blacks. *Journal of Psychiatric Research, 19*, 183-188.

Root, M. P. P., & Fallon, P. (1988). The incidence of victimization experiences in bulimic sample. *Journal of Interpersonal Violence, 3,* 161-173.

Rorty, M., Yager, J., & Rossotto, E. (1994). Childhood sexual, physical, and psychological abuse in bulimia nervosa. *American Journal of Psychiatry, 151,* 1122-1126.

Rosen, L.W., Shafer, C., Dummer, G., Cross, L., Deuman, G., & Malmberg, S. (1988). Prevalence of pathogenic weight-control behaviors among Native American women and girls. *International Journal of Eating Disorders, 7*(6), 807-811.

Rudofsky, B. (1972). *The unfashionable human body.* New York: Doubleday.

Russell, D. (1986). *The secret trauma: Incest in the lives of girls and women.* New York: Basic Books.

Rutherford, J., McGuffin, P., Katz, R.J., & Murray, R. M., (1993). Genetic influences on eating attitudes in a normal female twin population. *Psychological Medicine, 23,* 425-436.

Seid, R. P. (1994). Too "close to the bone": The historical context for women's obsession with slenderness. In P. Fallon, M. S. Katzman, & S. C. Wooley (Eds.), *Feminist perspectives on eating disorders* (3-16). New York: Guilford Press.

Selvini-Palazzoli, M.P. (1974). *Self-starvation: From individual to family therapy in the treatment of anorexia nervosa.* New York: Jason Aronson.

Shaw, R. , Lee, Y., & Steiner, H. (1994). *Temperamental dimensions in adolescent psychiatric patients.* Submitted for publication.

Silber, T. (1984). Anorexia nervosa in black adolescents. *Journal of the National Medical Association, 76,* 29- 32.

Smith, C., Feldman, S., Nasserbakht, A., & Steiner, H. (1993). Psychological characteristics and DSM-III-R diagnoses at 6-year follow-up of adolescent anorexia nervosa. *Journal of the American Academy of Child and Adolescent Psychiatry, 32*(6), 1237-1245.

Smith, C., & Steiner, H. (1992). Psychopathology in anorexia nervosa and depression. *Journal of the American Academy of Child and Adolescent Psychiatry, 31*(5), 841-843.

Steiger, H., Leung, F., & Houle, L. (1992). Relationships among borderline features, body dissatisfaction and bulimic symptoms in nonclinical families. *Addictive Behaviors, 17*(4), 397-406.

Steiner, H. (1990). Defense styles in eating disorders. *International Journal of Eating Disorders, 9,* 141-151.

Steiner, H., Smith, C., Rosenkrantz, R., & Litt, I.F. (1990a). The early care and feeding of anorexics. *Child Psychiatry and Human Development, 21,* 163-167.

Steiner, H., Rahimzadeh, P., & Lewiston, N. (1990b). Psychopathology in Cystic Fibrosis and anorexia nervosa: A controlled comparison. *International Journal of Eating Disorders, 9,* 675-683.

Steiner, H., Wilber, J.F., Prasad, C., Rogers, D., & Rosenkranz, R.T., (1989). Histidyl Proline Diketopiperazine (Cyclo [His-Pro]) in Eating Disorders. *Neuropeptides, 14,* 185-189.

Steiner-Adair, C. (1986). The body politic: Normal female adolescent development and the development of eating disorders. *Journal of the American Academy of Psychoanalysis, 14*(1), 95-114.

Striegel-Moore, R., Nicholson, T., & Tamborlane, W. (1992). Prevalence of eating disorder symptoms in preadolescent and adolescent girls with IDDM. *Diabetes Care, 15*(10), 1361-1368.

Strober, M. (1980) Personality and symptomatological features in young, nonchronic anorexia nervosa patients.*Journal of Psychosomatic Research, 24,* 353-359.

Strober, M. (1990). Family-genetic studies of eating disorders. *Journal of Clinical Psychiatry, 52*(10), 9-12.

Strober, M. (1991). Disorders of the self in anorexia nervosa: An organismic-developmental paradigm. In: C. Johnson (Ed.). *Psychodynamic treatment of anorexia nervosa and bulimia* (pp. 354-373). New York: Guilford Press.

Strober, M., & Katz, J.L.(1988). Depression in the eating disorders: A review and analysis of descriptive, family, and biological findings. In D. M. Garner & P. E. Garfinkel (Eds.). *Diagnostic issues in anorexia nervosa and bulimia nervosa* (pp. 80-111). New York: Brunner/Mazel.

Strober, M., Morrell, W., Burroughs, J., Salkin, B., & Jacobs, C. (1985). A controlled family study of anorexia nervosa. *Journal of Psychiatric Research, 19* (2,3), 239-246.

Strober, M., Salkin, B., Burroughs, J., & Morrell, W. (1982). Parental personality characteristics and family psychiatric morbidity. *Journal of Nervous and Mental Diseases, 170*(6), 345-351.

Strober, M., & Yager, J. (1985). A developmental perspective on the treatment of anorexia nervosa in adolescents. In D. M. Garner & P. E. Garfinkel (Eds.). *Anorexia nervosa and bulimia*. New York: Guilford Press.

Theander, S. (1970). Anorexia nervosa, a psychiatric investigation of 94 female patients. *Acta Psychiatrica Scandinivia,* [suppl]*214*, 1-194.

Thienemann, M., & Steiner, H. (1991). Family environment of eating disordered and depressed adolescents. *International Journal of Eating Disorders, 10*(6). 673-676.

Thornton, B. (1991). Gender role typing, the superwoman ideal, and the potential for eating disorders. *Sex Roles, 25*(7,8), 57-62.

Vande Wiele, R.L. (1980). Anorexia Nervosa and the hypothalmus. In D. Krieger & J. C. Hughes (Eds.). *Neuroendocrinology.* Sunderland, Mass: Sinauer Associates.

Vigersky, R.A.(ed).(1977) *Anorexia nervosa*. New York: Raven.

Waller, G. (1991). Sexual abuse as a factor in eating disorders. *British Journal of Psychiatry, 159,* 664-671.

Walters, E., Neale, M.C., Eaves, L.J., Heath, A.C., Kessler, R.C., & Kendler, K.S. (1992). Bulimia nervosa and major depression: A study of common genetic and environmental factors. *Psychological Medicine,* 22, 617-622.

Weissman, M.M., Fendrich, M., Warner, V. NAD, & Wickramaratne, P. (1992). Incidence of psychiatric disorder in offspring at high and low risk for depression. *Journal of the American Academy of Child and Adolescent Psychiatry, 31,* 640-648.

Weltzin, T.E., Fernstrom, M.H., Hansen, D., McConaha, C.& Kaye, W.H. (1991). Abnormal caloric requirements for weight maintenance in patients with anorexia and bulimia nervosa. *American Journal of Psychiatry, 148* (12), 1675-1682.

Worsley, A. (1981). In the eye of the beholder: social and personal characteristics of teenagers and their impressions of themselves and fat and slim people. *British Journal of Medical Psychology, 54,* 231-242.

Yager, J. (1982). Family issues in the pathogenesis of anorexia nervosa. *Psychosomatic Medicine, 44*(1), 43-60.

# Anorexia Nervosa and Depression: Results of a Longitudinal Study

*Beate Herpertz-Dahlmann and Helmut Remschmidt*

## 1 Introduction

In recent years investigators of eating disorders have given considerable attention to the co-occurrence of eating disorders and other psychiatric conditions. In anorexia nervosa affective and anxiety disorders have been the most frequently associated forms of psychiatric disturbances (Cantwell, Sturzenberger, Burroughs, Salkin, & Green, 1977; Altshuler & Weiner, 1985; Brewerton, Lydiard, Ballenger, & Herzog, 1993).

Several findings seem to suggest a relation between eating disorders and depression. Depressive symptoms have been frequently found in anorexia and bulimia nervosa (Strober & Katz, 1988). There is a high prevalence of mood disorders in families with an anorectic member (Strober, Lampert, Morrell, Burroughs, & Jacobs, 1990). Other observations have suggested the presence of biological markers for depression in eating disorders, for example, nonsuppression in the Dexamethasone Suppression Test (Herpertz-Dahlmann & Remschmidt, 1990), and last but not least, some reports have described mutual benefits from antidepressant medication (for a review see Kennedy & Shapiro, 1993).

One of the investigative approaches used to clarify whether the relation between eating and affective disorder are causative or chance is to study the course and outcome of the eating disorder. The following chapter reviews recent findings on the links between anorexia nervosa and depression during a long-term follow-up of adolescent anorectic patients. The aim of our study was to answer the following questions: Does depression parallel the ongoing course of the eating disorder or is it an independent phenomenon? Are depressive disorders more likely to develop in chronically ill patients, or do they also persist in subjects who recovered from their eating disorder? Does depression have predictive value that is prominent at the beginning of treatment for the later outcome of anorexia nervosa?

We chose a prospective study design that enabled us to examine depressive symptoms during acute presentation of anorexia nervosa and at follow-up. In comparison to most previous outcome studies we used the same diagnostic criteria at admission and follow-up and standardized psychometric instruments to avoid a subjective rating of the patients' psychopathology.

## 2 Method

### 2.1 Sample

The original sample (T1) consisted of 39 consecutively admitted adolescent inpatients (32 girls and 7 boys) who met DSM-III-R criteria for anorexia nervosa. Patients with bulimia were excluded. The sample was followed up approximately at three years (T2) (3,3 ± 0,3; Min.: 2,2; Max.: 4,3 years) and seven years (T3) (7,1 ± 0,5; Min.: 5,5; Max: 8,3 years) after discharge. All patients could be traced. Five patients (12%) refused to participate in the follow-up investigations, but for four of them reliable data could be obtained from their parents or therapists. The remaining 34 subjects could be assessed by personal interviews with no further drop-out at the second follow-up. The non-participants were compared to the cooperating subjects on all presentation variables (Fisher-test, *t*-test). No significant difference was found (Herpertz-Dahlmann, 1993). The main demographic and clinical features of the 34 personally assessed patients at the times of admission and follow-up are given in Table 1.

### 2.2 Procedure

Data were obtained from several assessment procedures: a) a structured psychiatric interview was used to assess mood disorder symptoms and specific eating disorder psychopathology, including DSM-III-R categories of major depression and eating disorders at admission and follow-up. At follow-up the interview also covered the Morgan-Hayward modification (Morgan & Hayward, 1988) of the Morgan-Russell-Assessment-Schedule (Morgan & Russell, 1975) to define the average

Table 1. Clinical Features of 34 Inpatients with Anorexia Nervosa (Personally Assessed Group)

|  | Admission | 3-Year Follow-up | 7-Year Follow-up |
|---|---|---|---|
| Age (years) |  |  |  |
| Mean | 16.2 (± 2.0) | 20.0 (± 2.0) | 23.7 (± 2.0) |
| Range | 10.3 - 20.9 | 13.7 - 24.7 | 17.7 - 28.6 |
| Onset of disease (years) |  |  |  |
| Mean | 14.9 (± 1.6) | — | — |
| Range | 9.4 -17.8 |  |  |
| Duration of illness prior to admission (years) |  |  |  |
| Mean | 1.4 (± 1.4) | — | — |
| Range | 0.2 - 8.4 |  |  |
| Duration of amenorrhea prior to admission (years) |  |  |  |
| Mean | 1.23 (± 1.5) | — | — |
| Range | 0.02[1] - 7.5 |  |  |
| Previous hospitalizations for anorexia nervosa |  |  |  |
| Number of patients | 20 (58.9%) | — | — |
| Length of inpatient treatment upon initial assessment (months) |  |  |  |
| Mean | 5.7 (± 3.8) | — | — |
| Range | 0.5 - 19.4 |  |  |
| Body mass index |  |  |  |
| Mean | 14.5 (± 1.6) | 19.2 (± 2.6) | 20.5 (± 2.9) |
| Range | 11.7 - 17.5 | 14.5 - 25.2 | 15.4 - 28.9 |
| Eating behavior |  |  |  |
| Vomiting, $n$ (%) | 4 (11.8%) | 4 (11.8%) | 4 (11.8%) |
| Purging | 6 (17.6%) | 4 (11.8%) | 3 ( 8.8%) |
| Binging[2] | 3 ( 8.8%) | 6 (17.6%) | 4 (11.8%) |
| Amenorrhea (females) | 29 (100%) | 11 (37.9%) | 4 (13.8%) |
| Length of follow-up period since onset of disease (years) | — | 5.0 (± 1.4) 3.7 - 12.2 | 8.9 (± 1.5) 7.5 - 16.1 |

[1] One patient became amenorrheal shortly after admission.
[2] At admission, frequency of binging was less than twice a week for three months.

outcome score (food intake, menstrual state, mental state, psychosexual state, socioeconomic state); b) an interview measure for depression (Hamilton Depression Rating Scale, HRSD, interview version, Williams, 1988); c) a self-report questionnaire for depression (Zung Scale, ZDS, Zung, 1972); d) at the

7-year follow-up, psychiatric comorbidity was examined by the Composite International Diagnostic Interview (CIDI) (WHO 1990) based on the Diagnostic Interview Schedule (Robins, Helzer, Groughon, & Ratcliff, 1981), from which lifetime and current diagnoses may be derived according to DSM-III-R and ICD-10. Any diagnoses during the previous 6 months were defined as current disorders.

## 3 Findings

### 3.1 Description and Analysis of Depressive Psychopathology in Anorectic Patients During Acute Presentation

It is well known that a wide range of depressive symptoms like depressive mood, emotional emptiness, social withdrawal, loss of libido, and low self-esteem are prominent in malnourished anorectic patients (Herpertz-Dahlmann, 1992; Strober & Katz, 1988). To assess depression in our sample during inpatient treatment we administered the Hamilton (Hamilton, 1960) and the Zung scale (Zung, 1972) three times: at admission, after weight gain (10-15% of the ideal body weight), and shortly before discharge when the patients had reached target weight.

At admission our patients displayed mild to moderate levels of depression on both the Hamilton and the Zung Scale. Parallel to weight gain we found a highly significant decrease of depressive symptoms (Figure 1).

These results are in accordance with those found by other authors. In comparison to patients with a primary affective disorder (e.g. major depressive disorder according to DSM-III-R criteria) patients with anorexia nervosa have significantly lower depression scores. This was confirmed by different psychometric instruments, for example, the Schedule for Affective Disorders and Schizophrenia, the Beck Depression Inventory, and the Hopkins Symptom Checklist (Herzog, 1984; Piran, Kennedy, Garfinkel, & Owens, 1985; Eckert, Goldberg, Halmi, Casper, & Davis, 1982). The depressive symptomatology in anorexia nervosa compared to genuine depression also seems to be different (Piran et al., 1985). Eating disorder patients describe less fatigue, less early awakening, and less retardation than patients with a genuine mood disorder. Eckert et al., (1982) demonstrated that the more depressed anorectic patients had more abnormal eating characteristics. They also found a reduction of depressive symptoms over treatment time.

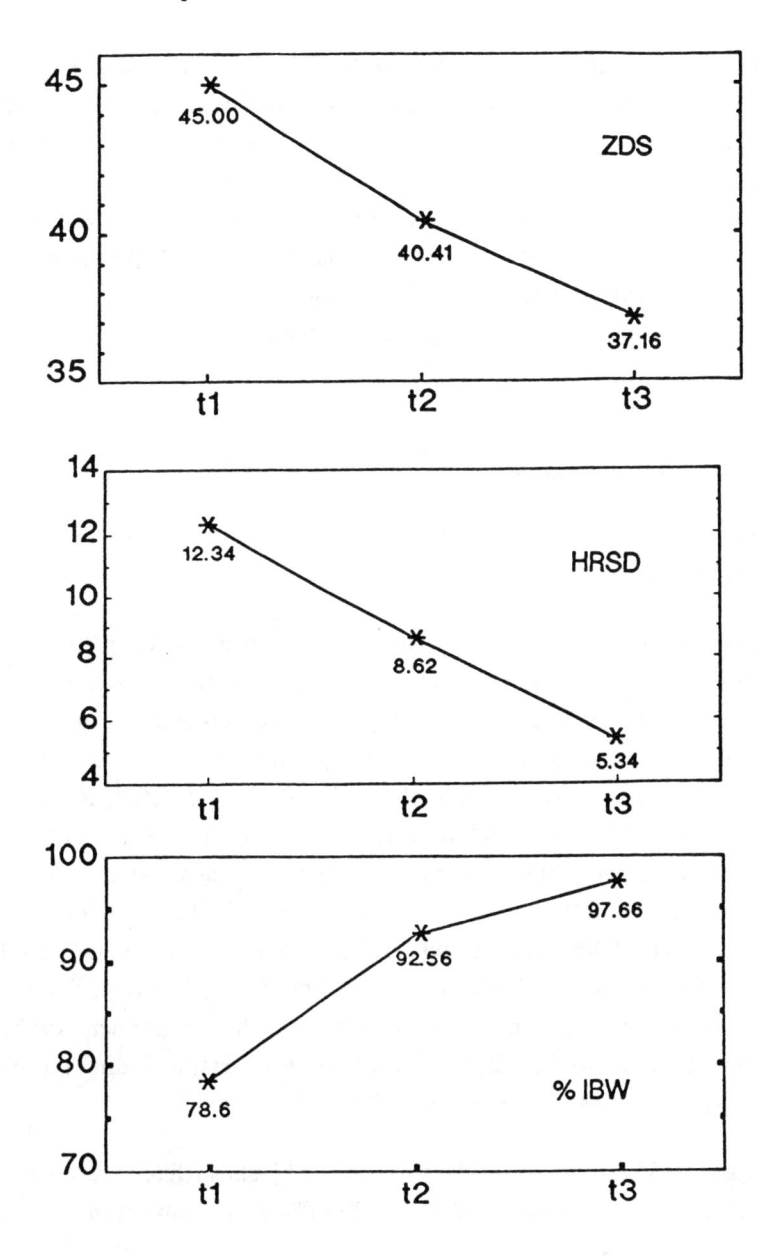

Figure 1. Depression scores and weight increase at three times (t1, t2, t3) during inpatient treatment. ZDS = Zung scale; HRSD = Hamilton scale; % IBW = % of ideal body weight

At admission 53% of our sample fulfilled DSM-III-R criteria for major depression. It is well known that the starvation process itself can provoke depressive reactions even in healthy, fasting subjects. Keys et al. (1950) were one of the first to note mental changes during semistarvation like emotional irritability, loss of libido, anhedonia, and difficulties in making decisions. For this reason, the discrimination of real depressive disorder and affective disturbances secondary to malnutrition in anorexic patients with severe weight loss might be impossible, which is an important aspect when discussing the predictive value of depression in one of the following sections.

## 3.2 Depression at Follow-up

### 3.2.1 Comorbidity of Affective Disorders in Anorexia Nervosa at Follow-up

Outcome studies reveal various psychiatric features in anorectic patients in later periods of life, apart from or in addition to the eating disorder. The most prevalent psychiatric disorders are anxiety (including obsessive compulsive disorder) and affective disorders. Depressive symptoms are prominent in 20% to 40% of the patients at follow-up (Morgan & Russell, 1975; Willi, Limacher, & Nussbaum, 1989; Remschmidt, Wienand, & Wewetzer, 1990). Unfortunately, very few of the outcome studies in anorexia nervosa have used defined criteria to classify diagnostic categories at follow-up; to our knowledge only five applied the DSM-III or DSM-III-R criteria (Hall, Slim, Hawker, & Salmond, 1984; Toner, Garfinkel, & Garner, 1986; Rosenvinge & Mouland, 1990; Halmi, Eckert, Marchi, Sampugnaro, Apple, & Cohen, 1991; Smith, Feldman, Nasserbakht, & Steiner, 1993). The observed prevalence rates of anxiety and affective disorders, including those of our 7-year follow-up investigation, are given in Table 2.

Hence, about 30-45% of the formerly anorectic subjects suffered from some kind of anxiety disorder at follow-up and about 20-40% from some form of affective disorder.

Certainly, it is advised to be cautious about comparing the results of the above-mentioned studies. There is a considerable range in age of the followed-up subjects, for example, the mean age of the sample by Rosenvinge and Mouland is significantly higher than that of the other outcome studies. The incidence of

Table 2. Prevalence Rates of Anxiety and Affective Disorder in Long-Term Outcome of Anorexia Nervosa

| Study | Number of patients | Mean age at follow-up (years) | Mean duration of follow-up (years) | Criteria | Anxiety disorders % | Affective disorders % |
|---|---|---|---|---|---|---|
| Hall et al., 1984 | 44 | 24 | 4 | DSM-III | not reported | 45.5 |
| Toner et al., 1986 | 55 | 28.2 | (5-14) | DSM-III | 47.4 | 33.5 |
| Rosenvinge & Mouland, 1990 | 30 | 38.9 | 14.4 | DSM-III | not reported | 23 |
| Halmi et al., 1991 | 62 | 29 | 10 | DSM-III-R | 33.9 | 29 |
| Smith et al., 1993 | 23 | 22.1 | 6 | DSM-III-R | 43.5 | 30.4 |
| This study | 34 | 23.7 | 7 | DSM-III-R | 41 | 18* |

*In addition to the 18% prevalence rate of affective disorders, one patient suffered from a current depressive episode in schizo-affective disorder, and another patient from organic mental brain syndrome with depressed mood and hallucinations after a severe suicide attempt.

affective disorder increases with advancing age so that in most of these studies final conclusions about the long-term prevalence of depression in former anorectic patients would be premature. Nevertheless, the prevalence rate in anorexia nervosa is higher than what would be expected in the general population. In an epidemiological survey by Robins, Helzer, Weissman, Orvaschel, Gruenberg, Burke, & Regier (1984) the lifetime prevalence of major depression in 18 to 24-year old female subjects was reported to be 7,5% and in 25 to 44-year old subjects to be 10,4%.

### 3.2.2 Relation Between Outcome of the Eating Disorder and Depressive Symptoms

The results of Hall et al. (1984) and Rosenvinge and Mouland (1990) suggest that the presence of depressive disorder at follow-up is associated with a poor outcome of the eating disorder. In the study by Halmi et al. (1991) there was no significant difference in the lifetime prevalence of affective disorders in the patients who were diagnosed at a 10-year follow-up with an eating disorder compared to those who recovered. However, subjects with diagnosed eating disorders had more current depression than those without an eating disorder.

One of the aims of the present study was to examine whether the severity of current depressive symptoms at follow-up was related to the outcome of the eating disorder. At both the 3-year (Herpertz-Dahlmann & Remschmidt, 1993 a) and 7-year follow-up (Herpertz-Dahlmann, Wewetzer, & Remschmidt, in press) there was a consistent and significant association (Spearman $r$) between the degree of depression measured by the Zung and the Hamilton scale and the quality of clinical outcome measured by the average outcome score. For the ZDS the correlation coefficients were $r = -0,4$ ($p = 0,023$) at the 3-year follow-up and $r = -0,75$ ($p = 0,0001$) at the 7-year follow-up. The respective coefficients for the HRSD were $r = -0,67$ ($p = 0,0001$) at the 3-year follow-up and $r = -0,81$ ($p = 0,0001$) at the 7-year follow-up (Figure 2). In summary, the worse the outcome of the eating disorder, the more depressed were the patients.

Multiple regression analyses indicated that the average outcome score was a significant predictor of depression rated either by the patients themselves or their therapists (Table 3). For the self-report questionnaire (ZDS) Scale E (socioeconomic state) had the most important single-effect at the 3-year and 7-year

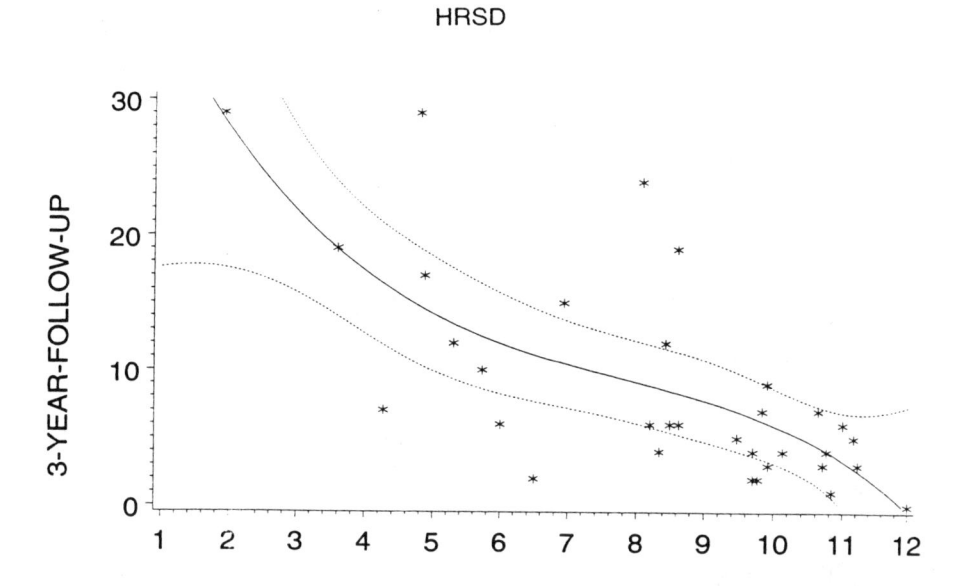

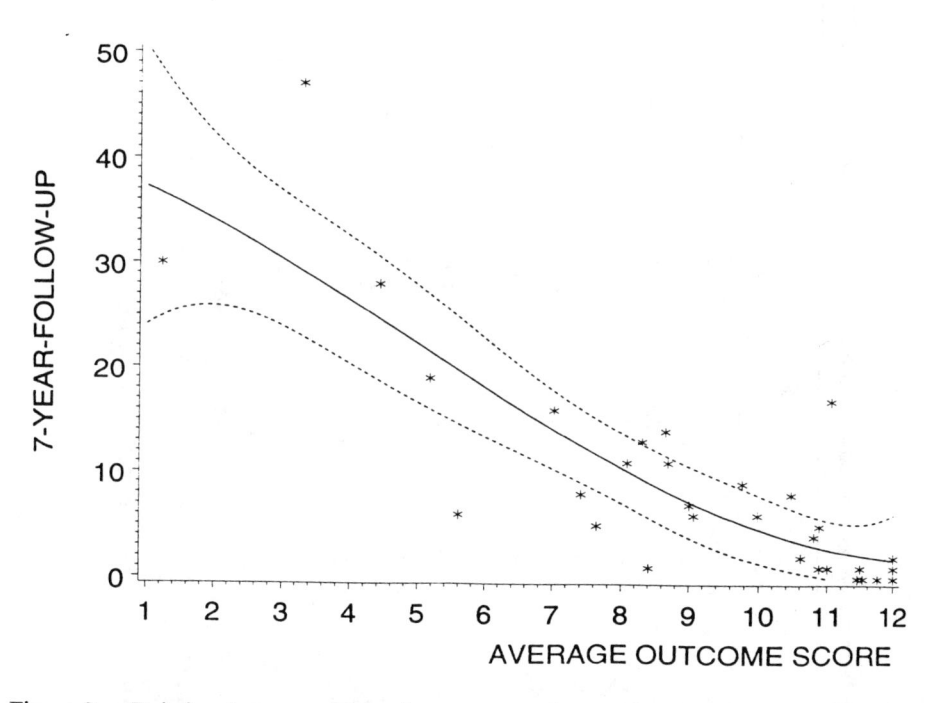

Figure 2. Relation between depression scores and average outcome score (Morgan & Hayward, 1988). HRSD= Hamilton scale

Table 3. Effects of Average Outcome Score Scales on Depression Scores (Multiple Regression) At 3-year And 7-year Follow-Up (N=34)

| | AOS-Scale[a] | Regression Coefficient ($\beta$) 3-year | 7-year | SD of $\beta$ 3-year | 7-year | $t$[b] 3-year | 7-year | $p$ 3-year | 7-year |
|---|---|---|---|---|---|---|---|---|---|
| ZDS | A | -0.35 | -0.56 | .48 | .62 | -0.73 | -0.88 | n.s. | n.s. |
| | C | -1.57 | -1.27 | .57 | .65 | 2.74 | -1.95 | ** | * |
| | D | 0.63 | 0.30 | .45 | .54 | 1.41 | 0.55 | n.s. | n.s. |
| | E | -1.56 | -2.08 | .74 | .81 | -2.10 | -2.55 | ** | ** |
| | $R^2$ | 0.52 | 0.63 | | | | | | |
| HRSD | A | -0.50 | 0.06 | .28 | .40 | -1.82 | 0.15 | * | n.s. |
| | C | -1.37 | -2.20 | .33 | .42 | -4.13 | -5.27 | **** | **** |
| | D | 0.13 | 0.40 | .26 | .34 | 0.52 | -1.16 | n.s. | n.s. |
| | E | -1.31 | -0.40 | .43 | .52 | -3.05 | -0.78 | *** | n.s. |
| | $R^2$ | 0.76 | 0.81 | | | | | | |

AOS = average outcome score; ZDS = Zung scale; HRSD = Hamilton scale; A = food intake; C = mental state; D = psychosexual state; E = socioeconomic state; $R^2$ = coefficient of multiple determination. *$p<0.05$ **$p<0.01$ ***$p<0.001$ ****$p<0.0001$.

Note: [a]In the regression model for the female subjects scale B (menstrual state) was a significant predictor only for the Zung scale at the 3-year follow up.
[b]For testing that the true coefficient is zero.

follow-up; for the clinician-rated scores (HRSD) this relationship was onlyapparent at the 3-year follow-up (the association between Scale C representing mental status and depression scores is a consequence of auto-correlation).

Thus, at least in the patients' view depression at follow-up was mostly related to "socioeconomic" dysfunction. According to Morgan and Hayward (1988), the socioeconomic status of the average outcome score comprises the relationship with the nuclear family and the individuation from the family as well as personal contacts, social activities, and employment record--in short, multiple aspects of social functioning. As now stated by our results, the poorer the social adaption of the patients the more depressed they feel. However, these results do not allow any statement about cause and effect in this interrelationship. Social dysfunctioning might just as well be a consequence of depression as poor social adaption might provoke depressive symptoms.

### 3.2.3 Depression in Anorectic Patients Compared to Healthy Controls

There are only very few studies that included a control group to draw a comparison between recovered and unrecovered anorectics in contrast to a healthy control group. In the follow-up study by Toner, Garfinkel, & Garner (1986) symptomatic anorectics displayed significantly higher levels of depression than improved anorectics and controls. In the Halmi et al. study (1991) significantly more former anorectic patients than controls had a current psychiatric diagnosis.

At the 3-year follow-up of our sample we compared the female patients to a control group matched for age, sex, and occupational status of subjects with no history of an eating disorder (Herpertz-Dahlmann & Remschmidt, 1993b). According to the general outcome by Morgan & Russell (1975), each subject was categorised in one of the three outcome groups: "good" (body weight within the range of 100 ± 15% of normal weight, regular menses), "intermediate" (weight not constantly sustained within 15% of average body weight and/or irregular menses) or "poor" outcome (low body weight causing concern in the patient or her attendants, absent or nearly absent menstruation).

According to the results of the HRSD, patients in the poor outcome group scored higher than those in the intermediate and good outcome group (Figure 3). Furthermore, patients with a good outcome had significantly higher depression scores than controls (overall differences by Brown-Mood Test, differences between subgroups by subsequent Median-Test, $p \leq 0.5$).

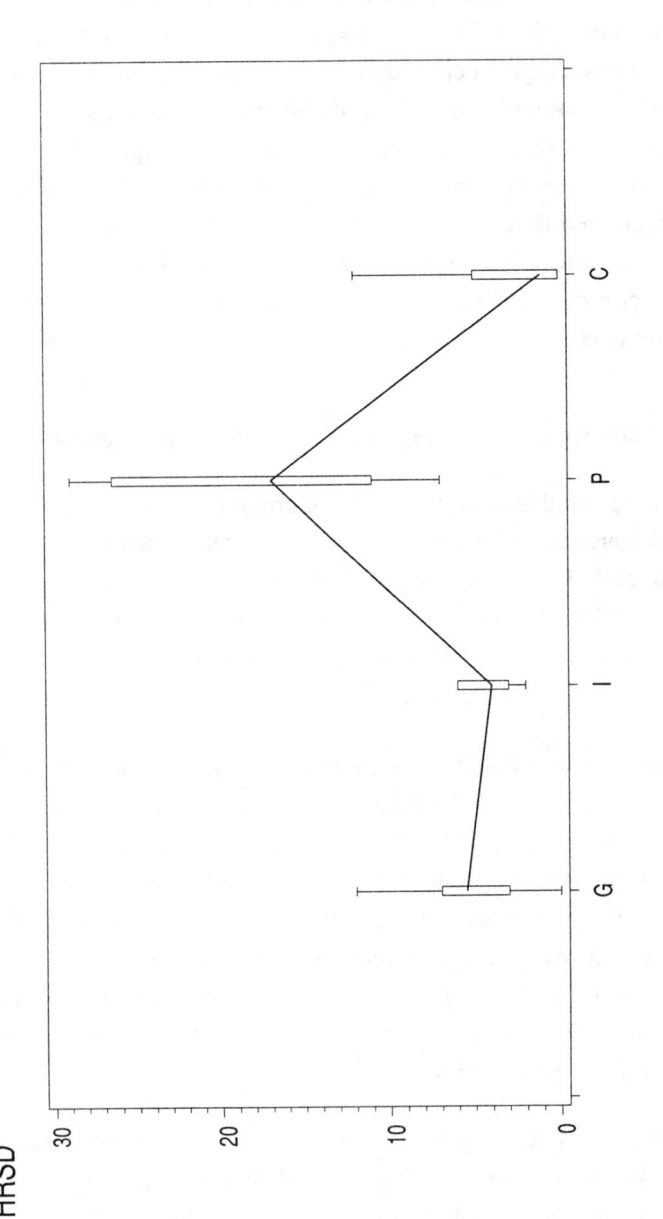

Figure 3. Differences between depression scores of patients with a good outcome (G), intermediate outcome (I), poor outcome (P) and controls (C) after three years of follow-up. HRSD = Hamilton scale

As already mentioned above, most follow-up studies describe higher levels of concomitant psychopathology in subjects who still have clinically relevant eating disorders compared to those who have recovered. A more striking observation is the difference between levels of depression in patients with a good outcome and in healthy controls, which might imply that depressive features belong to the "core personality disturbances" of at least some anorectic patients.

On the other hand, as Windauer, Lennerts, Talbot, Touyz, and Beumont (1993) point out, weight and menstrual functioning are probably insufficient criteria to define recovery of anorexia nervosa. Many of their patients with a so-called good outcome showed a wide range of the behavioural and attitudinal features of the eating disorder; nearly one third of their recovered sample also had marked to severe signs of depression measured by the Zung scale.

### 3.2.4 Psychosocial Functioning in Former Anorectic Patients Compared to Controls

Several studies have described poor social functioning in anorectic patients before the beginning of the illness and at follow-up (Burns & Crisp, 1984; Nussbaum, Shenker, Baird, & Saravay, 1985). To compare the patients' overall adjustment to those of healthy controls we tried to assess different psychopathological features that are associated with anorexia nervosa: nutritional habits, weight control methods, body perception, dependency on family, social contacts, partnership, psychosexual functioning, and educational or occupational adjustment.

Because of the small sample size, we combined the intermediate and poor outcome group to one group termed "unrecovered subjects". As shown in Figure 4, the unrecovered group had significantly worse scores in the eating disorder categories "nutrition" and "weight control methods" than the recovered and the control subjects. In the area "body perception" the unrecovered patients also scored lower, but the overall difference was no longer significant. Unrecovered patients, recovered patients, and healthy controls did not differ in the categories "dependency on family", "social contacts", and "occupational adjustment", but both the recovered and unrecovered former patients had significantly lower scores on psychosexual functioning than the controls.

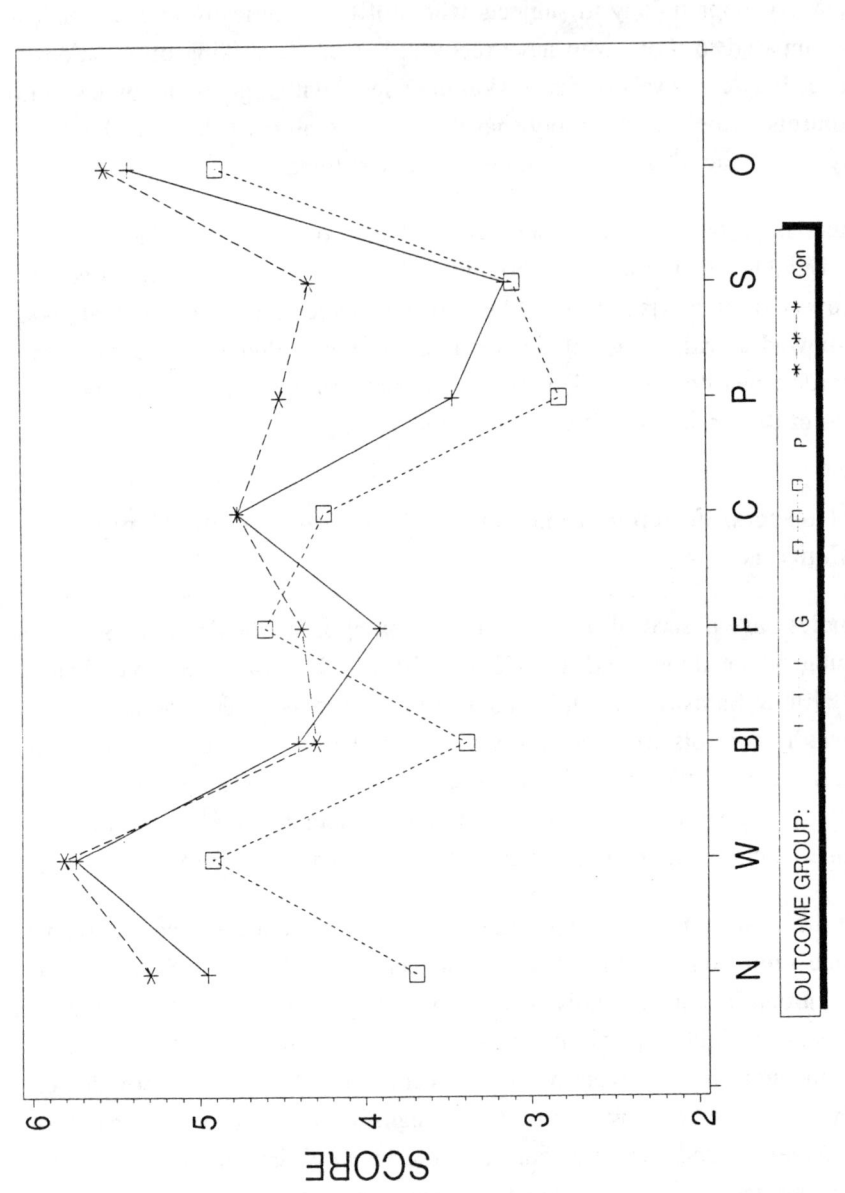

Figure 4. Differences between 2 outcome groups (female patients only, ≥18 years; G = good outcome group, n = 10; P = intermediate and poor outcome group, (n = 16) and controls (Con, n = 24) on parameters of disordered eating (N = nutrition, W = weight control methods, BI = body image) and of social functioning (F = dependency on family, C = social contacts, P = partnership, S = sexuality and O = occupational adjustment).

Persisting problems in the areas of heterosexual relationships and attitudes towards sexuality are well-known from other studies on adolescent anorexia nervosa (Steinhausen & Seidel, 1993; Windauer et al. 1993). Thirty-eight percent of the adolescent eating disordered sample of Steinhausen & Seidel (1993) showed a moderate to severe avoidance of active sexual behavior.

These observations support the notion that weight and menstrual functioning are not sufficient criteria for recovery in anorexia nervosa. As Steinhausen & Seidel (1993) point out, psychosocial functioning, including partnership and sexuality, are of great importance for assessing the course of the eating disorder and the wellness of the patients, although it has been neglected in research. It is also quite possible that continuing problems in heterosexual relationships add to feelings of low self-esteem and isolation that may reinforce depression.

## 3.2.5 Predictive Value of Depression

Because of the prospective character of our study, it was possible to assess the predictive value of depression during the acute presentation of the illness measured by HRSD and ZDS. We found no significant relationship between depression scores at admission and the outcome of the eating disorder defined by the average outcome score at the 3-year or 7-year follow-up (Table 4) (Herpertz-Dahlmann, Wewetzer, & Remschmidt, 1995).

Table 4. Correlations (Spearman $r$) between Average Outcome Score (AOS) and Zung (ZDS) and Hamilton (HRSD) Depression Scores

|  |  | AOS 3 years | AOS 7 years |
|---|---|---|---|
| ZDS | Admission | -0.03 n.s. | 0.03 n.s. |
|  | 3 years | -0.40 ** | -0.27 n.s. |
|  | 7 years |  | -0.75 *** |
| HRSD | Admission | -0.03 n.s. | 0.23 n.s. |
|  | 3 years | -0.67 *** | -0.45 *** |
|  | 7 years |  | -0.81 *** |

* $p < 0.05$; ** $p < 0.01$; *** $p < 0.001$

Thus, depression in the underweight anorectic had no predictive value for the outcome of the eating disorder. Other authors have already discussed the problems that arise in diagnosing depression in severely malnourished patients (Strober & Katz, 1988; Fichter & Pirke, 1990). Even in otherwise healthy subjects starvation-induced depressive psychopathology closely resembles DSM-III-R criteria of major depression, so that it is doubtful whether assessment of depression in anorectic patients with severe weight loss can have real significance. However, Spearman correlations calculated for the HRSD scores at the three year follow-up showed a significant association between the severity of depression three years after discharge and the outcome of the eating disorder after 7 years. Hence, beyond the period of acute malnutrition depressive symptomatology in anorectic seems to be more constant and, according to our results, of some prognostic importance for the outcome of the eating disorder.

## 4  Conclusions

The aim of the present investigation was to assess depression in the longitudinal course of adolescent anorexia nervosa by means of a prospective study design. Both at acute presentation and at follow-up, anorectic patients displayed a high prevalence of affective disorders, although there was a quantitative and qualitative difference in symptom phenomenology and severity compared to primary depression.

Depression on admission had no long-term predictive implications for the outcome of the eating disorder. In the underweight anorectic, starvation-induced depressive symptoms closely resemble DSM-III-R criteria of major depression so that the distinction between "true" depressive disorder and affective disturbances secondary to malnutrition may be impossible. Consequently, depression in acutely malnourished patients may not be a reliable prognostic indicator.

Beyond the period of acute malnutrition, symptoms of depression seem to be of more prognostic importance. Patients with depressive psychopathology after three years were likely to have a worse outcome of the eating disorder after seven years. Our results do not support the view that eating disorders are an alternative manifestation of affective disorders. Instead, there was a strong and consistent interrelation between the outcome of the eating disorder and concomitant depression. Patients with a chronic eating disorder displayed higher levels of depression than recovered patients. Thus, we might speculate that a successful treatment of the eating disorder also cures coexisting depressive symptoms.

## References

Altshuler, K.Z. & Weiner, M.F. (1985). Anorexia nervosa and depression: A dissenting view. *American Journal of Psychiatry*, 142, 328-332.
Brewerton, T.D., Lydiard, R.B., Ballenger, J.C., Herzog, D.B. (1993). Eating disorders and social phobia. *Archives of General Psychiatry*, 50(1), 70.
Burns, T. & Crisp, A.H. (1984). Outcome of anorexia nervosa in males. *British Journal of Psychiatry*, 145, 319-325.
Cantwell, D.P., Sturzenberger, S., Burroughs, J., Salkin, B., Green, J.K. (1977). Anorexia nervosa-an affective disorder? *Archives of General Psychiatry*, 34, 1087-1093.
Eckert, E.D., Goldberg, S.C., Halmi, K.A., Casper, R.C., Davis, J.M. (1982). Depression in anorexia nervosa. *Psychological Medicine*, 12, 115-122.
Fichter, M., Pirke, K.M. (1990). Psychobiology of human starvation. In H. Remschmidt, H., M.H. Schmidt (Eds.) *Anorexia Nervosa* (pp. 13-29). Toronto, Lewiston, New York, Bern, Göttingen, Stuttgart: Hogrefe & Huber Publishers.
Hall, A., Slim, E., Hawker, F., Salmond, C. (1984). Anorexia nervosa: Long-term outcome in 50 female patients. *British Journal of Psychiatry*, 145, 407-413.
Halmi, K.A., Eckert, E., Marchi, P., Sampugnaro, V., Apple, R., Cohen, J. (1991). Comorbidity of psychiatric diagnoses in anorexia nerovsa. *Archives of General Psychiatry*, 48, 712-718.
Hamilton, M. (1960). A rating scale of depression. *Journal of Neurology, Neurosurgery and Psychiatry*, 23, 56-62.
Herpertz-Dahlmann, B. (1992). Anorexia nervosa and depression. *Focus on Depression*, 3, 4-11.
Herpertz-Dahlmann, B. (1993). Eßstörungen und Depression in der Adoleszenz. In H. Remschmidt, A. Warnke (Eds.), *Beiträge zur Psychiatrie und Psychologie des Kindes- und Jugendalters*. Göttingen, Bern, Toronto, Seattle: Hogrefe.
Herpertz-Dahlmann, B. & Remschmidt, H. (1990). Anorexia nervosa and depression--a continuing debate. In: H. Remschmidt, M.H. Schmidt (Eds.): *Anorexia Nervosa* (pp. 69-84). Toronto Lewiston, New York, Bern, Göttingen, Stuttgart: Hogrefe & Huber Publishers.
Herpertz-Dahlmann, B. & Remschmidt, H. (1993a). Depression in anorexia nervosa at follow-up. *International Journal of Eating Disorders*, 14, 163-169.
Herpertz-Dahlmann, B. & Remschmidt, H. (1993b). Depression and psychosocial adjustment in adolescent anorexia nervosa. A controlled 3-year follow-up study. *European Child and Adolescent Psychiatry*, 2, 146-154.
Herpertz-Dahlmann, B., Wewetzer, Ch., Remschmidt, H. (1995).The predictive value of depression in anorexia nervosa. Results of a seven-year follow-up study. *Acta Psychiatrica Scandinavica*, 91, 114-119.
Herzog, D.B. (1984). Are anorexic and bulimic patients depressed? *American Journal of Psychiatry*, 141, 1594-1597.
Kennedy, S.H., Shapiro, C. (1993): *Medical management of the hospitalized patient*. In A.S. Kaplan, P.E. Garfinkel (Eds.), Medical Issues and the Eating Disorders (pp. 213-238). New York. Brunner/Mazel Publishers.
Keys, A., Brozek, J., Henschel, A., Mickelsen, O., Taylor, H.L. (1950). *The biology of human starvation*. University of Minneapolis Press: Minneapolis.
Morgan, H.G. & Hayward, A.E.(1988). Clinical assessment of anorexia nervosa--the Morgan-Russell outcome assessment schedule. *British Journal of Psychiatry*, 152, 367-371.
Morgan, H.G. & Russell, G.F.M. (1975) Value of family background and clinical features as predictors of long-term outcome in anorexia nervosa: Four-year follow-up study of 41 patients. *Psychological Medicine*, 5, 355-371.
Nussbaum, M., Shenker, R., Baird, D., Saravay, S. (1985). Follow-up investigation in patients with anorexia nervosa. *The Journal of Pediatrics*, 106, 835-840.
Piran, N., Kennedy, S., Garfinkel, P.E., Owens, M. (1985). Affective disturbance in eating disorders. *The Journal of Nervous and Mental Disease*, 173, 395-400.
Remschmidt, H., Wienand, F., Wewetzer, C. (1990). The Long-Term Course of Anorexia Nervosa. In H. Remschmidt, M.H. Schmidt (Eds.), *Anorexia Nervosa* (pp. 127-136). Toronto, Lewiston, New York, Bern, Göttingen, Stuttgart: Hogrefe & Huber Publishers.

Robins, L., Helzer, J., Groughon, I., Ratcliff, K. (1981). The NIMH diagnostic interview schedule: Its history, characteristics and validity. *Archives of General Psychiatry*, 38, 381-389.

Robins, L.N., Helzer, J.E., Weissman, M.M., Orvaschel, H., Gruenberg, E., Burke, J.D., Regier, D.A. (1984). Lifetime prevalence of specific psychiatric disorders in three sites. *Archives of General Psychology*, 41, 949-958.

Rosenvinge, J.H. & Mouland, S.O. (1990). Outcome and prognosis of anorexia nervosa--a retrospective study of 41 subjects. *The British Journal of Psychiatry*, 156, 92-98.

Smith, C., Feldmann, S.S., Nasserba Kht, A., Steiner, H. (1993). Psychological chracteristics and DSM-III-R diagnoses at 6-year follow-up of adolescent anorexia nervosa. *Journal of the American Academy of Child and Adolescent Psychiatry, 32,* 1237-1245.

Steinhausen, H.C. & Seidel, R. (1993). Short-term and intermediate-term outcome in adolescent eating disorders. *Acta Psychiatrica Scandinavica*, 88, 169-173.

Strober, M. & Katz, J. (1988). Depression in the eating disorders: A review and analysis of descriptive, family and biological factors. In D.M. Garner, P.E. Garfinkel (Eds.), *Diagnostic Issues in Anorexia nervosa and Bulimia*. New York: Brunner/Mazel.

Strober, M., Lampert, C., Morrell, W., Burroughs, J., Jacobs, C. (1990). A Controlled Family Study of Anorexia Nervosa: Evidence of Familial Aggregation and Lack of Shared Transmission with Affective Disorders. *International Journal of Eating Disorders*, 9, 239-253.

Toner, B.B., Garfinkel, P.E., Garner, D.M. (1986). Long-term follow-up of anorexia nervosa. *Psychosomatic Medicine*, 48, 520-529.

WHO, World Health Organisation (1990). *Computergestützte Diagnostik nach ICD-10 und DSM-III-R mit dem Composite International Diagnostic Interview (CIDI)*. Weinheim: Beltz Test GmbH, Psychologie Verlags Union.

Willi, J., Limacher, B., Nussbaum, P. (1989). 10-Jahres-Katamnese der 1973-1975 im Kanton Zürich erstmals hospitalisierten Anorexie-Fälle. *Schweizer Medizinische Wochenschrift*, 119, 147-155.

Williams, J.B.W. (1988). A Structured Interview Guide for the Hamilton Depression Rating Scale. *Archives of General Psychiatry*, 45, 742-747.

Windauer, U., Lennerts, W., Talbot, P., Touyz, S.W., Beaumont, P.J.V. (1993). How well are "cured" anorexia nervosa patients? An investigation of 16 weight-recovered anorexic patients. *British Journal of Psychiatry*, 163, 195-200.

Zung, W.W.K. (1972). The depression status inventory: An adjunct to the Self-Rating Depression Scale. *Journal of Clinical Psychology*, 28, 539-543.

# How Specific Are Body Image Disturbances in Patients With Anorexia Nervosa?

*Henning Flechtner, Christin Eltze, and Gerd Lehmkuhl*

## 1 Introduction

The perceptual and conceptual disturbances of patients with anorexia nervosa are gaining ever increasing scientific interest and attention because of their particular relevance regarding prognosis and therapy (Meermann, 1991). In this context, body perception and body experience are two very complex areas with cognitive as well as affective and conscious as well as unconscious elements.

Over the last years, a variety of empirical investigations concerning disturbances of body image in anorectic patients have been published (Meermann, 1991; Meermann & Fichter, 1982; Niebel, 1987), and yet, because of the partly contradictory results, Hsu (1982) questioned if there is, in fact, a specific body perception in anorexia nervosa. These critical objections are mainly related to the great methodological difficulties that are encountered by the experimental measurement of body image disturbances (Woerner, Lehmkuhl, & Woerner, 1989). According to Meermann and Fichter (1982), these concern on the one hand the different techniques of investigation, i.e., visual size estimation, image marking procedure, body image detection device, video and photography distortion techniques, silhouette selection method, and special questionnaires. On the other hand, objections are brought forward because of the often heterogeneous and hardly comparable samples of patients and control groups.

Table 1, shows a summary of experimental studies broken down into three different kinds of major results. The first group of studies showed a clear overestimation of body size in patients with eating disorders as compared to controls. The second group of investigations could not demonstrate any significant

Table 1. Summary of Studies on Body Image Changes in Anorexia Nervosa Patients, Bulimia Nervosa Patients, and Control Groups

| Anorexia nervosa | | | Bulimia nervosa | | |
|---|---|---|---|---|---|
| Authors | Methods | Groups | Authors | Methods | Groups |

*Overestimation in patients with eating disorders compared to controls*

| | | | | | |
|---|---|---|---|---|---|
| Slade & Russell 1973 | VSE | A (n=13), C (n=20) | Willmuth et al. 1985 | VSE | B (n=20), C (n=20) |
| Wingate & Christie 1973 | IMP | A (n=15), C (n=15) | Ruff & Barrios 1986 | BIDD | B (n=20), C (n=20) |
| Freeman et al. 1983, 1984 | VDT | A (n=19), B (n=27) | Freeman et al. 1983, 1984 | VDT | B (n=27), A (n=19) |
| | | N (n=9), C (n=15) | | | N (n=9), C (n=15) |
| | | | Freeman et al. 1985 | VDT | B with A phase before (n=23) |
| | | | | | B without A phase (n=24) |
| | | | | | A (n=17), P (n=18), C (n=33) |
| Garner & Garfinkel 1986 | VDT | A (n=23), C (n=12) | Collins et al. 1987 | VDT | B (n=24), A (n=78) |
| | | O (n=60) | | | O (n=15), C (n=60) |
| | | | Touyz et al. 1985 | VDT | B (n=19), A (n=31) |
| | | | Williamson et al. 1989 | SIL | B (n=108), K (n=423) |

*Overestimation of all groups (no significant differences between anorexia nervosa, bulimia nervosa, and controls)*

| | | | | | |
|---|---|---|---|---|---|
| Crisp & Kalucy 1974 | VSE | A (n=10), C (n=6) | Birtchell et al. 1985 | VSE | B (n=50), C (n=19) |
| Button et al. 1977 | VSE | A (n=20), C (n=16) | Norris 1984 | BIDD | B (n=12), A (n=12) |
| Casper et al. 1979 | VSE | A (n=79), C (n=130) | | | N (n=12), C (n=12) |
| Strober et al. 1979 | IMP | A (n=18), N (n=24) | | | |
| Ben-Tovim & Crisp 1984 | VSE | A (n=10), C (n=46) | | | |
| Norris 1984 | BIDD | A (n=12), B (n=12) | | | |
| | | N (n=12), C (n=12) | | | |

*Greater variability in the body size estimation of the patients with eating disorders*

| | | | | | |
|---|---|---|---|---|---|
| Garfinkel et al. 1979 | DPT | A (n=16), C (n=13) | | | |
| Touyz 1984 | VDT | A (n=15), C (n=15) | | | |
| Collins et al. 1987 | VDT | A (n=15), C (n=15) | | | |

A: Anorexia nervosa; B: Bulimia nervosa; N: Neurotics; P: Phobics; O: Obese; C: Healthy controls. BIDD: Body Image Detection Device; DPT: Distortion Photograph Technique; IMP: Image Marking Procedure; SIL: Silhouette-Selection-Method; VDT: Video Distortion Technique; VSE: Visual Size Estimation differences in estimation of body size between the various groups, and the third group found a greater variability of results in patients with eating disorders as compared to control groups (Casg & Brown, 1987; Slade, 1985). These results were obtained employing a variety of measurement techniques and again demonstrate the current difficulties in measuring body image and its changes in patients with eating disorders.

The available data especially underline the importance of patients' characteristics, age at onset of symptoms, and the time of measurement during the course of disease (Altabe & Thompson, 1993; Button, Fransella & Slade, 1977; Garner, Garfinkel, Stancer, & Moldofsky,1976; Halmi, Goldberg & Cunningham, 1977). Starting from the findings of Hilde Bruch (1962, 1973) who described body image disturbances, changes in the perception of affective and visceral stimuli, and a piercing feeling of ineffectiveness as cardinal symptoms of anorexia nervosa, an empirical approach of measuring different aspects of these psychological variables will be described in this chapter. Further therapeutic studies will have to establish their prognostic relevance.

## 2  Samples and Methods

In the following, the empirical results of three different investigations from independent samples of adolescent patients and control persons are comprehensively presented. The studies employed different methodological approaches regarding body perception and body image disturbances.

### 2.1  Study I

Using the Silhouette Selection Method, the body perception of 22 patients was assessed. These patients had received in-patient treatment for anorexia nervosa on average 5.1 years previous to follow-up. At the time of follow-up, they averaged 20;11 years of age and had a mean weight of 55,5 kg and a mean height of 165 cm. The obtained answers were compared with those from a control group of subjects with normal weight, corresponding age, and free of any psychiatric disorder. The patients were asked to select their actual and their ideal body size from 12 pictures showing images ranging from 75% up to 130% body size with 5% interval steps, as shown in Figure 1. Scores range from 1 (slim) to 12 (obese).

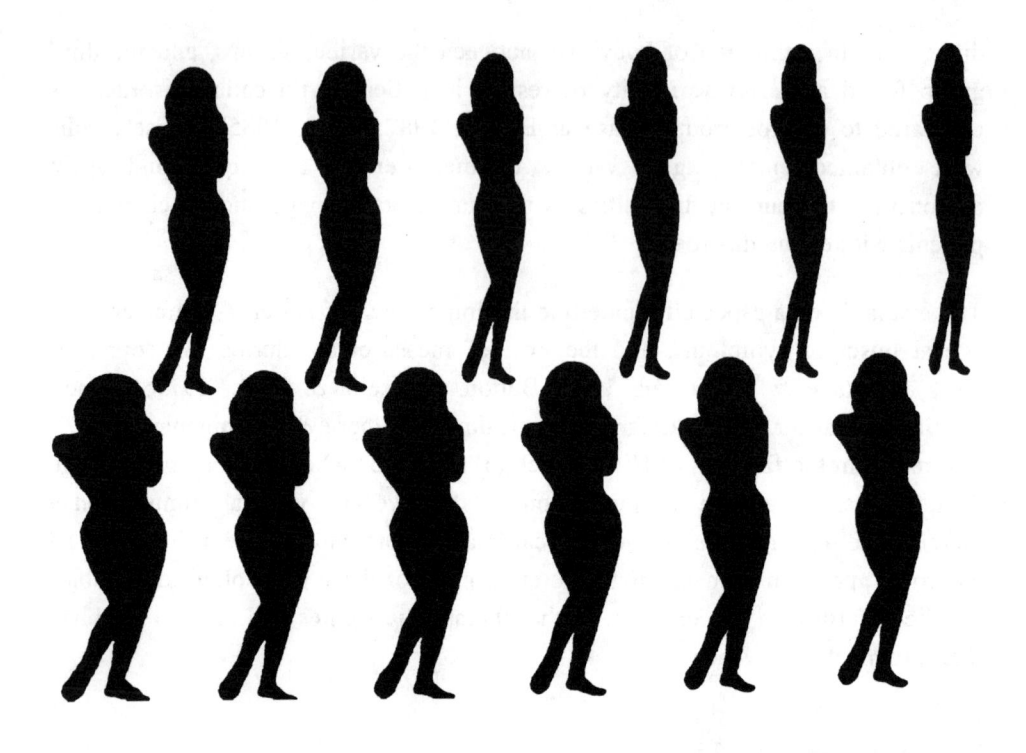

Figure 1.    „Silhouette-Selection-Method" for body size estimation

## 2.2   Study II

In a second investigation, 27 anorectic girls who were consecutively admitted to hospital were asked for their attitude towards their own body. The DSM-III-R diagnostic criteria for anorexia nervosa were met by all patients. Duration of symptoms prior to admission averaged 15.3 months. In most cases, previous ambulatory treatments had failed – seven adolescents had already received previous in-patient treatment. The mean weight loss was 15.7 kg and the weight at admission averaged 38.7 kg. Besides different methods for the evaluation of eating behaviour, family relations, and the course of therapy, the patient's attitude towards his or her own body was assessed using the questionnaire by Strauss and Appelt (1983). It consists of 52 items that were grouped by factor analysis into 3 separate scales: (a) insecurity/dysaesthesia, (b) attractiveness/self-confidence, and (c) accentuation of the body/sensitivity. The factor insecurity/dysaesthesia comprises expressions of lacking sensitivity as well as insecurity and rejection of appearance and bodily reactions. The items of the scale attractiveness/self-confidence describe a positive view of one's own body. Among expressions of satisfaction and identification, statements about one's own attractiveness, confidence in one's own body and its reactions belong to this second factor. The third scale labelled accentuation of the body/sensitivity, deals with the significance of body appearance and personal hygiene, judgements about the appeal of one's own body to others, sensitivity for appearance and bodily changes as well as concerns about one's own health and body performance.

## 2.3 Study III

The sample consisted of 19 anorectic and 10 bulimic patients and a control group of 95 subjects. The mean age was 16.9 years for the anorectic, 17.6 years for the bulimic, and 16.4 years for the normal subjects. A specific Picture Silhouette Test was developed during a comprehensive investigation that studied body image disturbances in patients with anorexia nervosa and bulimia nervosa. The picture of a female body in front view and profile was divided into three interchangeable parts in order to allow different body-part size estimations. The chest, the region of belly, hips, and thighs, and the lower legs were available as separate foldouts in the front view. In the profile view, the chest, the belly, the hips and thighs, and the lower legs can be assessed independently on the foldouts as shown in Figure 2. Depictions of each of the body regions are available in nine gradations ranging from extreme cachexia (Score 1) to extreme obesity (Score 9). Grade five represents the normal average ideal figure.

The patients with anorexia nervosa and the control persons without eating disorder were asked to carry out the assessments according to five different instructions: (a) how they rate themselves looking into the mirror (mirror image), (b) how they *think* their body looks, (c) how they *feel* their body looks, (d) how they wish their body to be (ideal self-image), (e) how they think that others perceive their body

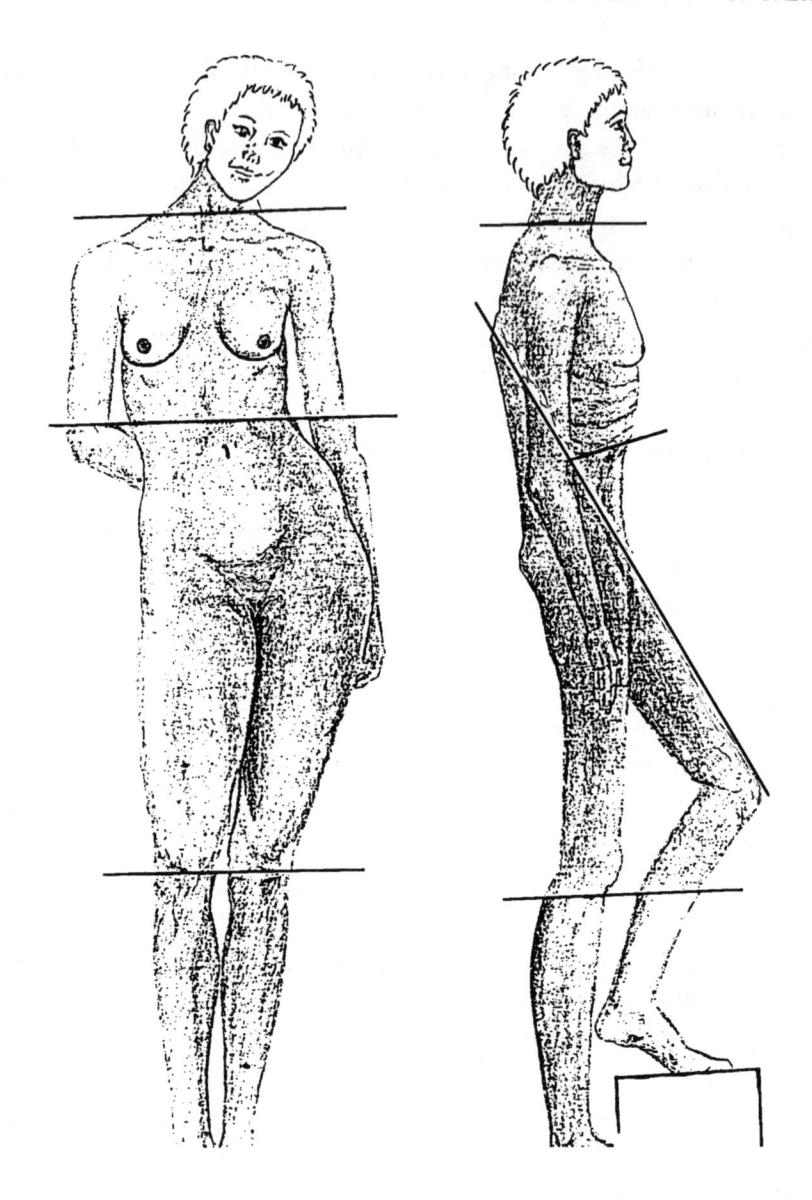

Figure 2. „Picture-Silhouette-Test" for body-part size estimation

(hetero-image). These instructions were used both with the Picture Silhouette Test and the Silhouette Selection Test. In addition to these two tests the following instruments were used: the Eating Disorder Inventory (EDI) (Garner, Olmstead, & Polivy, 1983) and the 34 item Body Shape Questionnaire (BSQ) (Cooper, Taylor, Cooper, & Fairburn, 1987). The BSQ is meant to cover the concern about the body shape – the experience of "feeling fat" – which is one of the typical signs of patients with anorexia and bulimia nervosa. Meanwhile, it was further developed and alternate short forms are also available (Evans & Dolan, 1993).

# 3 Results

## 3.1 Study I

The results based on the Silhouette Selection Method are summarised in Table 2. Almost two thirds of both the former anorectic patients and the normal weight controls wished to have a slimmer body image. As far as the discrepancy between real and ideal image were concerned no significant difference occurred between the two groups, the difference being 2.2 interval steps (11%) in the control group compared to 2.8 (14%) in the patient group.

Table 2. Study I - Body Perception as Assessed by the Silhouette Selection Method

|  | Anorexia Nervosa (N = 22) N    % | Control Group (N = 16) N    % |
|---|---|---|
| Real = ideal image | 5    23 | 5    31 |
| Real > ideal image | 14    63 | 11    69 |
| Real < ideal image | 3    14 | -    - |

## 3.2 Study II

The results from this study are summarised in Table 3. It is shown that the entire group of patients with anorexia nervosa express more uncertainty and a diminished sense of physical well-being in the Strauss and Appelt questionnaire in comparison to adolescents without an eating disorder. Correspondingly, the scores for the scale attractiveness/self-confidence, including satisfaction with one's own appearance,

Table 3. Study II - Questionnaire Findings in Anorectic Patients and Controls

| | Number of Items (N = 27) | Anorexia Nervosa Patients Total Group (N = 12) | Anorexia Nervosa Patients At Admission (N = 12) | Anorexia Nervosa Patients At Discharge (N = 27) | Normal Weight Control Group |
|---|---|---|---|---|---|
| **Body Attitudes Questionnaire** | | | | | |
| Insecurity/ dysaesthesia | 19 | 7.4 | 7.9 | 6.2 * | 4.9 ** |
| Attractiveness/ self-confidence | 13 | 3.9 | 3.3 | 4.9 * | 6.4 ** |
| Accentuation/ sensitivity | 20 | 12.4 | 13.3 | 13.3 | 10.8 * |

* $p < .05$   ** $p < .01$   *** $p < .001$

are significantly lower. The concern with the health of one's own body, in the sense of a hypochondriac-depressive preoccupation with appearance, is significantly more pronounced in anorectic patients than in the control group subjects.

A follow-up investigation was carried out in 12 patients at the end of in-patient treatment. The weight gain at that point in time averaged 10.3 kg. The self report showed significantly less uncertainty and dysaesthesia with regard to the experience of one's own body as well as a corresponding increase in the feelings of attractiveness and self confidence (see Table 3). However, significant differences remained in comparison to the control group. The hypochondriac-depressive preoccupation with one's own appearance did not change since the start of treatment. It was found that a slower weight gain was associated with an enhanced uncertainty with regard to body perception, whereas a more rapid and greater increase in weight was related to a significantly more attractive assessment of one's own body at the time of discharge from hospital.

## 3.3 Study III

In comparison to the controls, the anorectic patients showed significantly higher scores in four out of eight EDI scales, namely drive for thinness, interoceptive awareness, ineffectiveness, and interpersonal distrust. It is remarkable that no differences were found on the following subscales: bulimia, body dissatisfaction, maturity fears, and perfectionism (see Table 4).

Table 4.  Study III - Comparison of EDI Findings

| Scales | Anorexia Nervosa (N = 19) Mean | SD | Control Group (N = 95) Mean | SD | t-Test p |
|---|---|---|---|---|---|
| Drive for thinness | 8.0 | 5.7 | 2.9 | 3.6 | < .01 |
| Interoceptive awareness | 4.3 | 4.6 | 1.4 | 1.7 | < .05 |
| Bulimia | 0.9 | 1.6 | 0.7 | 1.2 | ns |
| Body dissatisfaction | 9.1 | 4.6 | 8.2 | 5.1 | ns |
| Ineffectiveness | 6.8 | 5.4 | 1.7 | 3.3 | < .01 |
| Maturity fears | 5.7 | 4.8 | 4.8 | 3.2 | ns |
| Perfectionism | 3.3 | 3.3 | 2.3 | 2.4 | ns |
| Interpersonal distrust | 5.5 | 3.5 | 2.2 | 2.6 | < .01 |

In the Body Shape Questionnaire (BSQ), the patients with anorexia nervosa showed a significantly more pronounced dissatisfaction with their physical appearance than the adolescent controls (mean score 100.3 versus 74.4, p < 0.05). With the help of the Silhouette Selection Method and the Picture Silhouette Test the body perception was investigated using different instructions. The results obtained with the Silhouette Selection Method are summarized in Table 5.

Table 5.    Study III - Comparison of Findings Using the Silhouette Selection Method

| Instructions | Anorexia Nervosa (N = 19) Mean | Bulimia Nervosa (N = 10) Mean | Control Group (N = 95) Mean |
|---|---|---|---|
| Mirror | 3.8 * | 7.9 | 7.0 |
| Thinking | 3.9 * | 8.1 | 7.2 |
| Emotions | 3.9 * | 8.7 | 7.1 |
| Ideal | 4.0 * | 5.5 | 5.7 |
| Other persons | 2.7 * | 7.5 | 6.9 |

* p < 0.1

The responses of the anorectic patients to all instructions differed from the responses of the control group and also from those of the bulimic patients in that they chose slimmer figures. However, a specific effect of the different test instructions with regard to the reported self-image was not found. Independently of the given instruction, anorectic patients perceived themselves as markedly more overweight compared to their estimation of how they were seen by others (see Table 6). They were obviously able to recognise the marked discrepancies between their own perception and the supposed assessments of other persons. The actual self assessment hardly deviated from the desired ideal image, thus indicating that the anorectic patients reached a state that came close to what they desired. Only in regard to the chest and the belly/hip/thigh regions was a clearly less slim figure reported as an ideal image. The differences regarding self perception and ideal figure in the group of bulimia nervosa patients and in the control group were, however, significant. They desired to have a much slimmer figure. With the Picture Silhouette Test it was possible to differentiate perceptions of the different parts of the body. For all these areas, self perception and the supposed assessment by others proved to be significantly different in patients with anorexia nervosa (see Table 6). This was not the case in the group of normal controls nor in the group of bulimia nervosa patients.

Table 6. Study III - Actual Assessment (Self Image) Compared to Ideal Image and Expected Estimation by Others (Hetero Image) in Patients and Controls (Picture Silhouette Test)

|  | Anorexia Nervosa Self Image versus | | Bulimia Nervosa Self Image versus | | Control Group Self Image versus | |
|---|---|---|---|---|---|---|
|  | Ideal (N=18) | Hetero (N=19) | Ideal (N=10) | Hetero (N=10) | Ideal (N=29) | Hetero (N=29) |
| | Front View | | | | | |
| Chest | 3.9 5.0** | 3.2** | 5.2 5.8 | 5.0 | 5.3 5.7* | 5.3 |
| Belly/hip/thigh | 3.4 4.0* | 2.9* | 4.8 3.9* | 5.0 | 4.5 4.0*** | 4.5 |
| | Profile | | | | | |
| Chest | 2.8 3.9** | 2.1** | 4.4 4.9 | 4.5 | 4.3 4.6 | 4.2 |
| Belly | 3.6 3.2 | 2.4** | 4.8 3.2* | 5.0 | 4.1 3.4*** | 4.2 |
| Hip/thigh | 3.9 4.1 | 3.2** | 5.9 4.4* | 5.5 | 5.1 4.5*** | 5.2 |

* $p < .05$; ** $p < .01$; *** $p < .001$

## 4  Discussion and Conclusions

Different samples and a variety of instruments were used to investigate and compare the body perception of patients with anorexia nervosa and bulimia nervosa with the body perception of adolescents that did not have an eating disorder. Our results indicate that the actual and ideal image of one's own body are also divergent in normal-weight adolescents just as they are in anorectic patients. In reference to Niebel (1987) and Collins and Plahn (1988), these findings can be interpreted to mean that developmental psychological and cultural factors play an important role in the judgement of one's own body (Altabe & Thompson, 1993). Particularly, because already in children and adolescents obesity and being overweight is associated with negative features and attributes in social situations. Because dealing with confronting the physical changes of one's own body is a specific developmental task in adolescence, being overweight leads to a specific vulnerability in adolescents. Concerning therapeutic approaches, it seems of utmost importance to conduct longitudinal studies showing how body image characteristics change within the therapeutic process (Haimovitz, Lansky, & O'Reilly, 1993).

The data of the second study also show that, in comparison with the subjects of the normal weight control group of the same age, the attitude towards one's own body and the estimation of the own attractiveness and self confidence of the body perception are disturbed and altered in adolescent anorectic patients.

This leads to the conclusion that body image disturbances are not solely perception disorders but refer to a subjectively negatively experienced body figure. This is also supported by the findings from the questionnaire for the assessment of the attitude towards one's own body by Strauss and Appelt (1983), in which patients with anorexia nervosa reported a higher level of uncertainty and dysaesthesia and a lower level of attractiveness and self confidence than the group without eating disorders.

In comparison to the investigation by Strauss and Appelt (1983), it can be stated that the differences in the attitude towards one's own body that exist between anorectic patients and normal-weight controls exist in adults as well as in adolescents. It is noteworthy that in neither the patient group nor the control group was a clear relation found between weight and age respectively, and the attitude towards one's own body as assessed by the questionnaire. This implies that weight does not directly correlate with the perception of one's own body. This finding can be interpreted to mean that, also in patients with anorectic symptoms, the subjective perception is not related to the real weight loss. These results can further be explained by assuming that the rather unconscious perception of the body and the conscious assessment of the body are possibly largely independent areas of body experience in the sense of Shontz (1974).

The results from the above-described third study also point in this direction. The differences in body estimation that arise when different instructions are given –i.e., mirror, thinking, and feeling – were found to be relatively small for both methods. The statistical analyses yielded no differences for the Silhouette Selection Method and significant differences only for a few body parts in the Picture Silhouette Test. In the latter, for instance, all groups chose as their ideal figure a larger shape than their actual estimation of the chest region. In the Silhouette Selection Method, similar to the Picture Silhouette Test, the adolescents of the control group chose a slimmer figure when instructed to choose their ideal image, whereas in patients with anorexia nervosa, the ideal image and their actual self assessment of their body (real image) matched. On the other hand, patients with eating disorders were in a position to realistically estimate their appearance. When instructed to assess how they are perceived by other persons, they reported a slimmer figure than that of their actual self assessment.

The results of the self report questionnaires indicate that adolescent patients with anorexia nervosa view themselves as being significantly less attractive and self confident when compared to the responses of the control group subjects. They expressed much more concern about their own body shape in the sense of a persistent feeling of being too fat.

In summary, it can be concluded that the disturbances of body image that are assumed to occur in patients with anorexia nervosa can be identified in a reproducible way by different methods, if the difference between self image and the expected assessment by others is considered as a measure for body image disturbance. Overall ideal image and actual self perception are not significantly different in patients with anorexia nervosa whereas they are in patients with bulimia nervosa and control group adolescents.

Since patients with anorexia nervosa generally rate themselves as less attractive and less self confident than adolescent controls, self concept and self perception in a broader sense also seem to be altered when changes in body image occur. These more general influences on self concept and self perception should also have implications for the development of future therapeutic approaches, like in the body orientated therapy developed by Vandereycken, Depreitere & Probst (1987) for anorectic patients with the aim of building up a realistic self concept, the experience of pleasure in one's own body, and strengthening of social competencies and abilities.

From the data that are currently available, it can be concluded that specific changes in body image and related areas do occur in patients with anorexia nervosa, but there is still great variability in the obtained results due to the applied methodology as well as other aspects of body image assessment that deserve further study. Although the observed changes in body image seem to be specific to the investigated groups of patients with anorexia nervosa as compared to patients with bulimia nervosa and controls, much additional information will be needed to classify and clarify the nature of these changes in body image and body perception in connection with psychopathology and symptomatology. It will be particularly important to more closely investigate the course of these psychological variables during treatment and to determine more precisely their influence on the development and outcome of these patients.

## References

Altabe, M., & Thompson, J. K. (1993). Body image changes during early adulthood. *International Journal of Eating Disorders, 13*, 323-328

Ben-Tovim, D. I., & Crisp, A. H. (1984). The reliability of estimates of body width and their relationship to current measured body size among anorexic and normal subjects. *Psychological Medicine, 14*, 843-846.

Birtchell, S. A., Lacey, J. H., & Harte, A. (1985). Body image distortion in bulimia nervosa. *British Journal of Psychiatry, 147*, 408-412.

Bruch, H. (1962). Perceptual and conceptual disturbances in anorexia nervosa. *Psychosomatic Medicine, 24*, 187-194.

Bruch, H. (1973). *Eating disorders, obesity, anorexia nervosa, and the person within.* New York: Basic Books.

Button, E. J., Fransella, F., & Slade, P. D. (1977). A reappraisal of body perception disturbance in anorexia nervosa. *Psychological Medicine, 7*, 235-243.

Casg, T. F., & Brown, T. A. (1987). Body image in anorexia nervosa and bulimia nervosa. *Behavior Modification, 11*, 487-521

Casper, R. C., Halmi, K. A., Goldberg, S. C., Eckert, E. D., & Davis, J. M. (1979). Disturbances in body image estimation as related to other characteristics and outcome in anorexia nervosa. *British Journal of Psychiatry, 134*, 60-66.

Collins, J. K., & Plahn, M. R. (1988). Recognition accuracy, stereotypic preference, aversion, and subjective judgement of body appearance in adolescents and young adults. *Journal of Youth and Adolescence, 17*, 317-334.

Cooper, P. J., Taylor, M. J., Cooper, Z., & Fairburn, Ch. G. (1987). The development and validation of the body shape questionnaire. *International Journal of Eating Disorders, 6*, 485-494.

Crisp, A. H., & Kalucy, R. S. (1974). Aspects of the perceptual disorder in anorexia nervosa. *British Journal of Medical Psychology, 47*, 349-361.

Evans, C., & Dolan, B. T. I. (1993) Body Shape Questionnaire: derivation of shortened alternate forms. *International Journal of Eating Disorders, 13*, 315-321.

Freeman, R. J., Beach, B., Davis, R., & Solyom, L. (1985). The prediction of relapse in bulimia nervosa. *Journal of Psychiatric Research, 19*, 349-353.

Freeman, R. J., Thomas, C. D., Solyom, L., & Hunter M. A. (1984). A modified video camera for measuring body image distortion: Technical description and reliability. *Psychological Medicine, 14*, 411-416.

Freeman, R. J., Thomas, C. D., Solyom, & Miles J. E. (1983). Body image disturbances in anorexia nervosa: A reexamination and a new technique. In P. L. Darby, P. E. Garfinkel, D.

M. Garner, & D.V. Coscina (Eds.), *Anorexia nervosa: Recent developments in research* (pp. 117-127). New York: Alan R. Riss
Garfinkel, P. E., Moldofsky, H., & Garner, D. M. (1979). The stability of perceptual disturbance in anorexia nervosa. *Psychological Medicine, 9*, 703-708.
Garner, D. M., Garfinkel, P. E., Stancer, H. C., & Moldofsky, H. (1976). Body image disturbances in anorexia nervosa and obesity. *Psychosomatic Medicine, 38*, 327-336.
Garner, D. M., Garner, M. V., & Rosen, L. W. (1993). Anorexia nervosa restricters who purge: implications for subtyping anorexia nervosa. *International Journal of Eating Disorders, 13*, 171-185.
Garner, D. M., Olmstedt, M. P., Bohr, Y., & Garfinkel, P. E. (1982). The eating attitudes test: Psychometric features and clinical correlates. *Psychological Medicine, 12*, 871-878.
Garner, D. M., Olmstedt, M. P., & Polivy, J. (1983). Development and validation of multidimensional eating disorder inventory for anorexia and bulimia. *International Journal of Eating Disorders, 2,* 15-34.
Haimovitz, D., Lansky, L. M., & O'Reilly, P. (1993). Fluctuations in body satisfaction across situations. *International Journal of Eating Disorders, 13*, 77-84.
Halmi, K. A., Goldberg, S., & Cunningham, S. (1977). Perceptual distribution of body image in adolescent girls: Distortion of body image in adolescence. *Psychological Medicine, 7,* 253-257.
Hsu, L. K. G. (1982). Is there a disturbance in body image in anorexia nervosa ? *Journal of Nervous and Mental Disease, 170*, 305-307.
Hundleby, J. D., & Bourgouin, N. C. (1993). Generality in the errors of estimation of body image. *International Journal of Eating Disorders, 13*, 85-92.
Levin, A. P., Kahan, M., Lamm, J. B., & Spauster, E. (1993). Multiple personality in eating disorder patients. *International Journal of Eating Disorders, 13*, 235-239.
Meermann, R. (1991). Body-Image-Störungen bei Anorexia und Bulimia nervosa und ihre Relevanz für die Therapie. In C. Jacobi, Th. Paul (Eds.), *Bulimia und Anorexia nervosa, Ursachen und Therapie* (pp. 69-85). Berlin-Heidelberg: Springer.
Meermann, R., & Fichter, M. (1982). Störungen des Körperschemas (body image) bei psychischen Krankheiten-Methodik und experimentelle Ergebnisse bei Anorexia nervosa. *Psychotherapie, Psychosomatik, medizinische Psychologie, 32*, 162-169.
Meermann, R., & Vandereycken, W. (1988). *Therapie der Magersucht und Bulimia nervosa.* Berlin: de Gruyter.
Niebel, G. (1987). Psychopathologische Aspekte gestörten Essverhaltens bei Frauen. *Zeitschrift für Psychotherapie und medizinische Psychologie, 37,* 317-330.
Norris, D. L. (1984). The effects of mirror confrontation on self-estimation of body dimensions in anorexia nervosa, bulimia, and two control groups. *Psychological Medicine, 14,* 835-842.
Rossiter, E. M., Agras, W. S., Telch, C. F., Schneider, J. A., & Cluster, B. (1993). Personality disorder characteristics predict outcome in the treatment of bulimia nervosa. *International Journal of Eating Disorders, 13,* 349-357.
Ruff, G. A., & Barrios, B. A. (1986). Realistic assessment of body image. *Behavioral Assessment, 8,* 237-251.
Shontz, F. C. (1974). Body image and its disorders. *International Journal of Psychiatry in Medicine, 5,* 461-472.
Slade, P. D. (1985). A Review of body-image studies in anorexia nervosa and bulimia nervosa. *Journal of Psychiatric Research, 19*, 255-265.
Slade, P. D., & Russell, G. F. M. (1973). Awareness of body dimensions in anorexia nervosa: Cross-sectional and longitudinal studies. *Psychological Medicine, 3,* 188-189.
Steinhausen, H.C., & Vollrath, M. (1993). The self-image of adolescent patients with eating disorders. *International Journal of Eating Disorders, 13,* 221-227.
Strauss, B., & Appelt, H. (1983). Ein Fragebogen zur Beurteilung des eigenen Körpers. *Diagnostica, 24*: 145-164.
Strober, M., Goldenberg, I., Green, J., & Saxon, J. (1979). Body image disturbances in anorexia nervosa during the acute and recuperative phase. *Psychological Medicine, 9,* 695-701.
Thompson, J. K., & Heinberg, L. J. (1993). Preliminary test of two hypotheses of body image disturbance. *International Journal of Eating Disorders, 14*, 59-63.
Touyz, S. W., Beumont, P. J. V., Collins, J. K., McCabe, M., & Jupp, J. (1984). Body shape perception and its disturbance in anorexia nervosa. *British Journal of Psychiatry, 144,* 167-171.
Touyz, S. W., Beumont, P. J. V., Collins, J. K., & Cowie, I. (1985). Body shape perception in bulimia and anorexia nervosa. *International Journal of Eating Disorders, 4*, 259-65.

Vandereycken, D. A., Depreitere, L., & Probst, R. (1987). Body-orientated therapy for anorexia nervosa patients. *American Journal of Psychotherapy, 61*, 252-259.

Williams, G. J., Power, K. G., Millar, H. R., Freeman, C. P., Yellowlees, A., Dowds, T., Walker, M., Campsie, L., Macpherson, F., & Jackson, M. A. (1993). Comparison of eating disorders and other dietary/weight groups on measures of perceived control, assertiveness, self-esteem, and self-directed hostility. *International Journal of Eating Disorders, 14*, 27-32.

Willmuth, M. E., Leitenberg, H., Rosen, J. C., Fondacaro, K. M., & Gross, J. (1985). Body size distortion in bulimia nervosa. *International Journal of ating Disorders, 4*, 71-78.

Wingate, B. A., & Christie, M. J. (1978). Ego strength and body image in anorexia nervosa. *Journal of Psychosomatic Research*, 22, 201-204.

Woerner, I., Lehmkuhl, G., & Woerner, W. (1989). Zur Beziehung von Körperwahrnehmung, Essverhalten und Körpergewicht bei anorektischen und normalgewichtigen Jugendlichen. *Zeitschrift für Klinische Psychologie, 18*, 19-331.

# Sexual Abuse and Psychological Dysfunctioning in Eating Disorders

*Johan Vanderlinden and Walter Vandereycken*

## 1 Introduction

Some early case studies stimulated interest in the possible relationship between serious traumatic experiences - especially physical and sexual abuse - and the development of an eating disorder (Goldfarb, 1987; McFarlane, McFarlane, & Golchrist, 1988; Schechter, Schwartz, & Greenfield, 1987; Sloan & Leigher, 1986; Torem, 1986; Wooley & Kearney-Cooke, 1986). These reports suggested that traumatic experiences are more frequently reported in bulimia nervosa patients than in anorexia nervosa patients (especially of the restricting type). If this impression is confirmed by systematic research, one may speculate about the relation between sexual abuse and the development of an eating disorder. Much of the ongoing discussion is centered around the specificity and the causal nature of the relation.

## 2 Review of the Literature

Several studies on large samples, both clinical and nonclinical, have been carried out. In probably the first systematic investigation of this issue, Oppenheimer, Howells, Palmer, and Chaloner (1985) mentioned astonishingly high figures: 70% of 78 female outpatients with an eating disorder reported sexual abuse during childhood and/or adolescence. These authors found no relation between a history of sexual abuse and the type of eating disorder. Finn, Hartman, Leon, and Lawson (1986) found a history of sexual abuse in 57% of 87 eating-disordered women. Comparisons of women with and without histories of sexual abuse did not reveal a clear association between the occurrence of an eating disorder and a history of sexual abuse. In a group of 75 bulimic women, Kearney-Cooke (1988) found that

58% had a history of sexual trauma. Root and Fallon (1988) reported on 172 eating disorder patients: 65% had been physically abused, 23% raped, and 28% sexually abused in childhood. Hall, Tice, Beresford, Wooley, and Hall (1989) found a history of sexual abuse in 50% of a group of 158 eating disorder patients versus 28% in a control group of 86 psychiatric patients. Bulik, Sullivan, and Rorty (1989) investigated childhood sexual abuse and family background in 34 bulimics and found 34.3% to have been sexually abused. Interestingly, when comparing abused with non-abused subjects, no differences were found on any of the subscales of the Eating Disorder Inventory (EDI; Garner, Olmsted, & Polivy, 1983).

Steiger and Zanko (1990) studied the prevalence of sexual abuse in 73 eating-disordered subjects, 21 psychiatric patients, and 24 "normal" women. Around 30% of the eating disorder group reported sexual abuse histories versus 33% in the psychiatric control group and 9% in the normal controls. Within the eating disorder group, restricting anorexia nervosa patients had significantly lower abuse rates (6%) than the other eating disorder subgroups. Palmer, Oppenheimer, Dignon, Chaloner, and Howells (1990) extended their first series (Oppenheimer et al., 1985) to a group of 158 patients: 31% reported childhood sexual abuse and another 27% mentioned other unpleasant or coercive sexual events. Again the investigators did not find a significant association between rates of abuse and a type of eating disorder. In a systematic study of 112 normal-weight bulimic women, Lacey (1990) found that only eight patients (7%) mentioned a history of sexual abuse involving physical contact; four of these (3.6%) described incest, but only in two cases (1.8%) did the incest occur during childhood. Lacey stressed that, based on his findings, sexual abuse had most frequently occurred in "multi-impulsive bulimics".

Waller (1991) reported sexual abuse in 50% of a series of 100 eating-disordered women. He also found that a history of abuse was associated with the type of eating disorder: bulimic women reported significantly higher rates of unwanted sexual experiences than restricting anorexics. Waller (1992) further showed that the frequency of bingeing and vomiting was significantly greater in women who reported sexual abuse that occurred within the family, before the age of 14 years, and involving physical force. According to another analysis of these findings, Waller (1993) suggested that the presence of a borderline personality disorder was often associated with the reporting of sexual abuse; this might be the mediating psychologial factor between sexual abuse and bulimic behavior. Folsom, Krahn, Nairn, Gold, Demitrack, and Silk (1993) compared rates of physical and sexual abuse in 102 women with an eating disorder and 49 female patients with a psychiatric disorder. No differences in abuse rates were found: sexual and physical abuse were reported in 69% and 51% respectively of the eating disorder sample, and in 80% and 56% of the psychiatric sample. No relation between a history of sexual abuse and scores on the Eating Disorder Inventory was found. However, within the eating disorder group, sexually abused subjects reported more severe psychiatric disturbances of an obsessive and phobic nature (assessed with the Hopkins Symptom Check List SCL-90; Derogatis, 1983) than non-abused subjects. The authors conclude that sexually abusive experiences, although related to increased psychological distress, do not induce more eating disorder symptoms.

Miller and McCluskey-Fawcett (1993) compared 72 bulimic women with 72 age-matched controls without eating problems on measures of sexual abuse and dissociation (assessed with the Dissociative Experiences Scale or DES; Bernstein & Putnam, 1986). Rates of reported sexual abuse after the age of 12 with an adult relative as the perpetrator were significantly greater among bulimic women: 15.3% versus 1.4% in normal controls. The clear difference in rates of sexual abuse prior to the age 12 was not statistically significant: 11.1% versus 1.4%. Dissociative experiences were significantly more common in bulimics, and the more so if they reported sexual abuse in their childhood.

Recently, Welch and Fairburn (1994) carried out a well-controlled study in four individually matched groups: 100 community controls without an eating disorder, 50 community cases of bulimia nervosa, 50 community controls with other psychiatric disorders (mostly depression), and 50 clinic patients with bulimia nervosa. Assessment of abuse histories before the onset of the eating disorder was established with an interview in the subject's own home. Significantly more community cases of bulimia nervosa had been abused before the onset of their eating disorder (26%) than the "normal" community controls (10%), but the rates of sexual abuse in the former closely resembled those in psychiatric controls (24%). A surprising result was the smaller number (16%) of bulimic inpatients who reported sexual abuse before the onset of the eating disorder. Welch and Fairburn (1994) concluded that childhood sexual abuse does increase the risk of psychiatric disorders, including bulimia nervosa, but that the increased risk is not specific to the eating disorder.

Besides these studies in clinical populations - except for the Welch and Fairburn (1994) study - others have been conducted exclusively in *non-clinical* populations. Calam and Slade (1989) administered the Eating Attitudes Test (EAT; Garner & Garfinkel, 1979) and the Sexual Events Questionnaire (Russell, 1983) to 130 female undergraduate students: 20% reported unwanted sexual experiences before the age of 14, 13% of which involved intrafamilial abuse. The experience of sexual events involving force was associated with higher EAT scores (except for the subscale "oral control"). Only unwanted sexual intercourse before the age 14 showed a significant correlation with the bulimia subscale of the EAT. Bailey and Gibbons (1989) studied the relationship between bulimia nervosa and abuse histories in a sample of 294 college students: 13% reported childhood sexual abuse, 11% rape, and 6% physical abuse. Only the latter correlated significantly with the diagnosis of bulimia. Smolak, Levine, and Sullins (1990) administered the EDI and a detailed questionnaire on sexual abuse to 298 undergraduate women: 23% reported sexual abuse in childhood. This subgroup showed significantly higher total EDI scores than the non-abused group; EDI scores were not related to severity of abuse, type of contact, or identity of the perpetrator.

## 3   Our Own Research Findings

In a first study (Vanderlinden, Vandereycken, Van Dyck, & Vertommen, 1993), the relation between traumatic experiences and dissociative phenomena was explored in 98 eating disorder patients using a self-report questionnaire on traumatic sexual experiences (Lange, 1990) and our own Dissociation Questionnaire (DIS-Q; Vanderlinden, Van Dyck, Vertommen, Vandereycken, & Verkes, 1993). Besides sexual abuse - including unwanted sexual intercourse and non-genital sexual contact between a child and a family member — the following situations were also considered as traumatic: physical abuse (e.g., repeated beating or torture), complete emotional neglect or abandonment in childhood, and the loss of a close family member. Only traumatic situations occurring before the onset of the eating disorder were assessed. The total (combined) trauma rate was 28%; 20% reported childhood sexual abuse, 8% of which was incest. Restricting anorexics had a significantly lower trauma rate (12%) than anorexia nervosa patients of the "mixed" type (who also binged, purged, or vomited), normal-weight bulimics, and atypical eating disorder patients (not fitting DSM-III-R criteria): 25%, 37%, and 58% respectively. Sexual abuse was significantly lower in the restricting anorexics (only 3%) than in the three other eating disorder subgroups (20%).

The trauma group scored significantly higher on the DIS-Q than the non-trauma group, with the sexually abused subjects having the highest scores, especially on the subscale "amnesia". The latter turned out to be the most specific characteristic for distinguishing sexually abused from non-abused patients. About 12 % of the eating disorder patients mentioned dissociative experiences to a degree as high as in a group of patients with dissociative disorders: 9 out of 12 of the former patients reported sexual abuse. These data suggest that trauma-induced dissociative experiences may play a role in the development of an eating disorder.

In a subsequent study, we investigated the relationship between childhood trauma and comorbidity (general neuroticism on the SCL-90) in 80 eating disorder patients; this study also included the EDI and the Eating Disorder Evaluation Scale (EDES; Vandereycken, 1993). Because patients often disclose traumatic experiences only after several months of psychotherapy, we also included information revealed during a six-month inpatient treatment together with the data from a self-report questionnaire about sexual experiences in the past (Lange, 1990) and from a clinical interview. Results showed an overall trauma rate of 53%, much higher than in our previous study: 20% reported sexual abuse (7% of which was incest), 35% emotional neglect, and 27% physical abuse. Sexual abuse was found to have occurred significantly more often among "mixed" anorexics (50%) and bulimics (18%) than among restricting anorexics (10%). The latter showed a similar rate (23%) of physical abuse as the "mixed" anorexics (21%), both being significantly lower than the rate in bulimics (37%).

Comparing the sexually abused patients (N=16) with the non-abused sample (N=64) on the EDI, EDES, and BAQ, only the bulimia subscale of the EDES showed a significant difference. When analyzing the results of the SCL-90, the sexually abused patients scored significantly higher on the total score ("general psychoneuroticism") and the subscales "anxiety" and "depression"; a significantly higher score was also found on the total DIS-Q score and on the subscales "identity confusion" and "amnesia". These data yielded by the DIS-Q confirmed the results of our first study, which showed the amnesia subscale to be the best for differentiating between sexually abused and non-abused patients. The vast majority of the eating disorder patients showing DIS-Q scores as high as patients with a dissociative disorder reported traumatic experiences (50% sexual abuse, 33% physical abuse). Only a small number (12%) of restricting anorexics belonged to this category.

## 4 Interpretation of Findings

It is very difficult to draw unequivocal conclusions from these studies reporting highly divergent rates of sexual abuse: from 7% in Lacey's (1990) study to 70% in the Oppenheimer et al. (1985) study. What factors are responsible for such remarkable divergence?

1. *Heterogeneity of the eating disorders.* Samples can vary considerably with respect to clinical features: type and severity of eating disorder, age of onset and duration, and comorbidity (additional diagnoses). Research data clearly suggest that sexual abuse may be related to higher levels of co-mordidity, in particular mood disorders, anxiety disorders, personality disorders (especially of the borderline type), and dissociative disorders.

2. *Definition of trauma and/or sexual abuse.* Some studies report only those sexually abusive experiences that took place before the onset of the eating disorder and with a perpetrator at least five years older than the victim. Some investigate only childhood sexual abuse, while other studies also include more recent traumatic experiences involving peers during adolescence or adulthood. We clearly need a consensus about definitions of sexual abuse.

3. *Severity of the abuse.* One important, although very complex, factor that has not been assessed in most studies is the severity and duration of the abuse. Research data (e.g., Boon & Drayer, 1993) show a relation between the degree of adult psychopathology and the severity of sexual abuse - for instance, abuse starting before the age of five years, abuse combined with violence or physical abuse, and abuse involving multiple perpetrators who are close relatives. Evaluation of severity remains, however, a difficult issue, because it concerns first and foremost the subjective experience of the victim. Furthermore, one must take into account the perceived response to (attempts of) disclosure. A lack of reaction or a hostile response may be at least as traumatic as the event itself (Waller & Ruddock, 1993).

4. *Assessment of sexual abuse.* Personal characteristics of the investigator (male or female, involved in the therapy or not), the timing of the assessment (before, during, or after therapy), and the methods of gathering information may have an impact on the results. Currently, no data are available that support the use of a specific assessment method, for instance self-report

questionnaire versus standardized interview. Moreover, there always remains the problem of memory distortion and induction, especially in this group of highly vulnerable, suggestible, and emotionally labile patients.

Next, suppose the data are somewhat reliable, what are the major findings then?

* Sexual abuse is reported by a substantial number of women with an eating disorder. Approximately 20 to 50 % report a history of childhood sexual abuse, but such rates have also been found in other psychiatric patients. Compared to the general female population, the rate of abuse appears to be higher in eating disorder patients (Welch & Fairburn, 1993).

* The rate of sexual abuse seems to be higher in patients with bulimic symptoms compared to restricting anorexics (Waller, 1992, 1993; Vanderlinden et al., 1993).

* Sexual abuse is more often associated with comorbidity, especially borderline personality disorder (Waller, 1992) and dissociative symptoms (Vanderlinden, 1993).

A specific and direct connection between sexual abuse (or other traumatic experiences) and the subsequent development of an eating disorder has not been demonstrated yet. But both the available research data and our own clinical experiences in therapeutic work with these patients seem to lead to at least one general conclusion: serious sexual and/or physical abuse in childhood and early adolescence puts the individual at special risk for developing psychological crises and even psychiatric disorders, including anorexia and bulimia nervosa.

## 5  Implications for Clinical Practice

Considering that an important subgroup of eating disorder patients reports pathological dissociative experiences in relation to childhood trauma, what are the implications of these findings for the therapeutic work with these patients? First, these data show that the therapist must carefully and routinely diagnose and assess both the possible presence of childhood trauma and dissociative symptoms in all eating disorder patients. Diagnosing anorexia and bulimia nervosa only on the basis of the eating pathology can be misleading. Here we want to recommend the use of standardized clinical interviews and questionnaires to assess the possible presence of childhood trauma and dissociative symptoms. A higher score on the dissociation questionnaire may indicate a history of trauma, especially high scores on the DIS-Q subscales "identity confusion" (> 2.9) and "amnesia" (> 2.5).

When a history of childhood trauma has been discovered, the question may arise: Do we have to treat the eating disorder first or the traumatic experience? We recommend first helping the patient gain better control over her eating behavior pattern. When a favorable development is noticeable in the eating/weight symptoms, in the second phase, the therapist may begin to explore the meaning and dynamics of traumatic memories and experiences. Hypnosis may be particularly useful in both exploring, identifying, and modifying traumatic memories and associated feelings (Vanderlinden & Vandereycken, 1990).

On reflection, many of the symptoms of the eating disorder may have a special meaning or function (see also Root & Fallon, 1989). Some examples:

1. Bingeing or fasting may be a way to anaesthetize intense negative feelings, such as anger, pain, anxiety, and powerlessness, that are associated with the trauma.

2. Vomiting/purging and/or fasting may serve to cleans oneself in a symbolic manner of negative sexual experiences.

3. By bingeing and/or fasting, the patient may be expressing her anger, feelings of hatred, guilt and inferiority; this frequently occurs in traumatized patients.

5. Bingeing and/or fasting may be viewed as attempts, in a very concrete manner, to render the body utterly unattractive sexually so as to construct a psychological and physical barrier or boundary and to keep other people at a distance.

6. Bingeing and/or fasting may be experienced as a way to relax and calm down, when particular traumatic events with accompanying feelings are relived.

The confrontation with traumatic experiences often brings about a serious emotional crisis and a relapse into the eating symptomatology. The therapist should prepare the patient for this. Sometimes, a short-term admission to a hospital may be indicated in order to be able to offer the patient sufficient security and protection. The main goal of the treatment is the integration of the traumatic memories and feelings into the patient's personality.

## References

Bailey, C.A., & Gibbons, S.J. (1989). Physical victimization and bulimic-like symptoms: Is there a relationship? *Deviant Behavior, 10*, 335-352.
Bernstein, E.M., & Putnam, F. (1986). Development, reliability and validity of a dissociation scale. *Journal of Nervous and Mental Disease, 174*, 727-735.
Boon, S., & Draijer, N. (1993). *Multiple personality disorder in the Netherlands: A study on reliability and validity of the diagnosis.* Amsterdam: Swets & Zeitlinger.
Bulik, C.M., Sullivan, P.F., & Rorty, M. (1989). Childhood sexual abuse in women with bulimia. *Journal of Clinical Psychiatry, 50*, 460-464.
Calam, R.M., & Slade, P.D. (1989). Sexual experiences and eating problems in female undergraduates. *International Journal of Eating Disorders, 8*, 391-397.
Connors, M.E., & Morse, W. (1993). Sexual abuse and eating disorders. *International Journal of Eating Disorders, 13*, 1-11.
Derogatis, L.R. (1983). *SCL-90: Administration, scoring and procedures manual.* Townson, MD: Clinical Psychometric Research.
Finn, S., Hartman, M., Leon, G., & Lawson, L. (1986). Eating disorders and sexual abuse: Lack of confirmation for a clinical hypothesis. *International Journal of Eating Disorders, 5*, 1051-1060.
Folsom, V., Krahn, D., Nairn, K., Gold, L., Demitrack, M.A., & Silk, K.R. (1993). The impact of sexual abuse and physical abuse on eating disordered and psychiatric symptoms: A comparison of eating disordered and psychiatric inpatients. *International Journal of Eating Disorders, 13*, 249-257.
Garner, D., & Garfinfel, P.E. (1979). The Eating Attitudes Test: An index of the symptoms of anorexia nervosa. *Psychological Medicine, 9*, 273-279.
Garner, D., Olmsted, M.P., & Polivy, J. (1983). Development and validation of a multidimensional eating disorder inventory for anorexia and bulimia. *International Journal of Eating Disorders, 2*, 15-35.
Goldfarb, L. (1987). Sexual abuse antecedent to anorexia nervosa, bulimia and compulsive overeating: Three case reports. *International Journal of Eating Disorders, 6*, 675-680.
Hall, R.C.W., Tice, L., Beresford, T.P., Wooley, B., & Hall, A.K. (1989). Sexual abuse in patients with anorexia nervosa and bulimia. *Psychosomatics, 30*, 79-88.
Kearney-Cooke, A. (1988). Group treatment of sexual abuse among women with eating disorders. *Women and Therapy, 7*, 5-22.
Lacey, J.H. (1990). Incest, incestuous fantasy and indecency: A clinical catchment area study of normal-weight bulimic women. *British Journal of Psychiatry, 157*, 399-403.
Lange, A. (1990). *A questionnaire on sexual experiences in the past.* Unpublished report, Free University of Amsterdam.
McFarlane, A.C., McFarlane, C., & Gilchrist, P.N. (1988). Post-traumatic bulimia and anorexia nervosa. *International Journal of Eating Disorders, 7*, 705-708.
Miller, D.A.F., & McCluskey-Fawcett, K. (1993). The relationship between childhood sexual abuse and subsequent onset of bulimia nervosa. *Child Abuse and Neglect, 17*, 305-314.
Oppenheimer, R., Howells, K., Palmer, L., & Chaloner, D. (1985). Adverse sexual experiences in childhood and clinical eating disorders: A preliminary description. *Journal of Psychiatric Research, 19*, 157-161.
Palmer, R.L., Oppenheimer, R., Dignon, A., Chaloner, D., Howells, K. (1990). Childhood sexual experiences with adults reported by women with eating disorders: An extended series. *British Journal of Psychiatry, 156*, 699-703.
Pope, H.G., & Hudson, K.I. (1992). Is childhood sexual abuse a risk factor for bulimia nervosa. *American Journal of Psychiatry, 149*, 455-463.
Root, M.P., & Fallon, P. (1988). The incidence of victimization experiences in a bulimic sample. *Journal of Interpersonal Violence, 3*, 161-173.
Russell, D. (1983). The incidence and prevalence of intrafamilial and extrafamilial sexual abuse of female children. *Child Abuse and Neglect, 7*, 133-146.

Schechter, I.D., Schwartz, H.P., & Greenfield, D.G. (1987). Sexual assault and anorexia nervosa. *International Journal of Eating Disorders, 6*, 313-316.

Sloan, G., & Leighner, P. (1986). Is there a relationship between sexual abuse or incest and eating disorders? *Canadian Journal of Psychiatry, 31*, 656-660.

Smolak, L., Levine, M., & Sullins, E. (1990). Are child sexual experiences related to eating-disordered attitudes and behaviors in a college sample? *International Journal of Eating Disorders, 9*, 167-178.

Steiger, H., & Zanko, M. (1990). Sexual traumata among eating-disordered, psychiatric and normal female groups. *Journal of Interpersonal Violence, 5*, 74-86.

Torem, M.S. (1986). Dissociative states presenting as an eating disorder. *American Journal of Clinical Hypnosis, 29*, 137-142.

Vandereycken, W. (1993). The Eating Disorder Evaluation Scale (EDES). *Eating Disorders, 1*, 115-122.

Vanderlinden, J. (1993). *Dissociative experiences, trauma and hypnosis: Research findings and clinical applications in eating disorders*. Delft: Eburon.

Vanderlinden, J., & Vandereycken, W. (1990). The use of hypnosis in the treatment of bulimia nervosa. *International Journal of Clinical and Experimental Hypnosis, 38*, 101-111.

Vanderlinden, J., Vandereycken, W., Van Dyck, R., & Vertommen, H. (1993). Dissociative experiences and trauma in eating disorders. *International Journal of Eating Disorders, 13*, 187-194.

Vanderlinden, J., Van Dyck, R., Vandereycken, W., Vertommen, H., & Verkes, R.J. (1993). The Dissociation Questionnaire: Development and characteristics of a new self-reporting questionnaire. *Clinical Psychology and Psychotherapy, 1*, 21-27.

Waller, G. (1991). Sexual abuse as a factor in eating disorders. *British Journal of Psychiatry, 159*, 664-671.

Waller, G. (1992). Sexual abuse and the severity of bulimic symptoms. *British Journal of Psychiatry, 161*, 90-93.

Waller, G. (1993). Sexual abuse and eating disorders: Borderline personality disorder as a mediating factor? *British Journal of Psychiatry, 162*, 771-775.

Waller, G., & Ruddock, A. (1993). Experiences of disclosure of childhood sexual abuse and psychopathology. *Child Abuse Review, 2*, 185-195.

Welch, S.L., & Fairburn, C.G. (1994). Sexual abuse and bulimia nervosa: Three integrated case control comparisons. *American Journal of Psychiatry, 151*, 402-407.

Wooley, S., & Kearney-Cooke, A. (1986). Intensive treatment of bulimia and body-image disturbance. In K.D. Brownell & J.P. Foreyt (Eds.), *Handbook of eating disorders* (pp.476-502). New York: Basic Books.

# Neurobiology of Eating Disorders in Adolescence

*Karl Martin Pirke and Petra Platte*

## 1 Introduction

Anorexia nervosa and bulimia nervosa are psychosomatic disorders characterized by various interactions between behavior and neurobiology. For example, permanent or intermittent starvation seen in eating disorders causes many endocrine alterations necessary for survival. On the other hand, starvation induces alterations of the neurotransmitter metabolism in the brain responsible for psychological disturbances. This is suggested by significant correlations between norepinephrine responses to orthostatic challenges and mood in anorectic patients studied longitudinally by Laessle et al. (1988).

Another example of psychosomatic interactions in eating disorders is the increase of cortisol secretion due to starvation. Hypercortisolism rapidly develops when the nutritional supply of carbohydrates is reduced beyond a critical threshold. An increased secretion of cortisol is needed for gluconeogenesis (the production of glucose from aminoacids produced during the breakdown of the proteins in muscle tissue). This process is necessary in order to supply glucose for the nutrition of the brain. Although 70% of the energy requirement of the brain can by substituted by betahydroxybutyricacids and acetoacetate, 30% of the energy requirement has to be supplied by glucose. However, the abnormality of cortisol secretion does have somatic and psychological consequences: we can assume that hypercortisolism contributes to the development of osteoporosis in eating disorders (Halmi, 1987). Laessle et al. (1990) have demonstrated cognitive deficits in patients with eating disorders, which correlated significantly with hypercortisolism. Hypercortisolism seems to play a role in the development of pseudoatrophy in the brain (Krieg et al., 1989), which can be regularly observed in patients with anorexia and bulimia nervosa. Additional studies are needed to evaluate the interactions between atrophy of the brain, cognitive deficits, and hypercortisolism. Also, it is currently unclear whether the cognitive impairments observed in laboratory experiments correlate with the impaired ability of eating disorder patients in every day problem solving.

The examples mentioned above underline the necessity of neurobiological studies in eating disorders. Three topics will be addressed in this chapter: (a) disturbance and maturation of the hypothalamicpituitary gonadal axis and its consequences; (b) the role of gastrointestinal hormones in eating disorders; (c) energy metabolism in eating disorders with special emphasis on the interactions between total energy expenditure and hyperactivity.

## 2 Maturation and Disturbances of the Hypothalamicpituitary Gonadal Axis and Consequences

The first endocrine manifestation of puberty in boys and girls is the so-called adrenarche. On the average, two years before the actual process of puberty, the adrenal gland starts to produce increasing amounts of androgen hormones such as DHEA (dehydroepiandrosterone). This weak androgen is, among others, responsible for the development of axillary hair. The prepubertal state is understood as a state of high sensitivity of the gonadal pituitary and the gonadal hypothalamic feedback system. During puberty this sensitivity decreases and gonadotropin secretion is no longer suppressed by the low circulating concentrations of androgens and estrogens characteristic of the immature state. The first significant increases of gonadotropin secretion occur only during sleep. At this time, the follicle stimulating hormone (FSH) response to gonadotropin releasing hormone is much greater than the luteinizing hormone (LH) response. During the next months, the episodic secretion of gonadotropins is no longer restricted to sleep but also occurs during the day. Response to gonadotropin releasing hormone (GnRH) becomes more mature, meaning that the LH increase becomes higher than the FSH increase.

When anorectic patients lose weight, they return to an infantile state of the hypothalamic pituitary gonadal axis. Even adrenarche is reversed, as indicated by low plasma concentrations of DHEA. During weight gain in anorectic patients, the pubertal development is repeated. As demonstrated in Figure 1, a pubertal LH

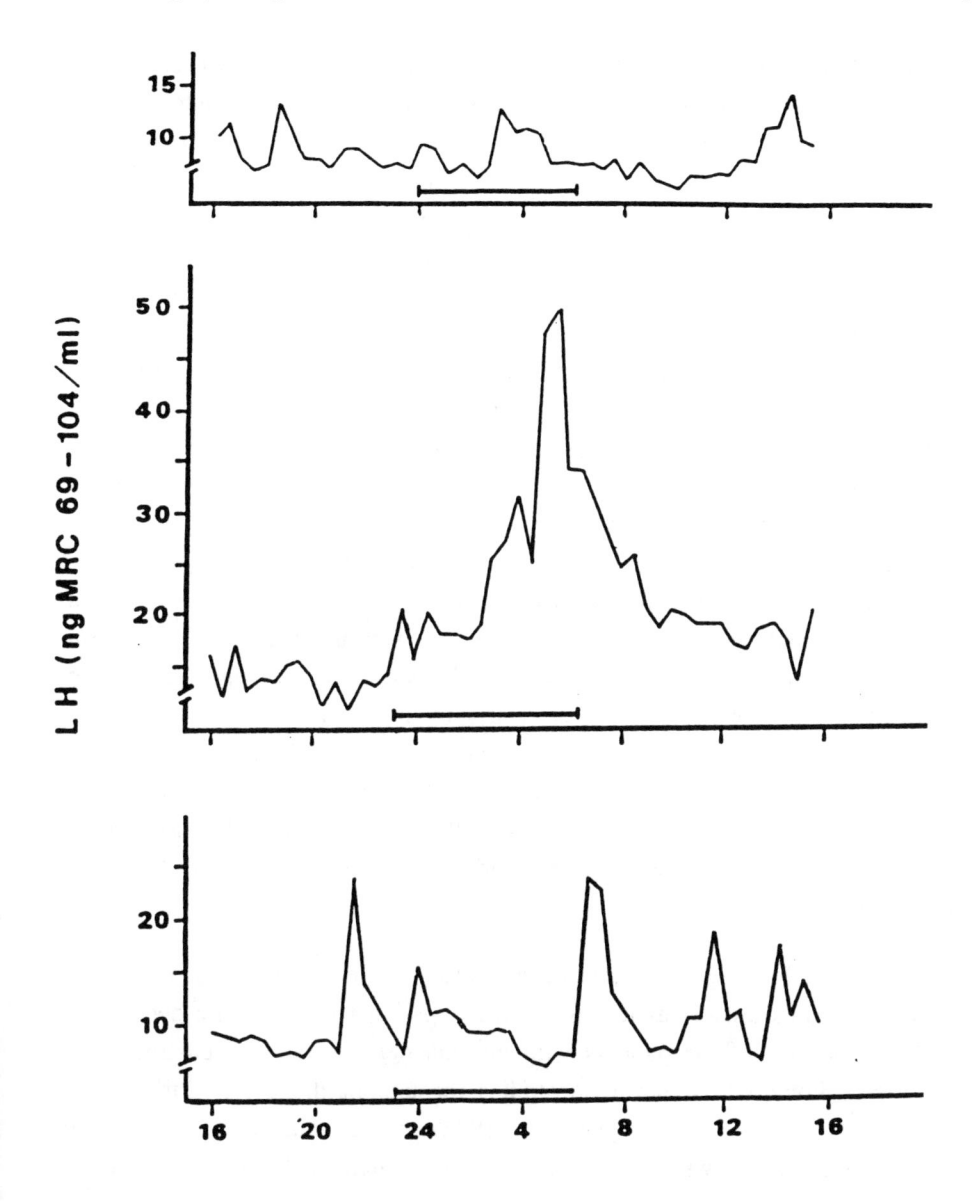

Figure 1.  LH secretion pattern in an 18 year old anorectic patient

Upper part:     prepubertal pattern at 66.2 % IBW
Middle part:    pubertal LH secretion pattern at 80 % IBW
Lower part:     adult LH secretion pattern at 83.2 % IBW

secretion pattern characterized by sleep-dependent increases can be observed. This pattern finally matures into an adult pattern in which the sleep dependence is lost and episodic gonadotropin secretions occur during night and day. As in normal pubertal development, the response to GnRH injection also normalizes, meaning that the FSH response slowly becomes smaller while the LH increase becomes greater. During this process, the ovary undergoes a polycystic state characterized by many small systems. Several studies have proven that this repeated pubertal development during weight gain is not only observed in patients with anorexia nervosa but can also be observed after weight loss and weight gain due to other causes (Vigersky & Loriaux, 1977). Although it is clear that low body weight or weight loss is responsible for the impairment of the hypothalamic pituitary gonadal axis, it is not clear which mechanisms are involved. It has been suggested that increased production of endorphins may be responsible. However, because it is not possible to stimulate normal LH and FSH secretion by endorphin antagonists such as nalaxone or naltrexone in low weight anorectics, this hypothesis appears unlikely. Menstrual cycles can be induced in low weight anorectics by injecting synthetic GnRH at 60 to 90 minutes intervals. This observation suggested that the hypogonadism in anorectic patients is clearly of hypothalamic origin. Numerous animal experiments in starved rats (Pirke & Spyra, 1981, 1982) gave no hint about which of the neurotransmitter or neuromodulator systems regulate the starvation-induced hypogonadism. The understanding of this problem would be, however, of greatest importance for the understanding of anorexia nervosa specifically and of pubertal development in general.

Whereas low body weight can explain menstrual cycle disturbances in anorexia nervosa, it remains unclear as to why so many patients with bulimia nervosa are infertile. About 1/3 of the patients with bulimia nervosa report menstrual cycle disturbances. Longitudinal hormone studies throughout the cycle (Pirke et al., 1987; Pirke et al., 1988; Schweiger et al., 1992) showed that more than 50 % of normal weight patients with bulimia nervosa have menstrual cycle disturbances. These disturbances can be divided into two categories. The more severe form of menstrual cycle disturbances is the unovulatory cycle as shown in the upper part of Figure 2. As judged from the consistently low estradiol values throughout the observation period, no follicular development occurred. Consequently, no follicle can be fertilized. This is a state of absolute infertility. A milder form of menstrual cycle disturbance is illustrated in the middle part of Figure 2. Seemingly normal development of the follicle judged from the increasing estradiol levels is shown.

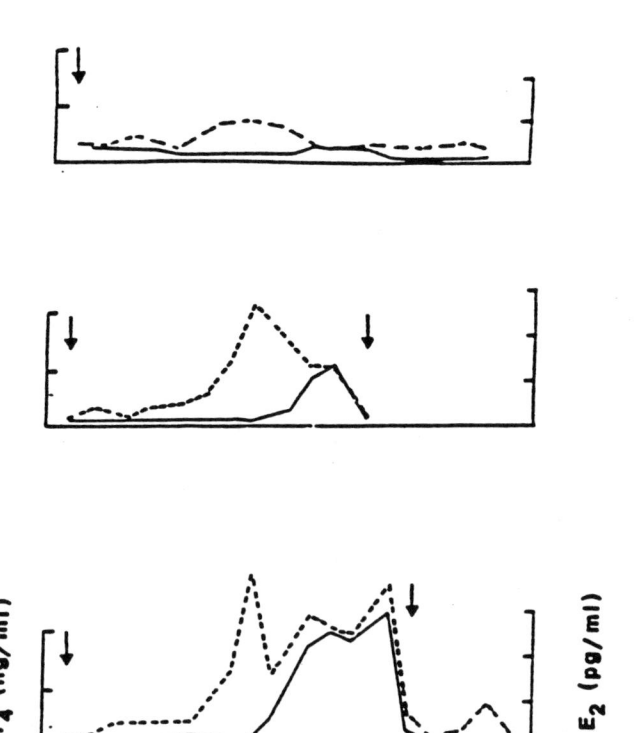

Figure 2. Estradiol ( ... ) and progesteron ( __ ) in patients with bulimia nervosa.

Upper part:  anovulatory cycle
Middle part: luteal phase defect
Lower part:  normal cycle

However, the progesterone values during the second part of the cycle are too low compared to a normal cycle (lower part of Figure 2). The luteal phase is shorter than normal. Luteal phase defects do not present states of absolute infertility. However, the chance of implantation for the fertilized egg is greatly reduced. The nature of infertility in bulimia nervosa became evident when episodic gonadotropin secretion was studied. Figure 3 shows that, in some patients with anovulatory cycles, the episodic secretion of LH is entirely absent. Some of the anovulatory bulimic patients, however, show apparently normal or only slightly disturbed patterns of episodic LH secretion (lower part of Figure 3). This probably means that other mechanisms acting on the level of the ovaries can also disturb menstrual cycle in bulimia nervosa. The nature of the hypothalamic and extra hypothalamic

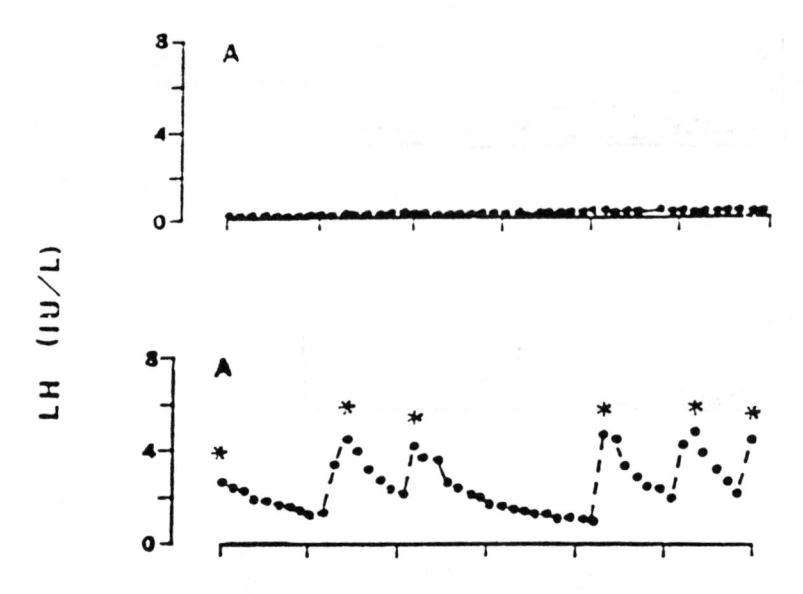

Figure 3. An anovulatory cycle

mechanisms responsible for the development of infertility in bulimia nervosa remains unclear. However, one observation seems to be relevant here. We observed that patients with anovulatory cycles had significantly higher cortisol plasma concentrations during the night in comparison with bulimic patients with normal cycles or luteal phase defects. Because it is well known that glucocorticoids can suppress the production of sex steroids in the gonads, we may speculate that hypercortisolism is an additional factor contributing to the development of infertility bulimia nervosa.

Dieting with minor or moderate weight loss has been shown to cause menstrual cycle disturbances (anovulatory cycles and luteal phase defects) in normal-weight, healthy young women (Pirke, Schweiger, Laessle, Dickhaut, Schweiger & Wachtler, 1986; Pirke et al., 1989; Schweiger et al., 1987). Frequent dieting with major weight fluctuations is observed in many patients with bulimia nervosa (Woell et al., 1989). We may speculate that these weight fluctuations are responsible for the occurrence of menstrual cycle disturbances in bulimia nervosa. This assumption however still has to be proven. The question of whether or not the intensity of weight fluctuationcorrelates with the development of anovulatory cycles in bulimia still has to be studied. The absolute body weight may also play a role. Being slightly overweight might protect patients from developing anovulatory cycles during weight fluctuations whereas weight at the lower end of the normal range may predispose bulimic patients for the development of anovulatory cycles. Unfortunately, bulimic patients with anovulatory cycles have not been followed up during treatment and normalization of eating behavior. We, therefore, do not know whether these patients undergo pubertal development of the hypothalamicpituitary gonadal axis as the much younger patients with anorexia nervosa do.

As is a case of anorexia, we do not have any information on the hypothalamic mechanism involved in the development of suppression of GnRH release in bulimia. From a biological point of view, it is important that fertility is suppressed when the availability of food is reduced. A women carrying a child would stand a much smaller chance of survival during a starvation period than a women not carrying a child. Thus, the rapid reduction of fertility during the periods of reduced availability of food seems to be important for the survival of the individuals and the human species. In the case of anorexia nervosa and bulimia, these mechanisms do have major disadvantages too. The suppression of gonadal hormone production rapidly causes osteoporosis which increases the risk of bone fracture. Osteoporosis has been demonstrated in both anorexia nervosa and bulimia nervosa. The lack of gonadal hormones may even have long term effects. It has been speculated that even after recovery from the eating disorders and the normalization of gonadal hormone secretion, the mineral content of the bone may remain too low so that during menopause, when there is a general loss of bone minerals, former anorectic and bulimic patients might end up with a greatly reduced mineral content of the bone that had occured during the initial mineral loosing period.

Clearly, osteoporosis is not only the consequence of low gonadal hormone productions. Other factors like prolonged hypercortisolism and pure nutritional intake of calcium and phosphate contribute to the development of osteoporosis. Therefore, we must assume that the prevention of osteoporosis in eating disorders can not simply be achieved by substituting estrogens and gestagens. A rapid and successful treatment of the eating disorders seems to be the most promising way to treat osteoporosis in eating disorders.

## 3   The Role of Gastrointestinal Hormones in Eating Disorders

Gastrointestinal hormones are secreted in different parts of the gastrointestinal tract as well as in the central nervous system. These hormones regulate many gastrointestinal functions. Like insulin, they are important for homeostasis. Because they are of great importance for the regulation of hunger and satiety, they have been studied in eating disorders in which a severe disturbance of hunger and satiety feelings can be assumed. In this section the role of insulin, somatostatin, and cholecystokinin will be discussed.

## 3.1 Insulin

It is a well known fact that food intake regulates insulin secretion. Food intake stimulates insulin production and the nutritional status determines basal insulin levels in plasma. In a hypocaloric state we observe low basal insulin concentrations. In a hypercaloric state we see increased insulin levels. It was, therefore, not surprising that low basal insulin concentrations were described in starving anorectic patients and in intermittently dieting persons with bulimia nervosa (Schreiber et al., 1991; Stordy et al., 1977). In contrast, obese subjects generally show elevated basal insulin secretion. When carbohydrate test meals were given to anorectic and bulimic patients, an exaggerated insulin secretion was observed. Considering the elevated insulin response, one would have expected a reduced or blunted glucose increase. This however, was not the case, despite increased insulin values, glucose concentrations after the test meal were higher in anorectic patients than in healthy controls. Similar observations were reported in patients with bulimia nervosa (Schweiger et al., 1987). These observations suggest that the effect of insulin at the receptor or post receptor site may be impaired. Insulin has been implicated in the regulation of satiety. However, because too little is known about the role of insulin in satiety and because the release and effects of insulin are altered in a rather complex way, as demonstrated above, it remains unclear whether insulin plays a role in hunger and satiety regulation in eating disorders.

## 3.2 Somatostatin

Somatostatin is a tetradecapeptide produced in many brain areas and in other tissues (Pearse et al., 1977). The majority of the somatostatin producing cells in the intestinal tract are located in the pancreas (D-cells) and in cells located in the gastric antrum (McIntosh et al., 1978). Most gastrointestinal hormones are inhibited by somatostatin (Lamers, 1987; Schusdziarra, 1988). The suppressing effect on insulin secretion is well documented. We have, therefore, hypothesized that somatostatin secretion should be elevated in anorectic patients with low basal insulin secretion.

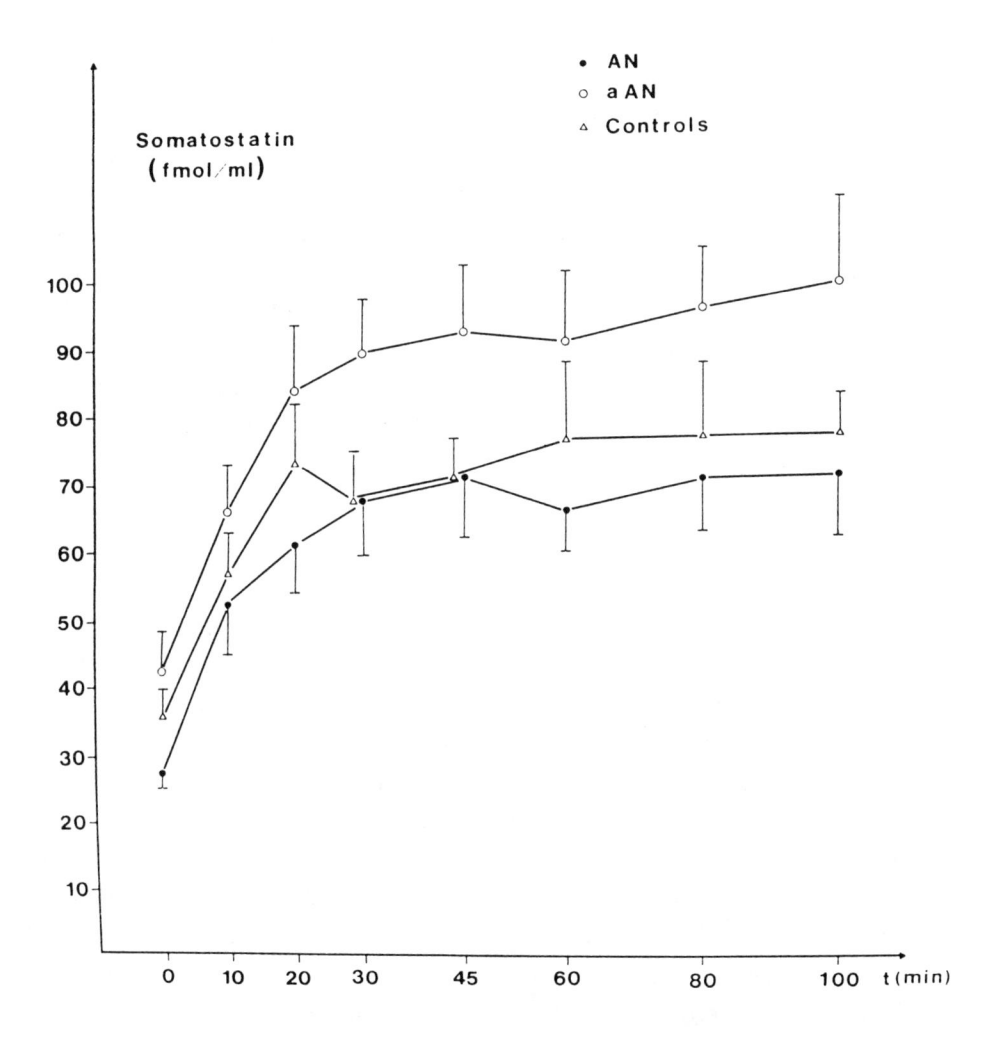

Figure 4. Plasma somatostatin before and after a standardized protein and fat-rich test meal: AN = weight-recovered anorectics; aAN = acutely ill anorectics.

Gastric emptying is inhibited by somatostatin (Creutzfeldt & Arnold, 1978). The impaired gastric emptying in anorectic patients, which has been described by many authors, could also be caused by an increase in somatostatin secretion.

We have measured somatostatin before and after a standardized fluid test meal of 800 kcal. The macronutrient composition was: 20 % protein, 40 % carbohydrates, and 40 % fat. Blood was sampled for up to 100 minutes. Somatostatin was analyzed by radioimmunoassay after extraction from plasma, as described in detail by Pirke, Friess, Kellner, Krieg & Fichter (1994). As demonstrated in Figure 4, the plasma concentrations of somatostatin were significantly elevated after the test meal in all three groups studied (anorectic patients, weight-recovered anorectics, and normal healthy controls). As predicted, there was indeed a significantly higher increase in somatostatin in the acutely ill anorectic group. Weight-recovered anorectics are, however, not different from controls, indicating that the elevated somatostatin release is state rather than trait dependent. Although the increased somatostatin response may be causally related to the impaired gastric emptying and to the suppression of basal insulin secretion, additional studies are needed to prove this relation.

### 3.3 Cholecystokinin (CCK)

Cholecystokinin, which circulates in peripheral blood in different molecular forms, was originally named after its ability to stimulate gall bladder contraction. It delays gastric emptying, however, it enhances small bowel utility, and it stimulates the secretion of pancreatic enzymes. Many studies in experimental animals and in man have suggested that CCK also plays a role in satiety (Gibbs & Smith, 1977). It is assumed that CCK bindes to receptors at the vagus nerve and that information on satiety is transported in this way to the hypothalamus. When we first studied CCK secretion in anorexia nervosa, bulimia, and in healthy controls, we employed a method in which different molecular forms of cholecystokinin were measured. In response to the test meal described earlier in the somatostatin study, CCK in anorectics was significantly higher than in bulimic patients and healthy controls. Separation of the different molecular forms of CCK showed that CCK-8-S was indeed lower in bulimic patients than in anorectics (Philipp et al., 1991). We later extended studies on CCK-8-S (Pirke, Kellner, Friess, Krieg & Fichter, 1994). In this experiment, the response of 18 anorectic and 17 bulimic patients and of 25 healthy controls was measured after the protein and fat rich test meal. As in the first study, bulimic patients had significantly lower responses than anorectic patients. However, the CCK-8-S responses of the normal controls (not studied in the first experiment) did not differ from those of the anorectic patients. This finding supports an earlier report by Geracioti & Liddle (1988), who measured CCK secretion using a bioassay. We may speculate that the reduced CCK-8-S response in bulimic patients causes reduced satiety and thus enables the bulimic patients to eat huge amounts of food during the binge attack. This is, however, in contrast to the subjective satiety ratings given by the bulimic patients during the same experiment. Bulimic patients gave higher satiety ratings after the test meal than did the normal controls.

In summarizing the results of the gastrointestinal hormone studies reported here, although abnormal secretion patterns have been found for all gastrointestinal hormones studied in either anorexia and bulimia nervosa, the consequences for the understanding of gastrointestinal function and of the regulation of hunger and satiety remain unclear. We hope that the use of agonists and antagonists of gastrointestinal hormones available now for clinical research may help to understand the interaction between gastrointestinal hormones and the regulation of eating in eating disorders.

## 4  Energy Metabolism in Eating Disorders

The energy needed to maintain a given body weight, i.e., total energy expenditure (TEE), consists of three parts: basal metabolic rate (BMR), diet induced thermogenesis (DIT), and energy requirement for physical activity (EA). The basal or resting metabolic rate - mainly influenced by the metabolic active lean body mass, the nutritional state, and the thyroid hormones - accounts for about 60% of the TEE. The second component is the DIT, i.e., the energy expended in the assimilation of food. This expenditure is mainly influenced by the composition of the food and accounts for about 10% of the TEE. The third component is the energy expended for physical activity and accounts for about 30% of the TEE. However, there is evidence that both BMR and DIT are adaptive, which means that they are influenced by current or antecedent energy balance. It is said that food restriction, for instance, can lead to down regulation of BMR, while intense athletic training can decrease DIT. The EA has a high variance and is, of course, determined by the level of physical activity. Energy metabolism can also be severely altered by smoking, coffee drinking, dieting, or exercising (Blackburn et al., 1989; Hofstetter et al., 1986; Poehlmann & Horton, 1989; Tuschl et al., 1991).

The caloric requirements necessary for patients with anorexia nervosa to gain weight were investigated in many studies. These studies showed a large variation in energy requirements within each study, and it is not clear why the variance is so great. High physical activity might contribute to the difficulty of weight gain in anorexia nervosa. Hyperactivity is frequently observed in anorectic patients and may to a great extent influence total energy expenditure. The knowledge of total energy expenditure is the basis for the development of appropriate strategies for treating anorexia nervosa. We did several studies to investigate the total energy expenditure in anorectic patients and controls using the doubly labeled water method. This technique provides a reliable and nonintrusive method for determining TEE in free living subjects. Its validity in humans was convincingly shown in a range of daily life activity levels (Schoeller et al., 1986). The rationale depends on the difference in turnover rates of the oxygen and hydrogen of body water. The stable isotopes D2 and O18 are given orally. They equilibrate within the body's water pool. D2 then leaves the body as water, mainly in the urine. Oxygen18 leaves the body as water and as respiratory carbon dioxide. Therefore, the rate of carbon dioxide production can be determined by the difference in elimination rates of the two isotopes. Energy expenditure is subsequently calculated from the carbon dioxide production rate by use of the standard formula of indirect calorimetry and an estimate of the respiratory quotient (De Weir, 1949). Basal or resting metabolic rate can be measured after an overnight fast using a ventilated hood system, an open circuit indirect calorimeter.

Many reports have been published on RMR (resting metabolic rate) in anorexia nervosa (for review, see Melchior et al., 1989). All reports found a reduced RMR, however some authors demonstrate that this effect is brought about by a reduction in lean body mass (LBM) only, whereas others show an additional reduction of RMR, presumably as a consequence of endocrine changes such as low triiodothyronine (T3) values or reduced norepinephrine secretion seen in most patients with anorexia nervosa (Heufelder et al., 1985). TEE has been studied either by recording caloric intake (Kaye, Gwirtsman, Obarzandek, George, Himmerson & Ebert, 1986) or by using the doubly labeled water method (Casper et al., 1991; Pirke et al., 1991). Pirke et al. (1991) found surprisingly high TEE values in anorectic patients, although the absolute values reported varied widely among research groups. High TEE in acute anorectics might be explained by the high physical activity. Some clinical reports comment that larger than normal quantities of food intake are required for weight gain in anorectics (Dempsey et al., 1984; Kaye, Gwirtsman, Obarzandek, George, Himmerson & Ebert, 1986). The study by Kaye, Gwirtsman, Obarzandek and George (1986) showed elevated caloric requirements during recovery from anorexia nervosa, with no difference in caloric intake compared with the controls after weight maintenance. The balance of total energy input and output governs weight development. The energy cost of exercise and diet induced thermogenesis contribute to TEE, as does the basal metabolic rate. Hyperactivity is frequently observed in anorectic patients (Kron et al., 1987) and may also influence TEE to a great extent.

Knowing the TEE is the basis for the development of appropriate strategies to treat eating disorders. Using the doubly labeled water technique and indirect calorimetry, we did two studies. In a first study we measured TEE in hyperactive anorectic patients and in controls. Anorexia nervosa was diagnosed according to DSM-III-R criteria (American Psychiatric Association, 1987). Four anorectics were restricters and four were vomiters. The normal weight healthy women were unrestrained eaters. They had to score three or less on the factor "cognitive restraint" of the Three Factor Eating Questionnaire of Stunkard and Messick (Stunkard & Messick, 1985). Table 1 gives the physical characteristics of the subjects of the first study.

Table 1.   Physical Characteristics of the Subjects

|  | Controls (N = 11) | Anorexia nervosa (N = 8) | p |
|---|---|---|---|
| Age (yr) | 24.5 ± 4.2 | 27.8 ± 5.2 | ns |
| Height (m) | 1.69 ± 0.05 | 1.68 ± 0.03 | ns |
| Weight 1st day (kg) | 57.5 ± 5.1 | 43.0 ± 5.6 | 0.00 |
| Weight 15th day (kg) | 57.3 ± 5.1 | 43.5 ± 5.8 | 0.00 |
| BMI (kg/m2) | 20.0 ± 1.3 | 15.2 ± 5.6 | 0.00 |
| Lean body mass (kg) | 43.6 ± 4.6 | 39.7 ± 2.6 | 0.05 |
| Lean body mass (% of body weight) | 71.6 ± 5.5 | 93.5 ± 8.4 | 0.00 |

All physical characteristics (with the exception of age and height) of the anorectic group are significantly different from those of the controls. In addition, the absolute amount of LBM and the relative amount of LBM are significantly different in the two groups. In the hyperactive group, 93% of body weight is represented as LBM. The total energy expenditure, triiodethyronine, and physical activity of both groups are given in Table 2. Activity diaries provide a rough indicator for physical activity. In this study, the hyperactive anorectics reported spending 115 minutes a day involved with physical activity. The control group reported spending 32 minutes a day in such activity. During the two week observation period, no group experienced any significant change in weight or body composition. The anorectic patients had a higher total energy expenditure than the controls but this difference is not significant. This study did not measure BMR or DIT.

Table 2.  Total Energy Expenditure, Triiodethyronine, and Physical Activity

|  | Controls (N=11) | Anorexia nervosa (N=8) | p |
|---|---|---|---|
| TEE (kcal/day) | 2357 ± 504 | 2899 ± 656 | ns |
| T3 (ng/ml) | 1.5 ± 0.2 | 0.9 ± 0.1 | 0.01 |
| Sports activity (min/day) | 32 ± 26 | 115 ± 52 | 0.00 |

Kaye et al. (1988) found a difference between vomiters and restricters with regard to energy requirement. We did not find this difference, probably because of the small sample size. The weight of the anorectic patients remained stable during the observation period. Although their body weight was, on the average, still 14.5 kg below that of the controls, their lean body mass was on the average only 3.9 kg lower, indicating that the remaining weight deficit was mainly due to lacking body fat. This is in agreement with earlier observations that, during weight gain, lean body mass is normalized more rapidly than fat in anorectics (Pirke, Pahl, Schweiger, Muenzing, Lang & Buell, 1986). Hyperactivity in anorexia has been widely documented (Kron et al., 1987) and is reflected in the activity diaries. Our activity diaries give only a rough indicator of the true activity, because only sport activities were recorded and the intensity of the activities were only subjectively rated. Activities such as fidgeting were not recorded so that, in reality, the total activity may be even greater than the diaries show. In this study, we have no information on the BMR. The decreased triiodethyronine values, however, suggest that the anorectic group might have had reduced energy expenditure under resting conditions, as described in the literature (Kaye, Gwirtsman, Obarzandek & Georg., 1986). Although a low BMR has been convincingly demonstrated in patients with eating disorders, the hyperactivity may determine the TEE in this anorectic group.

In the next study, BMR, DIT, and TEE were measured. Table 3 gives the physical characteristics of non-hyperactive anorectics, weight-gained anorectics, and controls. The anorectic patients were studied as inpatients in a hospital for behavioral medicine. Diagnoses were made according to the DSM-III-R criteria (American Psychiatric Association, 1987). Onset of anorexia nervosa occurred 10.3 (r 8.6) years before the start of this study. All patients had been hospitalized for at least 2 weeks. All patients were restricters. From a larger group of young women who had had an acute episode of anorexia nervosa (according to the DSM-III-R criteria) during the previous ten years, six women were selected as weight-recovered anorectics. The duration of illness in these six patients had been 2.8 (r 1.9) years. These former patients had a "good outcome" (normal weight and normal menstrual cycle) following an illness of 2.8 (r1.9) years duration, during which one patient showed bulimic episodes and the others were restricters. The normal subjects were unrestrained eaters who scored three or less on the factor "cognitive restraint" of the Three Factor Eating Questionnaire (Stunkard & Messick, 1985).

Table 3. Physical Characteristics of the Subjects

|  | Controls (N = 8) | Anorexia nervosa (N = 6) | Weight-gained anorectics (N = 8) |  |
| --- | --- | --- | --- | --- |
| Age (yr) | 25.2 ± 2.4 | 27.5 ± 7.8 | 24.6 ± 4.2 | ns |
| Height (m) | 1.68 ± .05 | 1.68 ± .05 | 1.71 ± .06 | ns |
| Weight 1st day (kg) | 59.9 ± 5.0 | 43.1 ± 4.5 | 60.8 ± 5.5 | <.05 [a,b] |
| Weight 15th day (kg) | 59.1 ± 5.2 | 43.6 ± 4.3 | 60.9 ± 5.9 | <.05 [a,b] |
| BMI (kg/m2) | 21.3 ± 1.9 | 15.2 ± 1.3 | 20.9 ± 1.8 | <.05 [a,b] |
| Lean body mass (kg) | 43.0 ± 3.0 | 36.5 ± 3.5 | 45.7 ± 3.8 | <.05 [a,b] |
| Lean body mass (% of body weight) | 72.0 ± 4.8 | 83.7 ± 6.0 | 75.3 ± 4.0 | <.05 [a,b] |

[a] controls versus anorexia nervosa,
[b] weight-gained versus anorexia nervosa

Height, weight, and body composition did not differ between the weight-gained anorectics and the control group. Patients with anorexia nervosa were significantly less heavy than controls and weight-gained anorectics. LBM and fat mass were also significantly lower in the anorectic group. Table 4 gives the data on RMR, TEE and activity. There was no difference in any component of the TEE between the weight-gained and the control groups. RMR and TEE were significantly lower in the acute anorectic group than in the control group. The reported daily time spent exercising did not differ between the groups. The difference between TEE and RMR, which mainly reflects energy used for physical activity, is slightly but not significantly higher in the weight-gained and control groups.

Table 4. Resting Metabolic Rate, Total Energy Expenditure, and Activity

|  | Controls (N = 12) | Anorexia nervosa (N = 6) | Weight-gained anorectics (N = 6) | p |
|---|---|---|---|---|
| RMR (kcal/day) | 1379 ± 146 | 1171 ± 113 | 1330 ± 131 | <.05 [a] |
| TEE (kcal/day) | 2596 ± 493 | 1946 ± 192 | 2692 ± 637 | <.05 [a] |
| TEE-RMR (kcal/day) | 1218 ± 437 | 755 ± 195 | 1273 ± 622 | ns |
| Exercise (min/day) | 42 ± 25 | 50 ± 24 | 38 ± 13 | ns |

[a] controls versus anorexia nervosa

In this study, RMR was significantly reduced in anorectic patients compared to controls. This is in agreement with many earlier studies reviewed by Keys et al. (1950). This difference disappeared after correcting RMR per unit of LBM: a) acute anorectics 32 ± 3.3 kcal/LBM (kg), b) weight-gained 29 ± 1.5 kcal/LBM (kg), c) controls 31 ± 1.8 kcal/LBM (kg). This finding is in agreement with the observation of Melchior et al. (1989) who concluded from their observations that RMR in anorectic patients is only reduced to the extent to which LBM is reduced. It is unclear why some authors observed the energy sparing effect in anorectic patients (Casper et al., 1991; Stordy et al., 1977) while others did not. Poehlmann and Horton (1989) have described the postexercise effect on RMR. This and other groups found that severe exercise increases RMR for up to one day. Because many anorectic patients are severe exercisers (Kron et al., 1987), we might speculate that the reduction of RMR, which we would expect in emaciated patients with anorexia nervosa, is compensated for by the postexercise effect on RMR. This is to our knowledge the third study of TEE measured by doubly labeled water method in acute anorectics. The paper by Casper et al. (1991) as well as our first study (Pirke et al., 1991) showed no difference between anorectics and controls. We have speculated that this effect was caused by the high level of physical activity that is often found in anorectics. This speculation is supported by the comparison of our two studies. In the first study we studied 8 anorectic patients who reported 115 (± 52) minutes of sports activity per day. They had an average TEE of 2899 ± 656 kcal/day. This very physically active group had a LBM of 39.7 (± 2.6) kg and a body weight of 43.0 (± 5.6) kg. In contrast to this group, the second group studied here had a lower LBM of 36.5 (± 3.5) kg, although their weight was not different from that of the first group 43.3 (± 4.5) kg. These patients reported a degree of sports activity that was less than half of the first group 50 (± 24) min/day and had a lower TEE 1946 (± 192) kcal/day.

The shortcomings of the method used to record sport activities are known. But the much higher LBM in our first study and the simultaneously elevated activity (assessed by the diaries) support the notion that activity diaries provide a valid but still rough categorization. Anorectics may use many calories in activities not considered as sport, such as fidgeting. Unfortunately, activity measurement is difficult to measure in anorectics because actometers do not give reliable results (unpublished results of our group), and more exact techniques like radar screening restrict subjects to a very limited room, and thus, interfere with activity. We may also speculate that the energy requirement for muscular work is altered in the anorectic patients, because biological changes were described in the muscle of anorectic patients (Russell et al., 1983). Our results suggest that it might be useful not only to influence the eating behavior in acute anorectic patients but also the activity behavior in order to normalize body weight.

## References

American Psychiatric Association. (1987). *Diagnostic and statistical manual of mental disorders* (3rd ed., revised). Washington, DC: American Psychiatric Press.

Blackburn, G.L., Wilson, G.T., & Kanders, B.S. (1989). Weight cycling: The experience of human dieters. *American Journal of Clinical Nutrition, 49*, 1105-1109.

Casper, R.C., Schoeller, D.A., Kushner, R., Hnilicka, J., & Trainer Gold, S. (1991). Total daily energy expenditure and activity level in anorexia nervosa. *American Journal of Clinical Nutrition, 53*, 1143-1150.

Creutzfeldt, W., & Arnold, R. (1978). Somatostatin and the stomach: Exocrine and endocrine aspects. *Metabolism, 27*, 1309.

Dempsey, D.T., Crosby, L.O., Pertschuk, M.J., Feurer, I.D., Buzby, G.P, & Mullen, J.L. (1984). Weight gain and nutritional efficacy in anorexia nervosa. *American Journal of Clinical Nutrition, 39,* 236-242.

De Weir, J.B.V. (1949). New methods for calculating metabolic rate with special reference to protein metabolism. *Journal of Physiology; 109,* 1-9.

Geracioti, T.D. Jr., & Liddle, R.A. (1988). Impaired cholecystoinin secretion in bulimia nervosa. *New England Journal of Medicine, 319,* 683-688.

Gibbs, J., & Smith, G.P. (1977). Cholecystokinin and satiety in rats and rhesus monkeys. *American Journal of Clinical Nutrition, 30,* 758-761.

Halmi, K.A. (1987). Anorexia Nervosa and Bulimia. *Ann. Rev. Med., 38,* 373-380.

Heufelder, A., Warnhoff, M, & Pirke, K.M. (1985). Platelet alpha-2-adrenoceptor and adenylate cyclase in patients with anorexia nervosa and bulimia. *Journal of Clinical Endocrinology and Metabolism, 61,* 1053-1060.

Hofstetter, A., Schutz, Y, Jequier, E, & Wahren, J. (1986). Increased 24-hour energy expenditure in cigarette smokers. *New England Jounral of Medicine, 314,* 79-82.

Kaye, W.H., Gwirtsman, H.E., George, T., Ebert, M.H., & Petersen, R. (1986). Caloric Consumption and activity levels after weight recovery in anorexia nervosa: a prolonged delay in normalization. *International Journal of Eating Disorders, 5,* 489-502.

Kaye, W.H, Gwirtsman, H.E., Obarzandek, E., & George, D.T. (1988). Relative importance of caloric intake needed to gain weight and level of physical activity in anorexia nervosa. *American Journal of Clinical Nutrition, 47,* 989-994.

Kaye, W.H., Gwirtsman, H.E., Obarzandek, E., George, D.T., Himmerson, D.C., & Ebert, M. H. (1986). Caloric intake necessary for weight maintenance in anorexia nervosa. Nonbulimics require greater caloric intake than bulimics. *American Journal of Clinical Nutrition, 44,* 435-443.

Keys, A., Brozek, J., Henschel, A., Mickelson, O., & Taylor, H.L. (1950). *The biology of human starvation.* Minneapolis: Minessota Press.

Krieg, J.C., Lauer, C., Leinsinger, G., Pahl, J., Schreiber, W., Pirke, K.M., & Moser, E.A. (1989). Brain morphology and regional cerebral blood flow in anorexia nervosa. *Biological Psychiatry, 25,* 1041-1048.

Kron, L., Katz, J.L., Gorzynski, G., & Weiner, H. (1987). Hyperactivity in anorexia nervosa. A fundamental clinical feature. *Comprehensive Psychiatry, 19,* 433-440.

Laessle, R.G., Bossert, S., Hanke, G., Hahlweg, K., & Pirke, K.M. (1990). Cognitive performence in patients with bulimia nervosa: Relationship to intermitent starvation. *Biological Psychiatry, 27,* 549-551.

Laessle, R.G., Kittl, S., Fichter, M.M., & Pirke, K.M. (1988). Cognitive correlates of depression in patients with eating disorders. *International Journal of Eating Disorders, 7:* 681-686.

Lamers, C.G. (1987). Clinical and pathophysiological aspects of somatostatin and the gastrointestinal tract. *Acta Endocrinology (Copenhagen), 286,* 19-25.

McIntosh, C., & Arnold, R. (1978). Gastrointestinal somatostatin in man and dog. *Metabolism, 27,* 1317.

Melchior, J.C., Rigaud, D., Rozen, r., Malon, D., & Apfelbaum, M. (1989). Energy expenditure economy induced by decrease in lean body mass in anorexia nervosa. *European Journal of Clinical Nutrition, 43,* 793-799.

Pearse, A.G.E., Polak, J.M., & Bloom, S.R. (1977). The newer gut hormones: Cellular sources, physiology, pathology and clinical aspects. *Gastroenterology, 72,* 746-761.

Philipp, E., Pirke, K.M., Kellner, M.B., & Krieg, H.C. (1991). Disturbed cholecystokinin secretion in patients with eating disorders. *Life Science, 48,* 2443-2450.

Pirke, K.M., Dogs, M., Fichter, M.M., & Tuschl, R.J. (1988). Gonadotrophins, oestardiol and progesterone during the menstrual cycle in bulimia nervosa. *Clinical Endocrinology, 29,* 265-270.

Pirke, K.M., Fichter, M.M., Chlond, C., Schweiger, U., Laessle, R.G., Schwingenschloegel, M., & Hoehl, C. (1987). Disturbances of the menstrual cycle in bulimia nervosa. *Clinical Endocrinology, 27,* 245-251.

Pirke, K.M., Friess, E., Kellner, M.B., Krieg, J.C., & Fichter, M.M. (1994). Somatostatin in Eating Disorders. *International Journal of Eating Disorders, 15,* 99-102.

Pirke, K.M., Kellner, M.B., Friess, E., Krieg, J.C., & Fichter, M.M. (1994). Satiety and Cholecystokinin. *International Journal of Eating Disorders, 15,* 63-69.

Pirke, K.M., Pahl, J., Schweiger, U., Muenzing, W., Lang, P., & Buell, U. (1986). Total body potassium, intracellular potassium and body composition in patients with anorexia nervosa during refeeding. *International Journal of Eating Disorders, 5,* 347-354.

Pirke, K.M., Schweiger, U., Laessle, R.G., Dickhaut, B., Schweiger, M., & Waechtler, M. (1986). Dieting influences the menstrual cycle: vegetarian versus non-vegetarian diet. *Fertility and Sterility, 46*, 1083-1088.

Pirke, K.M., Schweiger, U., Strowitzki, T., Tuschl, R.J., Laessle, R.G., Broocks, A., Huber, B., & Middendorf, R. (1989). Dieting causes menstrual irregularities in normal weight young women through impairment of episodic luteinizing hormone secretion. *Fertility and Sterility, 51*, 263-268.

Pirke, K.M., & Spyra, B. (1981). Influence of starvation on testosterone luteinizing hormone feedback in the rat. *Acta Endocrinologica (Kbh.), 96*, 413-421.

Pirke, K.M., & Spyra, B. (1982). Catecholamine turnover in the brain and the regulation of luteinizing hormone and corticosterone in starved male rats. *Acta Endocrinologica, 100*, 168-176.

Pirke, K.M., Trimborn, P., Platte, P., & Fichter, M.M. (1991). Average total energy expenditure in anorexia nervosa, bulimia nervosa and healthy young women. *Biological Psychiatry, 30*, 711-718.

Poehlmann, E.T., & Horton, E.S. (1989). The impact of food intake and exercise on energy expenditure. *Nutrition Review, 47*, 129-137.

Russel D.M., Prendergast, P.J., Darby, P.L., Garfinkel, P.E., Whitwell, & J. Jeejeebhoy, K.N. (1983). A comparison between muscle function and body composition in anorexia nervosa: the effect of refeeding. *American Journal of Clinical Nutrition, 38*, 229-237.

Schoeller, D.A., Ravussin, E., Schutz, Y., Acheson, K.J., Baertschi, P., & Jequier, E. (1986). Energy expenditure by doubly labeled water: Validity in humans and proposed calculations. *American Journal of Physiology, 250*, R823-R830.

Schreiber, W., Schweiger, U., Werner, D., Brunner, G., Tuschl, R.J., Laessle, R.G., Krieg, J.C., Fichter, M.M., & Pirke, K. M. (1991). Circadian pattern of large neutral amino acids, glucose, insulin and food intake in anorexia nervosa and bulimia nervosa. *Metabolism, 40*, 503-507.

Schusdziarra, V. (1988). Physiological significance of gastrointestinal somatostatin. *Hormone Research, 29*, 75-80.

Schweiger, U., Laessle, R.G., Pfister, H., Hoehl, C., Schwingenschloegel, M., Schweiger, M., & Pirke, K.M. (1987). Diet-induced menstrual irregularities: effects of age and weigt loss. *Fertility and Sterility, 48*, 746-751.

Schweiger, U., Pirke, K.M., Laessle, R.G., & Fichter, M.M. (1992). Gonadotropin Secretion in Bulimia Nervosa. *Journal of Clinical Endocrinology and Metabolism, 74*, 1122-1127.

Schweiger, U., Pöllinger, J., Laessle, R.G., Wolfram, G, Fichter, M.M., & Pirke, K.M. (1987). Altered insulin response to a balanced test meal in bulimic patients. *International Journal of Eating Disorders, 6*, 551-556.

Stordy, B.J., Marks, V., Kalucy, R.S., & Crisp, A.H. (1977). Weight gain, thermic effect of glucose and resting metabolic rate during recovery from anorexia nervosa. *American Journal of Clinical Nutrition, 30*, 138-146.

Stunkard, A.J., & Messick, S. (1985). The three factor eating questionnaire to measure dietary restraint, disinhibition and hunger. *Journal of Psychological Research, 29*, 71-83.

Tuschl, R.J., Platte, P., Laessle, R.G., Stichler, W., & Pirke, K.M. (1991). Energy expenditure and everyday eating behavior in healthy young women. *American Journal of Clinical Nutrition, 52*, 81-86.

Vigersky, R.A., & Loriaux, D.L. (1977). Anorexia nervosa as a model of hypothalamic dysfunction. In R.A. Vigersky (Ed.). *Anorexia nervosa* (pp. 109-122). New York: Raven Press.

Woell, C., Fichter, M.M., Pirke, K.M., & Wolfram, G. (1989). Eating behaviour of patients with bulimia nervosa. *International Journal of Eating Disorders, 8*, 557-568.

# Psychophysiology of Anorexia Nervosa

*Aribert Rothenberger, Claude Dumais-Huber, Gunther H. Moll, and Wolfgang Woerner*

## 1  Introduction

There is evidence of an *organic basis for anorexia nervosa* (AN) that involves a deficit at the level of subcortical structures such as the hypothalamus and the caudate nucleus (Vandereycken & Meermann, 1984; Herholz et al., 1987). However, it is an open question as to whether or not a cortical dysfunction in these patients exists. Indeed, the functional significance of the cortical pseudoatrophy that is observed in the CCT-scans of underweight anorectics and that fades away after weight gain remains, as yet, unexplained (Kohlmeyer et al., 1983; Rothenberger et al., 1991; Hentschel et al., 1994).

Surprisingly, the available methods for investigating the electrical brain activity have rarely been used in patients with anorexia nervosa (Pirke & Ploog, 1986), although they offer the advantage of good temporal resolution and provide a means for differentiating subcortical and cortical neuronal activities within the framework of evoked potential studies.

## 2  Standard EEG

In 1990, Hynek and Faltus visually evaluated the standard EEG tracings recorded in 77 adult patients who had received the clinical diagnosis of anorexia nervosa and in 76 patients suffering from a neurotic disorder. They looked at the usual frequency band activities, foci, paroxysms, reactivity to hyperventilation, and finally they classified the EEG tracings as normal, atypical, or abnormal. The relationship between clinical variables (e.g., weight gain) of the patient groups and the evaluated EEG criteria was not statistically significant. Thus, abnormalities in

Table 1. Abnormalities present in the standard EEG (given as percentages).

| GROUP | Vertex transients Non-periodic | Vertex transients Quasi-periodic | Paroxysmal dysrhythmia Present | Paroxysmal dysrhythmia Rare | Overall assessment Normal | Overall assessment Abnormal |
|---|---|---|---|---|---|---|
| Normal adults (N=98) | 8 | 6 | 1 | 0 | 94 | 6 |
| Healthy 13-year-olds (N=100) | 15 | 4 | 1 | 0 | 86 | 14 |
| Psychiatrically disordered children & adolescents (N=100) | 29 | 0 | 10 | 3 | 80 | 20 |
| Anorexia nervosa patients (N=100) | 71 | 58 | 22 | 8 | 44 | 56 |

standard EEG recordings reported in AN patients seem to be insensitive to gain in body weight.

To test this assumption in adolescents, we were prompted to analyze the standard EEGs recorded from normal adults, healthy 13-year-olds, adolescent patients with anorexia nervosa as well as children and adolescents with other psychiatric disorders (Table 1). Nearly 60% of the anorectic patients were found to have an atypical EEG (Figure 1). The observed abnormalities were mostly independent of body weight. Only the occurrence of paroxysmal dysrhythmia decreased in correspondence with an increase in body weight. What distinguishes our findings

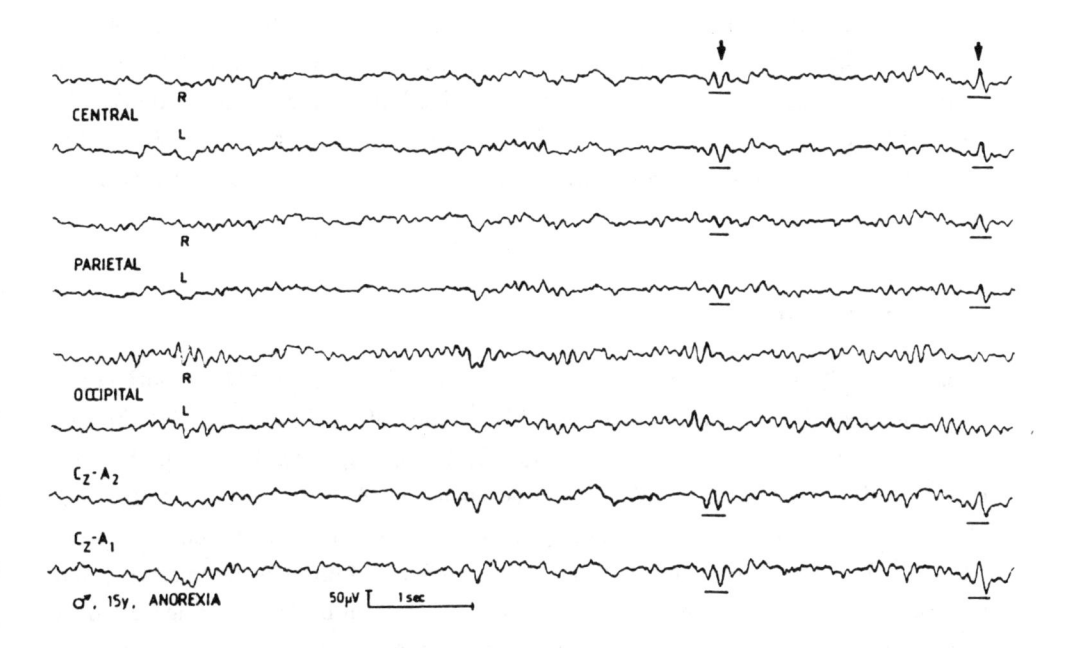

Figure 1: Routine EEG at rest (waking state) of an adolescent anorectic patient with an example of the vertex sharp wave which returns in cycles of about 3-6 seconds.

from previous reports is that in the group of anorectic patients we were able to detect particular graphoelements (so-called vertex transients) that occurred much more frequently than in other groups of subjects and that may be interpreted as signs of disinhibition. With increasing disinhibition these vertex transients can develop into 3-4/s sharp-slow waves. The origin of these graphoelements has been mainly attributed to subcortical areas but also partly to cortical regions (Niedermeyer & Lopez da Silva, 1982). A similar waveform known as vertex wave has been recorded under conditions of reduced vigilance and hence, low levels of neuronal inhibition. No description of the phenomenon has yet been reported for alert patients. If it is correct that patients with anorexia nervosa typically have an elevated level of vigilance as proposed by Herholz et al. (1987), but nevertheless frequently show such graphoelements in their standard EEGs, these vertex transients may be perceived as a stable indicator for an electrical vulnerabilty of the brain in the sense of a developmental deviation. Further, when we assessed the EEG soft signs taken as a whole (e.g., vertex transients, occipital transients, increased beta activity, tendency to synchronization of the theta rhythm), AN patients tended to show higher scores. However, the findings are not specific to the given psychopathology and can be observed in other child psychiatric disorders as well.

## 3.    Sleep-EEG

Another possibility to evaluate the central nervous activity of AN patients is the all-night sleep EEG. Especially because AN patients often show sleep disturbances and signs of depression related to their low body weight, it has been hypothesized that AN might be related to major affective disorders. A few studies (Walsh et al., 1985; Hudson et al., 1987; Lauer et al., 1988; Delvenne et al., 1992) compared the sleep EEG variables of adult/adolescent AN patients, bulimics, depressives, and normals. These results do not support a direct association between eating disorders and affective disorders like major depression. Nevertheless, AN patients showed some disturbances in their sleep cycle. They had longer duration of awakenings, lower sleep efficiency, and less REM sleep. Similar to waking EEG, sleep EEG characteristics were not significantly correlated to the Body Mass Index (Delvenne et al., 1992). Unfortunately, no longitudinal report concerning sleep EEG variables and body weight in AN exists, so no final statement can be formulated for the moment.

## 4  Auditory Evoked Potentials

Because spontaneous electrical brain activity seems to be relatively independent of changes in body weight in anorectic patients, we thought that stimulus-related processing of auditory information (i.e., a task that directly addresses the performance of a central nervous subsystem relevant for everyday situations) could possibly better demonstrate the influence of starving on electrical brain activity.

Thus, we resorted to the method of auditory evoked potentials (AEP) and their increase in amplitude with stimulus intensity, the so-called augmenting/reducing paradigm (Bruneau et al., 1985; Garreau, 1985). The arrival of the auditory input at the primary auditory cortex occurs, according to Vaughan and Arezzo's (1988) review, at about 9 ms after stimulus onset. Therefore, wave V of the AEPs derives from a subcortical origin and wave $N_1$ as well as wave $P_2$ (about 90-150 ms and 150-220 ms after stimulus onset, respectively) derive from cortical sources. In order to examine the subjects' modulation of sensory input, we recorded the AEPs at both CNS levels along the auditory pathway.

We examined (Rothenberger et al., 1986; Rothenberger et al., 1991) two groups of anorectic patients, each having only two male adolescents. In one group of 27 anorexia nervosa patients who were investigated only once, body weights of 32-51 kg (mean=42 kg) were measured. Patients with lower body weights had just started their treatment, whereas those with higher body weights were already showing some progress in response to therapy. In a second group of 12 anorectic adolescents who were examined twice, i.e., once during the first week of treatment and again after having reached and maintained the target weight for 2 weeks, mean body weight was 39 kg and 48 kg, respectively. In most cases, the weight set as the therapeutic goal lay within the normal range for the age group in question. All patients fulfilled the DSM-III criteria for anorexia nervosa and had normal hearing. As a control group for these 12 anorectic patients, 12 children (ten girls and two boys) diagnosed as having a "specific emotional disturbance" (corresponding to ICD-9 313, normal body weight, no eating disorder) were examined once.

All anorectic patients and the psychiatric controls were submitted to a recording of AEPs at each examination. All subjects had their body weight measured each time they were tested. Early and late AEPs were recorded over the vertex in response to a lower (55/50 dBHL) and a higher (75/70 dBHL) intensity of sound. Usually, amplitudes increase with increasing stimulus intensity (Garreau, 1985) (Figure 2).

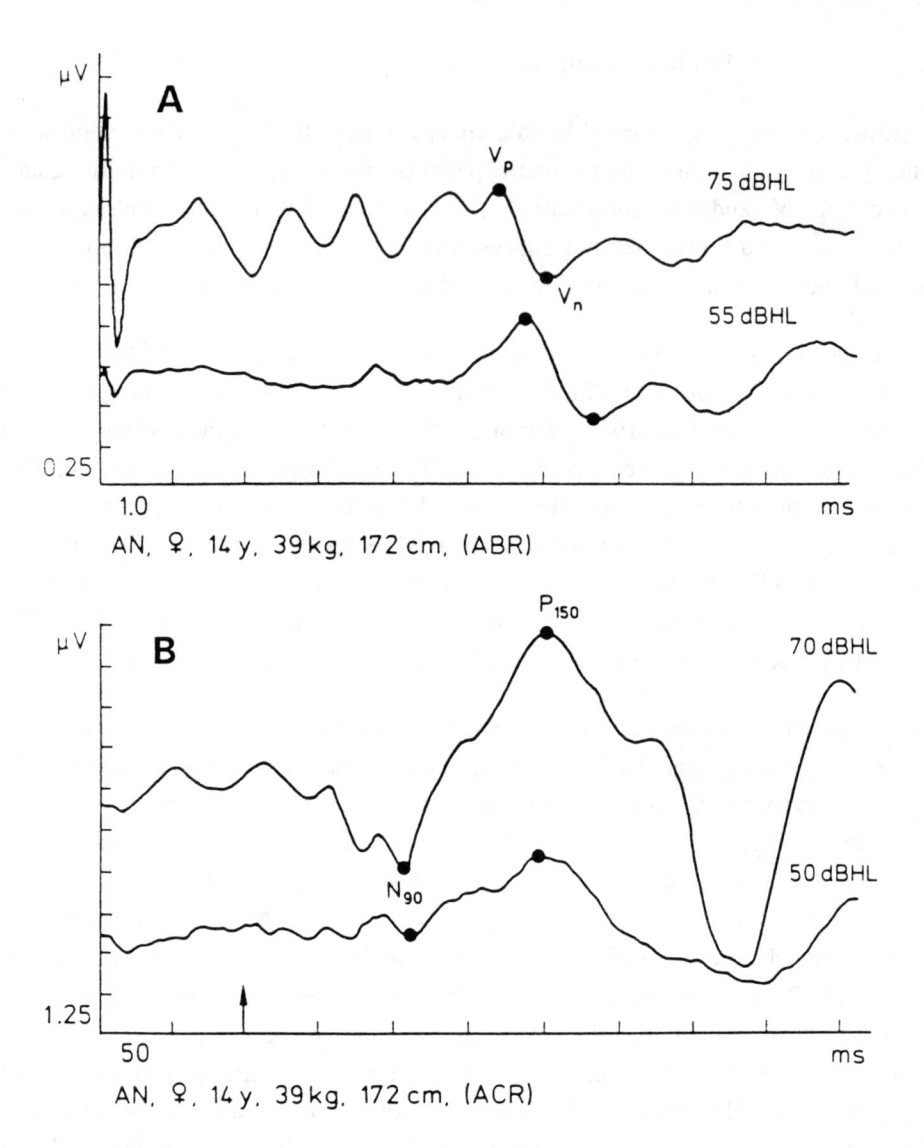

Figure 2. Auditory evoked potentials (AEP) in response to different stimulus intensities in a 14-year-old female anorectic patient with low body weight. A: Auditory brainstem responses recorded from Cz/M1, 11.3 stimuli/s. B: Auditory cortical responses from Cz/Fz, 0.8 stimuli/s. With increasing intensity of the stimuli the amplitude of AEP decreases at the brainstem level, whereas it clearly increases at the cortical level.

Our study indicated that anorectic patients, compared to psychopathological controls, had difficulties modulating the auditory stimuli adequately, even after weight gain. This applied particularly to the subcortical level of their central nervous pathways: Looking at the brainstem AEP amplitudes of wave V, this was reflected by a very small augmenting or even reducing pattern of responses to loud stimuli in anorectic patients as opposed to controls. When one considers that an active processing of stimuli in terms of a biofeedback already occurs at the level of the brainstem (Finley, 1984), one could assume that the small increments in amplitudes recorded subcortically with increasing stimulus intensity account for a poor modulation capacity in anorectic patients. Contrary to expectations, no significant differences in AEP amplitude changes to louder stimuli were observed between anorectic patients and controls at the cortical level (N90-P150). Nevertheless, the increase in amplitude of cortical responses (in contrast to subcortical AEP) tended to be higher (i.e., clear augmenting) in both groups of anorectic patients when their body weight was low.

Our assumption of a subcortical disturbance in anorectic patients is supported by the findings of Miyamoto et al. (1992). They recorded the auditory brainstem responses in 20 patients with AN (before and after weight gain) and 10 normal control subjects (investigated only once). Both groups of AN patients showed smaller amplitudes of wave V compared to the controls. In addition, underweight anorectics tended to exhibit amplitudes that were smaller than those of patients who had recovered body weight. The authors conclude that some dysfunction may exist at the level of the brainstem in AN patients even after a recovery in their body weight. Unfortunately, the authors did not report cortical AEPs, which would provide a basis for testing the cortical-subcortical interplay.

## 5    The Neuronal Decoupling Hypothesis

In our study, low weight anorectic patients showed diverging patterns with respect to cortical versus subcortical AEP responses (i.e., cortical augmenting vs. subcortical reducing of AEP amplitudes). This suggests a functional deficit arising from a decoupling (disconnection) of cortical and subcortical neuronal systems, possibly at the level of the thalamus. Our control group of psychiatrically disordered children as well as healthy subjects can be reported to be augmenters for early as well as late AEPs (Garreau, 1985; Rothenberger et al., 1987). Our interpretation of the AEP results may be seen in parallel to the topographical mapping of the late AEPs (P300) of Malloy (1987) in obsessive-compulsive patients. He hypothesizes a frontocortical-subcortical disconnection syndrome with a disturbance at the orbitomedial part of the frontal cortex. Because anorectic patients often exhibit obsessive-compulsive behavior, this line of research might prove fruitful. The latter might also include the idea that stimulation of arousal at the level of the hippocampus may relate to the onset of compulsive behavior in AN (Mills, 1985).

Additionally, the PET studies by Herholz et al. (1987) have indeed shown that the metabolic rates do not significantly change in the frontal lobe regions of anorectic patients despite the observation of increased metabolic activity in the caudate nucleus when these patients have low body weights. Considering that damage to both the frontal lobes and the caudate nucleus may lead to the same sort of functional disorders, it follows that our experimental approach for studying a possible frontocortical-subcortical dysfunction in anorectic patients should be pursued in future research.

## 6   P300 Wave

The aforementioned group of 27 AN adolescents were also submitted to a standard auditory oddball P300 paradigm (infrequent tone of 2000 Hz in 20% of the stimuli as target; frequent tone of 1000 Hz in 80% of the stimuli as non-target). We expected that low body weight AN patients would be unable to activate enough cortical neuronal resources to process such information adequately. Against predictions, neither low body weight, high number of cortical sulci in CCT, nor cortisol level seem to influence the general EEG activity at rest and/or the cognitive P300 component recorded during a standard oddball paradigm. It might be that this psychophysiological method is not appropriate for uncovering neuronal disturbances prevailing in AN (Rothenberger et al., 1986).

AN patients have difficulties with their body image, and this symptom is tightly bound to the emotional state of these patients. Therefore, we may anticipate that AN patients in contrast to healthy controls will activate their neuronal networks in a different way when female silhouettes with high body weight are presented as target stimuli. To test this hypothesis, Seeger and Lehmkuhl (1993) examined 10 adolescent anorectics and 10 age and "cognitively" matched normal controls using the following experimental design: An oddball paradigm involved two runs, (a) the first one corresponding to the presentation of "emotional" stimuli - i.e., two female silhouettes appearing in a random sequence (target: thick, non-target: slim); (b) in the second run, two squares were chosen as "neutral" stimuli that were also randomly presented (target: red, non-target: blue).

The main result reported by these authors was that AN patients, when compared to normals, showed shorter reaction times, prolonged latencies of P300 at left frontocentral leads, and greater area measures for P300-waves at left centro-temporal leads when the emotionally high-loaded stimulus (thick female silhouette) was presented as a target. Other comparisons were statistically non-significant. Given the fact that P300-latency reflects the time needed for stimulus evaluation and updating, low weight AN patients may show a body image related deficit of neuronal processing at the level of frontocortical areas (i.e., reduced ability for emotional control, prolonged and incomplete updating) when there is a high affective load of the stimulus, although they try to resolve this task by mobilizing electrical brain activity as seen by the large surface area under the P300-wave (Figure 3).

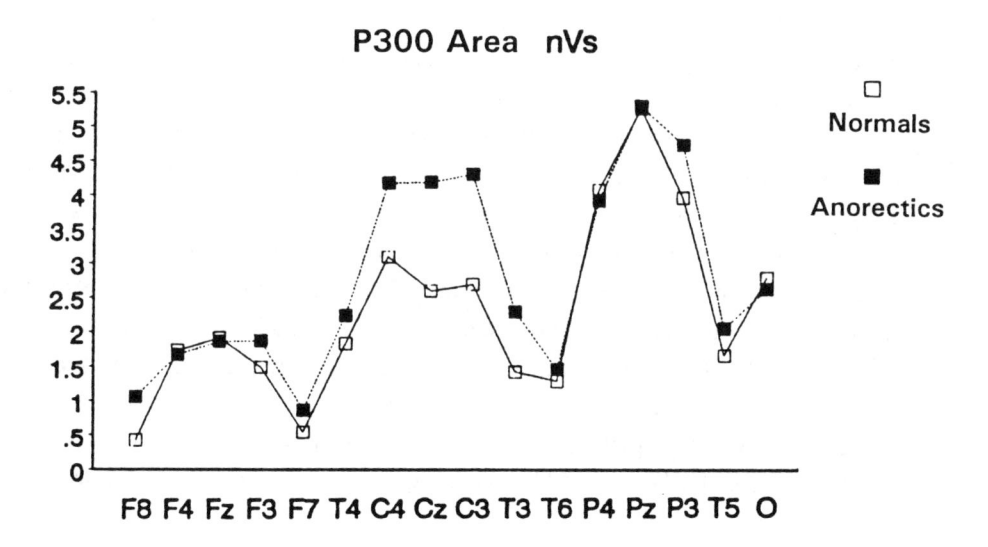

Figure 3. P300 to the visually presented target stimulus (silhouette of a fat woman): area below the curve in 10 normals (open squares) and in 10 anorectics (black squares). (From Seeger & Lehmkuhl, 1993).

A further sign of divergent information processing in AN adolescents may also be the high amplitude of a slow negative wave observed after the P300 component. Whether this reflects a higher arousal level in AN patients that might explain their shorter reaction times remains an issue to be further debated.

In addition to these findings and without overestimating the value of neurophysiological indicators, other tasks could be helpful to test the assumption of a neuronal impairment that would be tightly bound to weight changes and would have its site in the cortex. Some of these approaches will be discussed in the remainder of this report.

## 7  Contingent Negative Variation and Post-Imperative Negative Variation

Therefore, we resorted to the so-called S1-S2-R paradigm, which makes it possible to measure the contingent negative variation (CNV) and the post-imperative negative variation (PINV). The CNV is a slow cortical potential shift developing in a paired stimuli reaction time task (the so-called S1-S2-R paradigm); it has proved to be a valuable electrophysiological measure of cognitive functioning. The PINV appears sensitive to emotionally-loaded features of stimuli in the sense that it can be induced in normals by introduction of a stress situation (e.g., labyrinthine stimulation) during the interstimulus interval (Gauthier & Gottesmann, 1977) or after the imperative stimulus as a punishment for incorrect response (Peters & Knott, 1976). In this context, it has been suggested that PINV mirrors to some extent a state of anxiety and uncertainty towards the experimental situation, especially when the latter is being manipulated in such a way that it becomes ambiguous and difficult to resolve (e.g., when S2 is made uncontrollable) (Bolz & Giedke, 1981; Delaunoy et al., 1978; Birbaumer et al., 1986). In this case, the development of a PINV under stress situations is to be interpreted as a consequence of inadequate processing of contingencies and not as a correlate of anxiety per se; the latter would simply represent a perturbing factor for a given subject.

We set out to illuminate the cognitive functions subserving behavioral control in *anorectic patients* (Table 2) in the expectation to further potentiate our hypothesis

Table 2. Psychopathological characteristics of anorectic patients compared with healthy controls.

|  | Anorectics (N=20) | Controls (N=20) | U-test p |
|---|---|---|---|
| AGE (yrs;months) | 15;1 | 15;2 | ns |
| IQ (full-scale PSB) | 121 | 121 | ns |
| CONNERS - Scale | 9.8 | 3.2 | *** |
| CBCL | | | |
| *T-values:* | | | |
| -Total | 65.7 | 47.7 | *** |
| -Externalizing | 55.9 | 48.9 | * |
| -Internalizing | 67.3 | 48.3 | *** |
| *Raw scores:* | | | |
| -Anxiety | 3.6 | 0.7 | *** |
| -Depression | 7.5 | 1.3 | *** |
| -Somatic disorder | 3.1 | 1.7 | ** |
| -Withdrawal | 7.7 | 1.7 | *** |
| -Obsessiveness | 6.2 | 0.8 | *** |
| -Schizoid tendencies | 4.5 | 0.2 | *** |
| -Aggressivity | 5.7 | 3.3 | (*) |
| -Attention disorder | 3.2 | 1.3 | * |
| -Delinquent behavior | 0.5 | 0.5 | ns |
| Severity (psychopathology) | 3.4 | 0.2 | *** |
| Interview of parents (MEI) | | | |
| FAI | 0.5 | 0.3 | ns |
| SES | 3.3 | 4.0 | (*) |
| Axis V of DSM-III | 3.4 | 2.1 | *** |
| CGAS (0-100) | 45.3 | 89.8 | *** |
| Body height (cm) | 158 | 165 | NS |
| " weight (kg) | 36 | 54 | ** |
| ideal body weight | 46 | 52 | NS |
| % ideal body weight | 78 | 103 | ** |

(*) p<.1, *p<0.05, **p<0.01, ***p<0.001 (ns = not significant)
CBCL = Child Behavior Checklist ; MEI = Mannheimer Eltern-Interview;
FAI = Family Adversity Index ; SES = socioeconomic status; CGAS = Child Global Assessment Score

on the recruitment of frontocortical neuron assemblies developed in experiments with tic patients and ADHD children (Rothenberger, 1990; Dumais-Huber & Rothenberger, 1992). In the case of AN, however, the nature of the underlying deficits has been less explored.

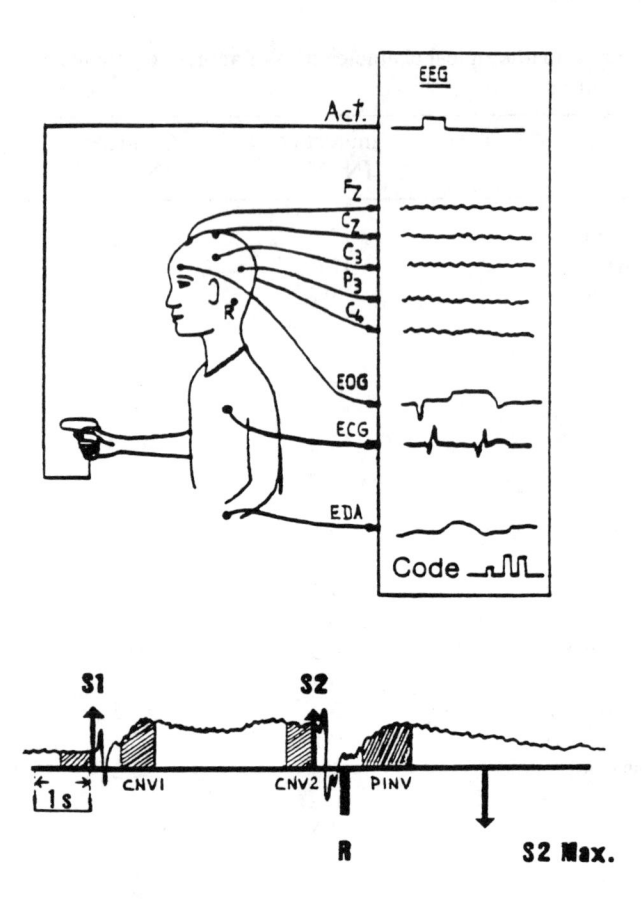

Figure 4. Schematic illustration of experimental set up (at the top) used to record EEG activity during a paired stimuli reaction time task. S1=warning signal, 1000 Hz sine tone, 4 sec duration, 70 dB above hearing level; S2=imperative signal, aversive white noise, 70 dB. The time windows chosen for amplitude measures of slow cortical potentials, i.e. CNV1, CNV2, and PINV are shown at the bottom with the 500 ms pre-S1 baseline also indicated by a shaded area.

Our two-stimulus paradigm implied an active participation of the subjects who had to control the auditory stimuli, a situation that contrasted with the passive attitude of subjects submitted to an augmenting/reducing paradigm (see above). To test the effect of stimulus controllability, the experiment was run under 2 conditions (control [C] and non-control [NC], see experimental set up, Figure 4), whereby S2 lasted 3 seconds during NC trials, as it could not effectively be terminated by button press in this condition. Using a relatively long interstimulus interval (such as our choice of ISI=4 seconds) makes it possible to identify both early and late components of the CNV, which are respectively found to reflect *orienting* and *anticipatory functions*. At shorter ISIs, these two CNV components would not be readily dissociated because they would likely be confounded in a single monophasic wave form under these conditions (Rohrbaugh & Gaillard, 1983). This dissociation of components which is expected to occur in our paradigm, may thus help us in "segmenting" the described children's performance at the task into more discrete units. The use of psychophysiological measures in paradigms inspired by the chronometric approach (such as our forewarned reaction time task) is well suited to extend the information derived from reaction times (*overt* response) and should provide indicators of both (a) cognitive (*covert*) processes occurring during the foreperiod (e.g., stimulus evaluation, anticipation, preparation) as well as during the time period between the imperative stimulus and the overt response (e.g., response selection) and (b) *contingency evaluation*. The interpretation of these psychophysiological markers should in turn be guided by multiple stage information processing models, so that a finer resolution in the temporal organization of cognitive functions can be achieved when attempting to localize the operative step(s) that is (are) critically impaired in a given psychiatric disorder. For this purpose, recording the chosen slow cortical potentials, namely CNV and PINV, is a relevant non-invasive means to better characterize group differences in the cognitive strategies adopted by the children under examination. Applied to AN, the acquisition of CNV and PINV data (Dumais-Huber, 1993) may contribute to a better understanding of the psychopathology and assist clinicians in taking decisions for a more adequate therapy.

## 7.1  Orienting (CNV1) and Anticipation (CNV2)

With respect to topography, the data gathered in AN patients did not substantiate the hypothesis of a frontal lobe deficit that would be manifested by the lack of frontal predominance for the CNV1 component. Indeed, anorectic patients exhibited a CNV1 that was largest over Fz, just like their healthy controls did. In addition, the prediction that was made concerning the topographical distribution of CNV2 (i.e., a central dominance in all children) was not supported in the case of AN patients (Figure 5).

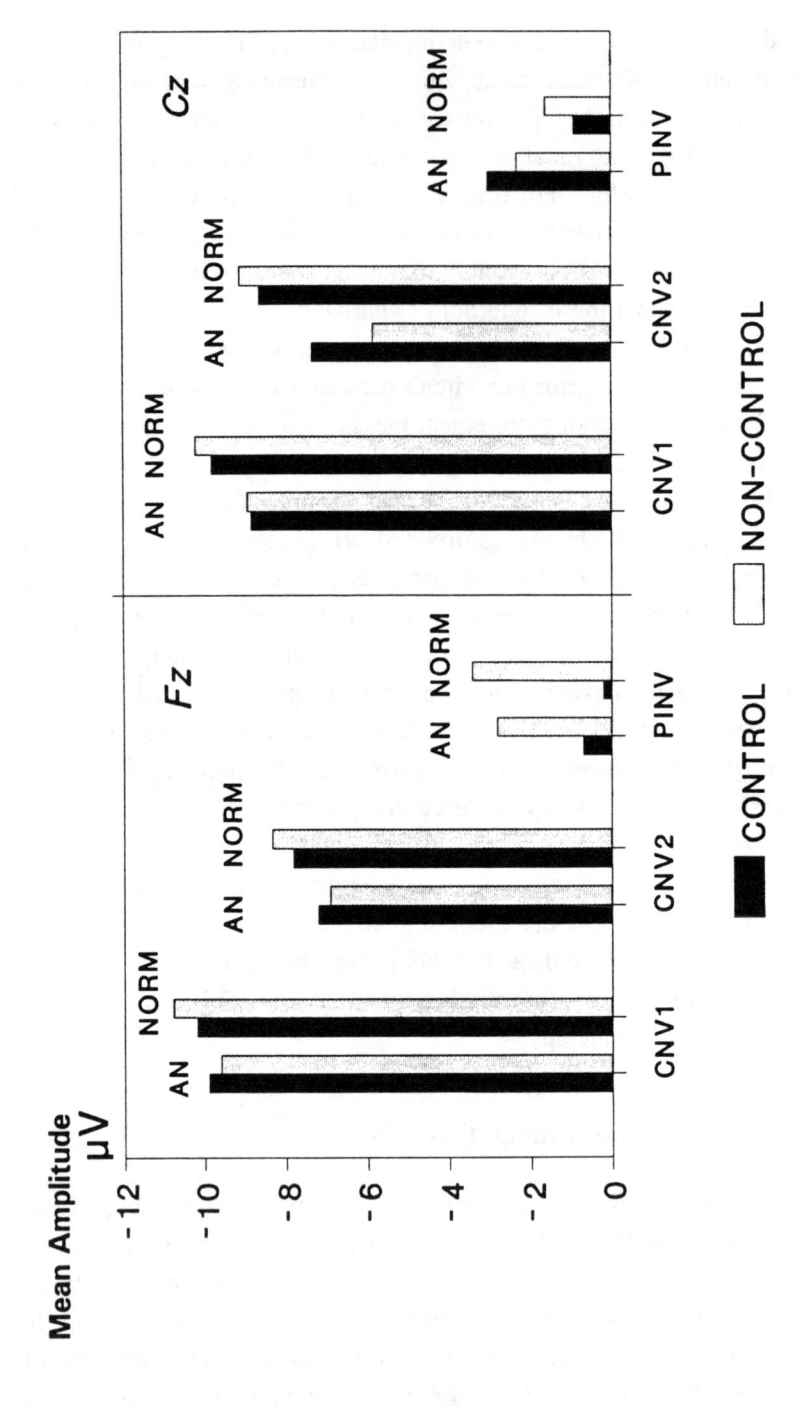

Figure 5. Mean amplitude values of slow cortical potentials (CNV1, CNV2, and PINV) recorded over Fz and Cz in 20 anorectic patients (AN) and 20 healthy controls (NORM) matched for age, sex and IQ. Measures made under control (C, dark bars) and non-control (NC, light bars) conditions.

According to expectation, the amplitudes of CNV1 and CNV2 were found to be smaller in AN patients than in healthy controls; however, these differences between the two groups did not reach significance level. The reduction in CNV amplitudes was particularly marked for the CNV2 developing in the NC condition. This observation is reminiscent of an overload effect such as the one described in ADHD children for the CNV1 component. Because the deficit found in AN patients seems to affect the late component of CNV (CNV2) more than its early component and, given that CNV2 amplitudes are normally highest over the vertex, it is understandable that the differences in CNV2 amplitudes between AN patients and healthy controls are observed mostly for the Cz derivation. Even though AN patients, in contrast to healthy adolescents, did not exhibit a central dominance of CNV2, this is not to say that they achieved a good activation of frontocortical areas. As a matter of fact, the CNV2 amplitudes recorded in AN patients were about equally distributed over Fz and Cz in the C condition and they showed no compensatory recruitment of frontocortical neural networks in the NC condition as the CNV2 amplitudes at Fz were also affected by the reported disfacilitation (reduced cortical negativity), although to a lesser degree than the ones at Cz.

Thus, our CNV1 results suggest that orienting processes are practically intact in AN patients. However, CNV2 results indicate that AN patients have difficulty in establishing a preparatory set for motor response. Presumably, some psychopathological features play an important role in interfering with ongoing task-related cognitive processes: Being obsessed by their fear of overeating and gaining weight, AN patients may be disturbed in their performance as their attentional resources are directed away from the experimental task. Already in the early paper of McCallum & Walter (1968), the effect of "internal distraction" on CNV has been described in anectodal terms in a few cases of lower than usual amplitudes shown to arise in the examined subjects when they were particularly worried about business or personal matters.

## 7.2 Contingency Changes (PINV)

Our results attest to the anticipated condition effect on PINV amplitudes: Indeed, an increase in PINV activity was observed over Fz in adolescents of both groups during NC trials (Figure 5). According to our expectations, AN patients exhibited PINV activity in both C and NC conditions, whereas healthy controls did develop PINV activity only in the NC condition. Regarding topography however, our data failed to support the predicted manifestation of a frontal lobe deficit in AN patients in a way that would have prevented the appearance of a PINV maximum over Fz; if anything, this frontal predominance observed in anorectics was simply weaker than the one found in healthy adolescents.

Because the central predominance of PINV reported in the C condition was minimal in healthy controls (PINV amplitudes of about -0.5 µV +/-0.3 µV), the frontal maximum found in the NC condition corresponds to an *increase in cortical activation* restricted to the frontocortical areas. On the other hand, because the recruitment of frontocortical networks observed in AN patients in the NC condition was accompanied by some reduction of the large PINV activity generated at Cz, so that no significant increase in the overall PINV activity was documented, one may speak of a *shift* in PINV activity. However, looking at the distributional pattern of PINV activity over the frontocentral areas (Cz-Fz), it appears that this shift was not sufficient to yield a clear frontal dominance of PINV.

### 7.3 Pathophysiological Models

If the cortical-subcortical disconnection hypothesis (including a deficit of some sensory modulation) put forward by Rothenberger et al. (1991) on the basis of data gathered by means of an augmenting/reducing paradigm were really present in anorectics, it would consequently impede the pre-setting of the excitability thresholds of cortical networks. In other words, *a disturbance dissociating subcortical and cortical structures would prevent the inhibitory influence of basal ganglia from exerting its regulatory role on the cortex*. This might be the reason why a tendency for hyperaugmenting of AEPs at the cortical level (although not statistically significant) was documented in underweight anorectics together with a reducing at subcortical level in the above-mentioned study (Rothenberger et al., 1991). In light of the critical comments of Connolly (1987) on the theoretical foundations of EP augmenting/reducing processes, it is suggested that part of the observed cortical augmenting might have been attributable to tonic mesencephalic reticular formation (MRF)-related arousal, even though most of the cortical activity recorded after averaging is mediated by phasic thalamic disinhibition. The question may then be raised as to whether a similar MRF-mediated activation of sensory non-specific cortical areas could account for the large PINV amplitudes measured at the vertex in AN patients during C trials. It is very difficult (if not impossible) to bring supportive arguments for resolving this issue if we refer ourselves only to the empirical data of the present work.

In contrast to the shorter reaction times of AN patients reported in the P300 experiment of Seeger & Lehmkuhl (1993), slightly increased reaction times were found in the AN patients submitted to our task. This slowing down in working speed was particularly marked when uncontrollable trials were to be dealt with, a result which may be related to the overload effect already discussed in the interpretation of the reduced CNV2 developing in the NC condition. This manifestation of deficit viewed as a disturbance in motor preparation may also account for the fact that the lengthening of reaction times prevailed *across all NC trials* in anorectics, as they were not capable of speeding up their reactions again like the healthy adolescents did.

## 7.4 CNV/PINV and Weight Gain

The follow-up data we gathered in 14 AN patients to assess the effect of gain in body weight on CNV and PINV indicated a normalization of SCPs at the second evaluation (Dumais-Huber, 1993). As shown in Figure 6, this took the form of a disinhibition of CNV1 and CNV2 (i.e., increase in amplitudes) and, to a lesser extent, of an inhibition of PINV (i.e., decrease in amplitudes). This CNV enhancement was attributed to therapy because the change essentially went against the developmental trends observed in this particular age group. In contrast, a maturational effect could not be completely excluded in the case of PINV attenuation, because the modification in PINV amplitudes documented at the second evaluation basically occurred in the same direction as the age-related amplitude changes. Overall, results suggest a positive influence of weight gain on the ability of AN patients to modulate external stimuli. Apparently, recovery in body weight contributed to make more neuronal resources accessible to the AN patients for behavioral control.

The paucity of psychophysiological studies in anorectics precludes the comparison of our SCP data with the literature, on the one hand, but it also justifies the need to continue doing research along these lines, on the other hand. In this respect, a multi-level investigation appears well suited to elucidate the multifaceted behavioral features of AN patients and to lay down the foundation for an integrated view of this particular psychiatric disorder.

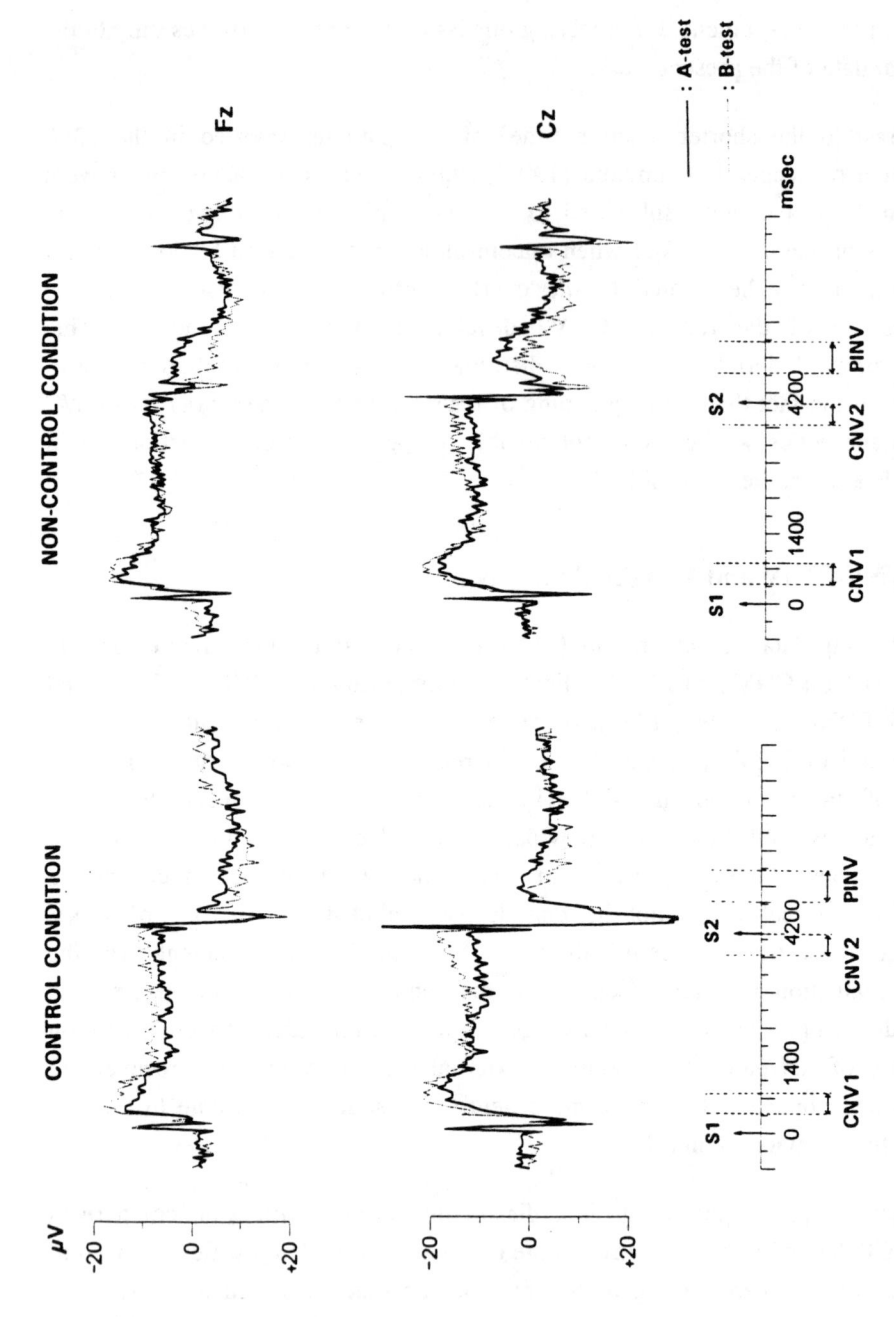

Figure 6. Influence of gain in body weight on slow cortical potentials: Recordings of CNV1, CNV2, and PINV are given for the Fz and Cz derivations (control and non-control conditions) and grand averages are computed over 14 AN patients according to the time of examination, i.e., *before* (A-test, dark curves) and *after* (B-test, dashed curves) therapy.

## 8    Heart Rate and Electrodermal Activity

*Cardiac function* is an important factor during AN illness. Marcus et al. (1989) described the results of somatic examinations in 94 adolescent anorectics (age range 12-18 years). About 60% had a heart rate below 60 beats/min., about 80% had a systolic blood pressure under 110 mm Hg, and about 60% had a diastolic blood pressure under 70 mm Hg; in addition, an abnormal ECG was recorded in 35% of the cases.

Several studies (Moodie & Salcedo, 1983; Moodie, 1987; Nakagawa et al., 1985; Nudel et al., 1984; Brunner et al., 1989; George et al., 1990; Kaye et al., 1990) reported abnormal cardiac responses to exercise, stress and drugs in AN patients and abnormal working capacity with a reduction in left ventricular muscle mass. Hemodynamic studies generally revealed a lowered cardiac index, most likely secondary to the small size of the heart and the reduction in stroke volume. Under stress, there seems to be a slight increase in heart rate and a small decrease in diastolic blood pressure (often accompanied with ST-segment depression), but a failure of stressed AN patients to lower their systolic blood pressure to baseline levels as controls did. Thus, cardiac function should be carefully controlled because the reduced performance of AN patients at exercising may reflect abnormal sympathetic responses as a risk for cardiovascular decompensation especially under refeeding therapy (Kahn et al., 1991). Even after weight gain, it takes a long time until normalization of the cardiovascular modulation capacity occurs (see Pirke,1990; Rothenberger et al., 1990).

This is probably due to the complicated interaction between vagal tone and sympathetic activity for cardiac regulation. During AN illness, bradycardia is an effect of hypervagal activity coupled with reduced sympathetic activity (Kennedy & Heslegrave, 1989). Months of therapy and rehabilitation are needed to rebalance this interplay. This may possibly be related to altered regulation and slowly developing normalization of presynaptic beta-adrenergic receptor activity, an important modulation of vascular and metabolic function (Kaye et al., 1990).

So far, available data concerning cardiovascular reactivity and central nervous responses in AN reveal the existence of a deficit in modulation. Whether this also holds true for electrodermal activity is as yet unknown. We are not aware of any paper discussing this topic. This is rather amazing when one considers that a lowered thyroid function (reduced T3 hormone) is sometimes observed in these patients together with dry skin and low skin temperature.

Here, it seems informative to introduce an *analysis of autonomic responses* (Figure 7) carried out by members of our research group (Moll & Rothenberger, 1993) on the same data set as the one that has been the object of the previously mentioned electrophysiology study : When considering the transition between C and NC trials (6 trials before and 6 trials after the condition change), both AN patients and healthy controls exhibited a skin conductance response (SCR) much more frequently after S2 than after S1. In subjects of both groups, this electrodermal activity (EDA) increased in the NC condition. Within each condition, however, the augmentation of EDA following S2 was much less frequent in AN patients than in healthy adolescents. Conversely, a larger increase in spontaneous vertical eye movements and in heart rate (HR) following S2 relative to their respective levels preceding S2 was found in AN patients. These results do not provide any clear-cut information to substantiate or else reject the hypothesis of an increased arousal in anorectics. Presumably, these measures of the autonomic nervous system (ANS) functioning tap different categories of neurophysiological mechanisms; further, the EDA responses habituated across NC trials, whereas no such habituation occurred for EOG and ECG activities (electrooculogram and electrocardiogram, respectively). This is consistent with the views of Duffy (1972) who stresses that *"the organism does not react as a massive undifferentiated whole"*, so that an interchangeable use of psychophysiological measures such as EEG, EDA and HR to assess arousal is not warranted. Along these lines, models of *fractionation of ANS arousal measures* according to which different emotional responses were attributed to distinct arousal systems have been put forward: Fowles (1980) proposed that EDA responses are to reflect the activity of a "Behavioral Inhibition System" (BIS), whereas HR changes are to be linked to a "Behavioral Activation System" (BAS). Although there is a consensus among scientists as to the relevance of establishing such a distinction between different ANS arousal measures, the nature of their particular relationships to the hypothesized arousal systems is still questioned. Wilde & Barry (1992), for instance, reported that both EDA and HR measures would be respectively associated (but probably in a different manner) with the so-called BAS and BIS, a finding that goes against the predictions of Fowles.

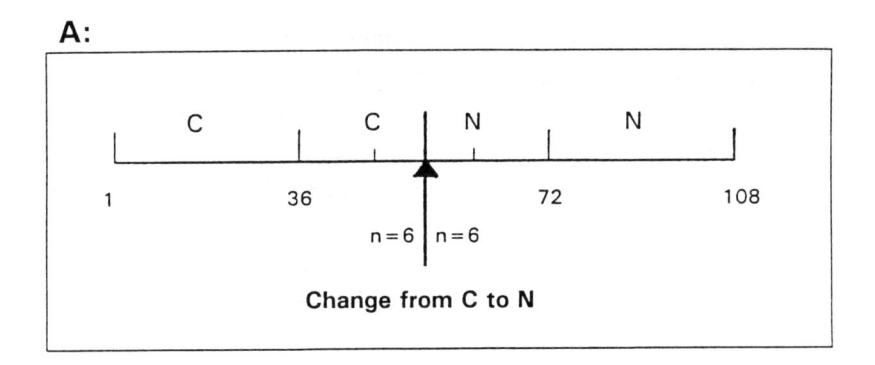

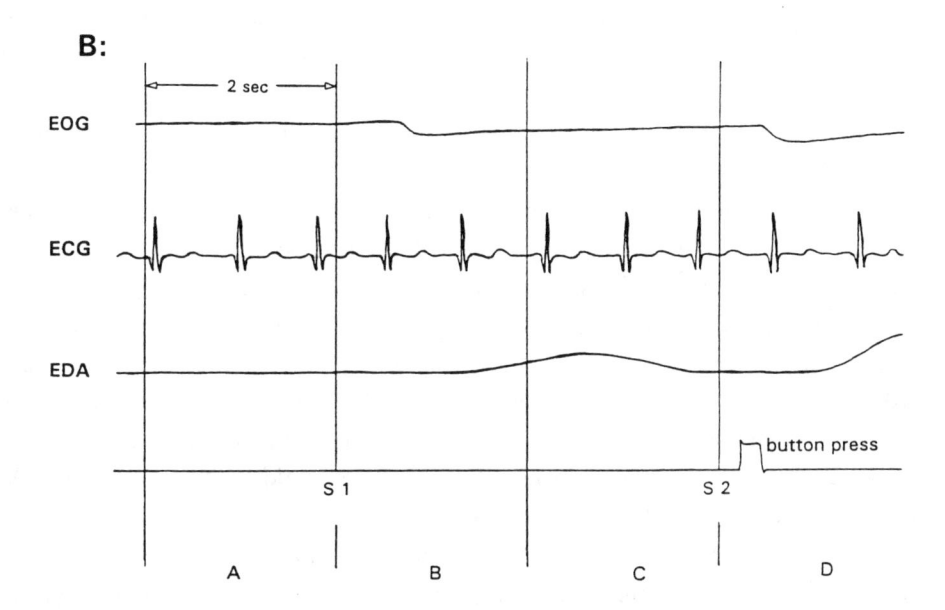

Figure 7. Experimental setting and parameters for the assessment of autonomic responses. A: Design of the stimulus sequence with change in condition (C=control versus N=non-control). Analysis was centered on 12 trials selected before (C1 to C6) and after (N1 to N6) this change, whereby the first non-controllable trial (N1) was excluded because the subject could only have recognized the lack of control *after* motor response. B: Selected channels include spontaneous vertical eye movements (EOG), electrocardiogram (ECG) and electrodermal activity (EDA). Auditory signals S1 and S2 are displayed together with motor response (button press). A, B, C and D refer to the time intervals of two seconds each used for measures.

In our experiment, however, Fowles' expectations were partly supported in that the observed post-S2 SCR response increased in the NC condition (i.e., a situation which presumably involves the BIS as "anxiety system"), whereas HR measures did not show any difference between C and NC conditions. These last considerations may provide a theoretical framework for the changes in ANS measures occurring when trials become uncontrollable, but they give no explanation as to the meaning of the changes in ANS measures that were observed upon the presentation of S2 regardless of the condition.

Irrespective of the experimental condition, AN patients appeared to have *difficulty in modulating the auditory input* presented to them in that they were *hyporesponsive to the aversive noise (S2) in terms of EDA activity*, but *hyperresponsive to S2 in terms of HR and EOG activity*. Thus, one cannot generally say that AN patients are characterized by higher arousal levels (Herholz et al., 1987). Here, a short excursus on the physiological mechanisms at stake would help us gain more insight into the matter: EDA may be perceived as a rough indicator of sympathetic arousal, although this response must be considered as a special case of sympathetic nervous system activity since postganglionic fibers innervating the sweat glands are cholinergic, thereby contrasting with most other postganglionic sympathetic endings that are noradrenergic. Expressed in a simple fashion, SCR can be said to be a phasic measure of the eccrine glands to external stimuli and stress-related situations. However, needless to say that a detailed account of this system mediating the SCR response would be much more complex and would include an intricate network of neural pathways within the CNS (Edelberg, 1972). In the particular case of anorexia nervosa, one often encounters a disturbance in bodily homeostasis including symptoms such as hypothermia and bradycardia. In this psychopathological state, the deficit in the hypothalamus-mediated thermoregulation corresponds to a decrease in peripheral blood supply (a vasoconstriction elicited by sympathetic activation), which may have the effect of

reducing the development of EDA response. In addition, when considering HR regulation, we have to consider the influence of both parasympathetic and sympathetic nervous systems as the predominance of their respective activities varies according to situations. As a matter of fact, a bradycardia was observed in AN patients *prior* to S2, reflecting parasympathetic activation. The post-S2 HR acceleration then found in AN patients would be a sign of the prevalence of sympathetic activity for energy mobilization during active coping. It must be clearly stated that even if HR and spontaneous eye movements are peripheral measures reflecting ANS activity, the neural mechanisms responsible for their generation are by no means restricted to the brainstem. In both cases, descending influence of the CNS cannot be ignored. Indeed, the mechanisms of cardiac control reach a high level of sophistication as they involve the sensorimotor cortex as well as the lateral and posterior hypothalamus, MRF, and parts of the cingulate, septum and amygdala (Gunn et al., 1972). Interestingly, within the framework of an operant conditioning of SCPs, the withdrawal of feedback and reinforcement caused the pre-S2 HR deceleration (usually observed under biofeedback conditions) to disappear in patients with bilateral frontal lobe damage (Rockstroh et al., 1989): This finding demonstrates a clear cortical-cardiac interaction wherein the frontal lobe is an essential component to the regulation of the event-related cardiac response as indexed by the HR. Finally, the structures that are activated to elicit spontaneous eye movements also attest to a complex pattern of innervation as they engage the frontal and occipital cortical areas, the superior colliculi, the pretectal area, the oculomotor nuclei, the paramedian pontine reticular formation as well as the abducens nucleus (Barr & Kiernan, 1983).

*Taken as a whole*, empirical data indicate that AN patients may operate at higher arousal levels, but at the moment, however, further investigation is required in order to gather sufficient evidence (a) for drawing a differentiated picture of the way energy would be released in various physiological systems in a model of activation inspired by Duffy (1972), and (b) for describing how the different measures of arousal relate to one another. It is important to note that the apparently inconsistent EDA responses of AN patients observed *within* and *between* conditions (lower reactivity of SCR to S2 within each condition in comparison with healthy controls and SCR increase from C to NC condition) may parallel the observations of Papakostopoulos & McCallum (1973). These authors reported that two distinct patterns of autonomic changes — often opposite in direction — were to be recognized in the course of their experiment: A phasic or short-lived change (e.g., HR deceleration within the trials of a given experimental condition such as during the interstimulus interval) and a tonic or sustained change depending on the stage of the experiment (e.g., HR acceleration when passing from a no-response to a response situation). Although the most convincing evidence for their statement was derived from HR measures and not from EDA activity, it seems reasonable to extrapolate this distinction between phasic and tonic autonomic changes to account for the data gathered in AN patients during our S1-S2-R task.

## 9 Discussion and Conclusion

As demonstrated in the present paper, the field of psychophysiology of AN is a small one but it deserves attention and should be enlarged by future studies. Surprisingly, the cognitive functioning of AN patients has not been well investigated so far. In contrast to thousands of publications on different aspects of AN, there exist only about ten articles on the IQ of patients of this group (Blanz et al., in press) and its relationship to low body weight and to other symptoms of AN. Studies on differentiated *neuropsychological functioning* are scarce. Recently, Casper and Heller (1991) hypothesized that anorectic symptomatology might be related to atypical hemispheric lateralization. They used visual-constructive tasks to test right hemisphere (RH) involvement and verbal fluency tasks to test left hemispheric (LH) activity; further, a chimeric face task (Heller & Levy, 1981; Levine & Levy, 1986) was administered. A left bias on the chimeric faces is taken to indicate activation or involvement of the right hemisphere. Similarly, leftward placement/drawing of items/figures within pictures is assumed to reflect a greater engagement of the right hemisphere. Results are suggestive of a decreased cognitive functioning in AN and a relationship between anorectic symptomatology and asymmetric brain activation, i.e., a lower body weight and more pronounced/severe symptoms were associated with increased LH activation. Weight gain, greater awareness of negative affect, and overestimation of body parts correlated with an increase in RH activation. The authors speculate that a decreased RH function contributes to a tendency to suppress or ignore negative affect during acute AN. With weight gain, increasing RH activity may be associated with enhanced processing of emotion. Furthermore, increased activity of the right frontal regions appears to be linked to increased negative affect (Davidson, 1984). In an analogous manner, the increased capacity to acknowledge negative affect observed by Casper and Heller (1991) in anorectics during weight gain may thus be interpreted as reflecting an overall enhanced activation of the right hemisphere relative to the LH activity level.

Our preliminary data on frontal lobe sensitive executive functions point to a possible deficit in cognitive impulse control in low weight AN patients as measured by means of the Matching Familiar Figures Test (MFFT) of Kagan and Kogan (1970), whereas other executive functions like interference control, cognitive flexibility, and time estimation seemed to be preserved. Among the subjects described in Table 1 (20 AN patients and 20 healthy controls), anorectics made more errors and responded faster than healthy controls when performing the MFFT (errors: 3.8 in AN patients vs 2.8 in healthy controls, p=not significant; time:165.7 sec in AN patients vs 196.8 sec in healthy controls, p<0.1). Until now, psychophysiological data did not report on laterality effects, but it would be easily manageable to evaluate this aspect by topographical analysis with brain mapping like it was done in a first step by Seeger and Lehmkuhl (1993). At this moment, anterior-posterior distribution and cortical-subcortical interaction of neuronal activity was the focus of interest. In this context, it could be shown that AN patients have a *reduced capacity to modulate* incoming stimuli. This applies mainly to the subcortical level (e.g., auditory brainstem response [ABR], autonomic nervous system [ANS] ). Adolescent AN patients seem to have little control over more complex neuronal regulatory systems (e.g., auditory cortical response [ACR], ECG) and might "overcontrol" simple systems like auditory brainstem responses and EDA. Furthermore, there is some evidence for a reduction of frontal lobe functions during the low weight phase of AN, as shown by the P300 data of Seeger and Lehmkuhl (1993), the report of Casper and Heller (1991), as well as our preliminary data on the MFFT. This neurodynamic view seems promising because it is known from animal studies that the orbitofrontal cortex is highly involved in the interaction with subcortical structures (e.g., hypothalamus and brainstem) to regulate eating behavior, sexuality, aggressiveness as well as heart rate, blood pressure, respiration, and skin temperature (Fuster, 1989). Thus, it can be speculated that adolescent anorectics may suffer from some transitory frontal lobe deficit combined with a transitory functional discoupling of cortical and subcortical neuronal assemblies. At least, a differential functional discoupling of subcortically regulated autonomic neuronal systems (e.g., ECG vs EDA) has to be taken into consideration, either as a basic trait variable and/or as a long-term state variable resulting from starvation and dieting.

Finally, because most (if not all) mentioned neuronal deficits are closely related to body weight and eating behavior, the therapeutic objective must be to increase body weight in due time by adequate eating behavior if the full capacity for modulating somatic and mental functions is ever to be restored. This would provide a sound basis for increasing the abilities of these patients for self-regulation of behavior — a prerequisite for developing a normal life and a healthy personality as members of our society.

## References

Barr M. L., & Kiernan J. A. (1983). *The human nervous system: An anatomical viewpoint* (4th edition). Philadelphia: Harper & Row.
Birbaumer N., Elbert T., Rockstroh B., & Lutzenberger W. (1986). On the dynamics of the post-imperative negative variation. In W. C. McCallum, R. Zappoli & F. Denoth (Eds.). *Cerebral psychophysiology: studies in event-related potentials* (EEG Suppl. 38, pp 212-219). Amsterdam: Elsevier.
Blanz B., Detzner M., Lay B., Rose F., & Schmidt M. H. (in press). The intellectual functioning of adolescent eating disorder patients is above-average. *European Child and Adolescent Psychiatry*.
Bolz J., & Giedke H. (1981). Controllability of an aversive stimulus in depressed patients and healthy controls: a study using slow brain potentials. *Biological Psychiatry*, 16, 441-452.
Bruneau N., Roux S., Garreau B., & Lelord G. (1985). Frontal auditory evoked potentials and augmenting/reducing. *Electroencephalography and Clinical Neurophysiology*, 62, 364-371.
Brunner R. L., Maloney M. J., Daniels S., Mays W., & Farrel M. (1989). A controlled study of type A behavior and psychophysiologic responses to stress in anorexia nervosa. *Psychiatry Research*, 30, 223-230.
Casper R. C., & Heller W. (1991). "La douce différence" and mood in anorexia nervosa: neuropsychological correlates. *Progress in Neuropsychopharmacology and Biological Psychiatry*, 15, 15-23.
Connolly J. F. (1987). Commentary: ERPs suggest the importance of subcortical mechanisms in activities typically associated with cortical functions. In: R Johnson, J. W. Rohrbaugh & R. Parasuraman (Eds.), *Current trends in event-related potential research* (EEG Suppl. 40, pp. 635-644). Amsterdam: Elsevier.
Davidson R. J. (1984). Affect, cognition, and hemispheric specialization. In C. E. Izard, J. Kagan, R. Zajouc (Eds.), *Emotion, cognition and behavior* (pp. 320-365). New York: Cambridge University Press.
Delaunoy J., Gerono A., & Rousseau J. C. (1978). Experimental production of post-imperative negative variation in normal subjects. In D. A. Otto (Ed.), *Multidisciplinary Perspectives in Event-Related Brain Potential Research* (pp. 355-357). Washington, DC: US Government Printing Office.
Delvenne V., Kerkhofs M., Appelboom-Fondu J., Lucas F., & Mendlewicz J. (1992). Sleep polygraphic variables in anorexia and depression: a comparative study in adolescents. *Journal of Affective Disorders*, 25, 167-172.
Duffy E. (1972). Activation. In N. S. Greenfield & R. A. Sternbach (Eds.), *Handbook of psychophysiology* (pp. 577-622). New York: Holt, Rinehart & Winston.
Dumais-Huber C. (1993). *Electrical brain activity and stimulus control. A study on the regulatory processes of the frontal cortex in psychiatric disordered children*. Doctoral thesis, University of Heidelberg, Germany.
Dumais-Huber C., & Rothenberger A. (1992). Psychophysiological correlates of orienting, anticipation and contingency changes in children with psychiatric disorders. *Journal of Psychophysiology*, 6(3), 225-239.
Edelberg R. (1972). Electrical activity of the skin: Its measurement and uses in psychophysiology. In N. S. Greenfield & R. A. Sternbach (Eds.), *Handbook of psychophysiology* (pp. 367-418). New York: Holt, Rinehart & Winston.
Finley W. W. (1984). Biofeedback of very early potentials from the brainstem. In T. Elbert, B. Rockstroh, W. Lutzenberger & N. Birbaumer (Eds.), *Self-regulation of the brain and behavior* (pp. 143-163). Berlin, Heidelberg, New York: Springer.
Fowles D.C. (1980). The three arousal model: Implications of Gray's two factor learning theory for heart rate, electrodermal activity, and psychopathy. *Psychophysiology*, 17, 87-104.
Fuster J. M. (1989). *The prefrontal cortex* (2nd ed.). New York: Raven Press.
Garreau B. (1985). *Etude des activités évoquées du tronc cérébral et de la région frontale chez l'enfant autistique*. Diplôme, Université P. et M. Curie, Paris.
Gauthier P., & Gottesmann C. (1977). Study of post-imperative negativity induction. *Electroencephalography and Clinical Neurophysiology*, 43, 534-535.
George D. T., Kaye W. H., Goldstein D. S., Brewerton T. D., & Jimerson D. C. (1990). Altered norepinephrine regulation in bulimia: effects of pharmacological challenge with isoproterenol. *Psychiatry Research*, 33, 1-10.

Gunn C. G., Wolf S., Block R. T., & Person R. J. (1972). Psychophysiology of the cardiovascular system. In N. S. Greenfield & RA Sternbach (Eds.), *Handbook of psychophysiology* (pp. 457-489). New York: Holt, Rinehart & Winston.

Heller W., & Levy J. (1981). Perception and expression of emotion in right-handers and left-handers. *Neuropsychologia*, 19, 263-272.

Hentschel F., Woerner W., & Rothenberger A. (1994). Hirnvolumenschwankungen bei Anorexia nervosa. *Klinische Neuroradiologie*, 4, 19-26.

Herholz K., Krieg J. C., Emrich H. M., Pawlik G., Beil C., Pirke K. M., Pahl J. J., Wagner R., Wienhard K., Ploog D., & Heiss W. D. (1987). Regional cerebral glucose metabolism in anorexia nervosa measured by positron emission tomography. *Biological Psychiatry*, 22, 43-51.

Hudson J. I., & Pope H. G. (1987). Newer antidepressants in the treatment of bulimia nervosa. *Psychopharmacology Bulletin*, 23, 52-57.

Hynek K., & Faltus F. (1990). An EEG study in anorexia nervosa and an attempt to use it for prognostic prediction (Czech). *Ceskoslovenska Psychiatrie*, 86, 369-374.

Kagan J., Kogan N. (1970). Individual variation in cognitive processes. In P. H. Mussen (Ed.), *Carmichael's manual of child psychiatry* (3rd ed.). New York: Wiley.

Kahn D., Halls J., Bianco J. A., & Perlman S. B. (1991). Radionuclide ventriculography in severely underweight anorexia nervosa patients before and during refeeding therapy. *Journal of Adolescent Health*, 12, 301-306.

Kaye W. H., George D. T., Gwirtsman H. E., Jimerson D. C., Goldstein D. S., Ebert M. H., & Lake C. R. (1990). Isoproterenol infusion test in anorexia nervosa: assessment of pre- and post-beta-noradrenergic receptor activity. *Psychopharmacology Bulletin*, 26, 355-359.

Kennedy S. H., Heslegrave R. J. (1989). Cardiac regulation in bulimia nervosa. *Journal of Psychiatric Research*, 23, 267-273.

Kohlmeyer K., Lehmkuhl G., & Poustka F. (1983). Computed tomography of anorexia nervosa. *American Journal of Neuroradiology*, 4, 437-438.

Lauer C., Zulley J., Krieg J. C., Rieman D., & Berger M. (1988). EEG sleep and the cholinergic REM induction test in anorexic and bulimic patients. *Psychiatry Research*, 26, 171-181.

Levine S. C., & Levy J. (1986). Perceptual asymmetry for chimeric faces across the life span. *Brain and Cognition*, 5, 291-306.

Malloy P. (1987). Frontal lobe dysfunction in obsessive-compulsive disorder. In E. Perecman (Ed.), *The frontal lobes revisited* (pp. 207-223). New York: IRBN Press.

Marcus A., Blanz B., Lehmkuhl G., Rothenberger A., & Eisert H. G. (1989). Somatische Befunde bei Kindern und Jugendlichen mit Anorexia nervosa. *Acta Paedopsychiatrica*, 52, 1-11.

McCallum W. C., & Walter W. G. (1968). The effects of attention and distraction on the contingent negative variation in normal and neurotic subjects. *Electroencephalography and Clinical Neurophysiology*, 25, 319-329.

Miyamoto H., Sakuna K., Kumaga K., Ichikawa T., & Koizumi J. (1992). Auditory brainstem response (ABR) in anorexia nervosa. *Japanese Journal of Psychiatry and Neurology*, 46, 673-679.

Mills I. H. (1985). The neuronal basis of compulsive behavior in anorexia nervosa. *Journal of Psychiatric Research*, 19, 231-235.

Moll G. H., & Rothenberger A. (1993). Magersucht im Jugendalter - mangelnde Modulation autonomer vegetativer Systeme? In P. Baumann (Ed.), *Biologische Psychiatrie der Gegenwart* (3. Drei-Länder-Symposium für Biologische Psychiatrie, Lausanne, Sept. '92, pp. 380-383). New York: Springer.

Moodie D. S. (1987). Anorexia and the heart. Results of studies to assess effects. *Postgraduate Medicine*, 81, 46-55.

Moodie D. S., & Salcedo E. (1983). Cardiac function in adolescents and young adults with anorexia nervosa. *Journal of Adolescent Health Care*, 4, 9-14.

Nakagawa K., Akikawa K., Namioka M., Kubo M., & Matsubara M. (1985). Responses to epinephrine in patients with anorexia nervosa. *Endocrinologia Japonica*, 32, 845-849.

Niedermeyer E. & Lopez da Silva F. (1982). *Electroencephalography*. Munich: Urban & Schwarzenberg.

Nudel D. B., Gootman N., Nussbaum M. P., & Shenker J. R. (1984). Altered exercise performance and abnormal sympathetic responses to exercise in patients with anorexia nervosa. *Journal of Pediatrics*, 105, 34-37.

Papakostopoulos D., & McCallum W. C. (1973). The CNV and autonomic change in situations of increasing complexity. In W.C. McCallum & J. R. Knott (Eds.), *Event-related slow potentials of the brain: their relations to behavior* (EEG Suppl. 33, pp. 287-293). Amsterdam: Elsevier.

Peters J. F. & Knott J. R. (1976). CNV and post-response negativity with stressful auditory feedback. In W.C. McCallum & J. Knott (Eds.), *The Responsive Brain*.(pp. 52-54) Bristol: Wright.

Pirke K. M. (1990). The noradrenergic system in anorexia and bulimia nervosa. In H. Remschmidt & M. H. Schmidt (Eds.), *Anorexia nervosa* (pp. 30-44), Toronto: Hogrefe and Huber.

Pirke K. M., & Ploog D. (1986). Psychobiology of anorexia nervosa. In R. J. Wurtman & J. J. Wurtman (Eds.), *Nutrition and the brain:* (Vol. 7, pp. 167-198). New York: Raven.

Rockstroh B., Elbert T., Canavan A., Lutzenberger W., & Birbaumer N. (1989). *Slow cortical potentials and behaviour*. Baltimore: Urban & Schwarzenberg.

Rohrbaugh J. W., & Gaillard A. (1983). Sensory and motor aspects of the contingent negative variation. In A. W. K. Gaillard & W. Ritter (Eds.), *Tutorials in Event Related Potential Research: Endogenous Components* (pp. 269-310). Amsterdam: Elsevier.

Rothenberger A. (1990). The role of frontal lobes in child psychiatric disorders. In A. Rothenberger (Ed.), *Brain and Behavior in Child Psychiatry* (pp. 34-58). Berlin, Heidelberg: Springer.

Rothenberger A., Blanz B., & Lehmkuhl G. (1991). What happens to electrical brain activity when anorectic adolescents gain weight? *European Archives of Psychiatry and Clinical Neuroscience*, 240, 144-147.

Rothenberger A., Müller H. U., & Müller W. E. (1990). Central versus peripheral disturbance in the norepinephrine metabolism of adolescents with anorexia nervosa. In H. Remschmidt & M. H. Schmidt (Eds.), *Child and Youth Psychiatry: European Perspectives* (Vol. 1, pp. 45-53). Toronto: Hogrefe and Huber.

Rothenberger A., Reiser A., Grote I., & Woerner W. (1987). Modulation of sensory input in infants at different psychosocial and organic risk. In M. Kutas & B. Renault (Eds.), *ICON IV Conference Proceedings. LENA* (pp. 85-88). Paris: Dourdan.

Rothenberger A., Lehmkuhl G., Kohlmeyer K., Blanz B., Reiser A., & Grote I. (1986). Anorexia nervosa (AN) in adolescents - evoked potentials help to elucidate the biological background. In V. Gallai (Ed.), *Maturation of the CNS and evoked potentials* (pp. 375-384). Amsterdam: Elsevier.

Seeger G., & Lehmkuhl G. (1993). Hirnelektrische Korrelate der Verarbeitung affektiver versus neutraler Reize bei Jugendlichen mit Anorexia nervosa. In P. Baumann (Ed.), *Biologische Psychiatrie der Gegenwart* (3. Drei-Länder-Symposium für Biologische Psychiatrie, Lausanne, September 1992, pp. 375-379). New York: Springer.

Vandereycken W., & Meermann R. (1984). *Anorexia nervosa*. Berlin:Walter de Gruyter.

Vaughan H. G. Jr., & Arezzo J. C. (1988). The neural basis of event-related potentials. In T. W. Picton (Ed.), *Human event-related potentials* (EEG handbook, revised series, Vol. 3). Amsterdam: Elsevier.

Wilde K. M., & Barry R. J. (1992). *Fractionation of arousal measures: A test of Fowles' hypothesis*. Paper presented at the Sixth International Congress of Psychophysiology, September 1992, Berlin.

Walsh B. T., Goetz R., Roose S. P., Fingeroth S., & Glassman A. H. (1985). EEG-monitored sleep in anorexia nervosa and bulimia. *Biological Psychiatry*, 20, 947-956.

# Part III

# Management and Treatment

# Medical Assessment and the Initial Interview in the Management of Young Patients with Anorexia Nervosa

*Pierre J.V. Beumont, Kitty Lowinger, and Janice D. Russell*

## 1 Introduction

Anorexia nervosa is unique among illnesses in that it consists of two equally important components: a pervasive behavioural and attitudinal disturbance associated with deep-seated psychological and interpersonal problems; and a complex medical disorder, partly the effect of nature's attempt to compensate for a state of longstanding undernutrition and partly the result of complications brought about by the various behaviours that were used to bring about weight loss. Our task in this chapter is to address two issues. First, we will describe the medical assessment of these patients, presenting our views on the medical evaluation of anorexia nervosa in general and then focussing attention on some aspects that are of special importance to prepubertal children and young adolescents. Second, we will set this assessment within the context of the initial interview with the patient and family, emphasizing the importance of dealing with the psychological as well as the physical in understanding the problem and in the initiation of treatment.

## 2 Medical Assessment

Although it has often been trivialized in the past, there is now general acceptance that anorexia nervosa is indeed a serious health problem. Not only does it affect large numbers of girls and young women (it is 5 times as common as insulin dependent diabetes mellitus in this section of the population (Lucas et al., 1991)) and cause great psychological distress to patients and their families, but it is also the cause of varied and often severe physical morbidity leading to a mortality rate approaching 20% at 20 year follow-up (Theander, 1985), by far the highest of any functional psychiatric illness. Physical morbidity may persist even in those patients who appear to have recovered from the illness, as manifested in stunting of growth, reproductive failure, and premature osteoporosis. At the same time as these long-term deleterious effects are coming to be recognized, however, there is an increasing trend for the treatment of anorexia patients to pass from psychiatrists and physicians to psychologists, dietitians, occupational and family therapists, and social workers. This is especially likely in the case of prepubertal and young adolescent patients. While these professionals may be well trained to deal with the psychological and social aspects of the illness, they are not equipped to assess and treat the physical disorder. Hence there is a real danger that the physical morbidity will be overlooked. For that reason it is important that all medical practitioners - including family doctors or general practitioners - become better informed about the illness and more confident in their ability to treat it. They will often be required to do the preliminary medical examination of the patient, or even to take overall care for the medical management, while the psychological treatment is undertaken by a non-medical colleague.

## 2.1 The Basis of the Physical Disorder

A primary physical cause was long sought for anorexia nervosa, and numerous theories were advanced proposing an underlying endocrine or hypothalamic pathology. Few modern authorities would countenance such suggestions, and there is now general consensus among persons working in the area that the physical disturbances are all epiphenomena, the result of undernutrition and of the behaviours used to induce it (Beumont, 1984a). Indeed, many of the most characteristic physical features of the illness can be reproduced in healthy persons subjected to experimental starvation (Fichter & Pirke, 1984).

The effects of starvation depend on the kind of dietary deficiency from which it arises. Because the anorexia patient has not gone through a prior phase of protein and vitamin deprivation and of parasitic infestation before entering negative energy balance, the nutritional disturbance, at least in the early phase of illness, is usually more benign than that found in a victim of protein-calorie malnutrition or famine with equivalent weight loss. To some extent, it resembles the nutritional states associated with spontaneous hypophagias in animals, such as those found in birds during incubation or in hibernating mammals (Beumont, 1984b). At first, the anorexia patient chooses a diet low in energy-dense foods but relatively high in protein and other essential nutrients (Beumont et al., 1981). This type of diet, together with the characteristically high levels of activity, exerts a nitrogen sparing effect so that the initial weight reduction is due mainly to loss of fat (Beumont, 1986). Malnutrition, as opposed to undernutrition, is relatively mild.

Normally, the body's immediate energy requirements are met by glucose, and glucose is the preferred energy substrate for the brain. As weight loss becomes more severe in the patient who persists with anorexic behaviour, the glucose stored in glycogen deposits in the muscles and liver is rapidly exhausted and fat reserves are mobilized, leading to the formation of ketone bodies. They account for the sweet smell of acetone on the breath of emaciated patients. In order to accommodate to the state of semi-starvation, gluco-neogenesis is stimulated and protein tissue is broken down (Pirke & Ploog, 1987). This leads to protein depletion and water loss from the intracellular compartment. Electrolyte imbalance and metabolic complications ensue, including severe hypoglycemia which may be asymptomatic. These abnormalities become aggravated as the patient further decreases her nutritional intake to the point of total starvation.

By this time the patient is severely undernourished and may go on to a weight of only 50% or even less of normal body weight. Buccal fat pads are lost and the patient's appearance is skeletal. Skin turgor is reduced, and the patient has sunken eyes, ketotic halitosis, bradycardia, hypotension, and poor peripheral circulation. The skin is dry and rough with overgrowth of lanugo hair, the ribs protrude, and the teeth may be eroded from gastric acid during vomiting. Secondary sexual characteristics are often underdeveloped.

Fortunately, the purely nutritional effects of anorexia nervosa are reversible if the patient resumes healthy eating and regains weight. Total body protein is replenished (J.D. Russell et al., 1994), electrolyte imbalance is corrected, and normal hydration and a normal state of nutrition are restored. However, some medical complications may become irreversible and persist despite the improvement in nutritional status.

## 2.2 Medical Complications

The medical complications of anorexia nervosa are varied and often serious (Bhanji & Mattingly, 1988), accounting for the high prevalence of physical morbidity and the alarming mortality rate of the illness, which may be as high as

10% in the short term, depending on the availability of effective medical management. The long term mortality is reported to be about 20% (Theander, 1985).

There are some important differences between the presentation of anorexia nervosa in prepubertal and early adolescent patients as compared to those who are older. First, the sex distribution is more even, with about 30% of younger patients being male (Bryant-Waugh, 1993), rather than only about 5%. Clinically, dehydration is more frequent and more severe, because of the larger proportion of total body water in the body composition of the young child, and because vomiting is more likely to be part of the repertoire of weight losing behaviours than in older patients. Also, the condition of the young patient may deteriorate very rapidly, with severe emaciation and depression occurring early in the clinical course (Fosson et al., 1993).

There is an important distinction between those symptoms that are indicative of compensatory mechanisms to cope with the state of undernutrition, on the one hand, and those that result directly from the behavioural disturbance on the other. In the former group are phenomena such as anovulatory infertility, which helps prevent a young woman from conceiving at a time when she is grossly undernourished; a state of functional hypothyroidism, a means of conserving scarce energy resources; and an elevation of circulating growth hormone levels, which is part of the mechanism by which glucose levels are preserved in the face of semi-starvation and inadequate protein intake (Beumont, 1984a). To attempt to reverse these processes prior to restoration of a normal state of nutrition is both unnecessary and unwise. By setting aside such physiological readjustments, one merely exposes the patient further to the effects of energy depletion. In contrast, conditions such as dehydration and electrolyte imbalance, often the result of self-induced vomiting or purgation, demand immediate attention. If neglected they may lead to even more serious complications. So too, longterm effects such as growth retardation in the young patient, or the insidious development of osteoporosis, are matters of major concern and appropriate intervention.

## 2.3 History Taking and Psychoeducational Counselling

The first requirement of medical management is an accurate evaluation of the patient's physical condition. This comprises history taking, physical examination, and the necessary laboratory investigations. It is usefully combined with an educational intervention directed at providing the patient with information concerning the nature of the physical complications of her illness. The principles of the psychoeducational approach have been well enunciated in the literature (Garner et al., 1985), and the doctor undertaking the initial physical examination of the patient is a most appropriate person to provide this important component of treatment.

Young anorexia nervosa sufferers seldom present of their own volition, but are brought by concerned relatives, either both parents or the mother by herself. Many parents recall the struggle they had with the family doctor before the diagnosis was made. All too often, the doctor dismissed the parents' fears as groundless and attributed the patient's incipient anorexia to "normal adolescent dieting". Just as with reports by relatives that a patient is drinking alcohol to excess, so too with a dieting adolescent patient, it is probably best to assume that the parents are correct in their observations and not be misled by the young person's protestations that there is nothing the matter.

This confusion may be fostered by being too scrupulous about the issue of confidentiality. Certainly, patients have the right to be interviewed on their own, but so must parents be allowed to express their concerns. We find it useful to ask the patient's permission for the parents to come into the early part of the interview, explain what they are worried about in front of their child, and then leave the room so that patient and doctor may explore the matter further. Conducting the dual interview with parents and child requires sincerity and sensitivity. On the one hand the parents should be empowered to speak frankly about their concerns. On the other, confrontation must be avoided as that would reduce the ability of both doctor and parents to help the patient abandon the abnormal behaviours.

## 2.4 Dieting History

A comprehensive dietary history is important. What exactly is the patient eating? Is the diet balanced, or is there a selective avoidance of energy-dense foods and an inadequate intake of dietary protein? Vegetarianism is extremely common among anorexia patients and contributes to their nutritional deficiency. Of course, the patient may deliberately set out to deceive the examiner, but more often gives accurate responses, which are then defended by saying that it is "enough for me".

The mother's account of her child's eating practices must also be elicited. How does the child behave at table: fly into a rage when pressed to finish the meal? Or is there is any indication that the patient is disposing of food? Friends and acquaintances from school often observe patients throwing away their school lunches and report such behaviours to their teachers or directly to the parents.

Both the patient's and the mother's knowledge about nutritional matters should be explored. What do they really know about food, diet, and health? Frequently they hold beliefs that are untrue and extreme, such as the belief that 1,200 or 1,500 calories a day is sufficient for a growing girl, or the conviction that all fat should be avoided. They should be made aware of the need for a reasonable energy intake, 2,000 or more calories a day for an active girl (even more for a boy), and the relationship of adequate energy intake to physical activity and well-being.

## 2.5 Purging Behaviours

Because purging behaviours such as self-induced vomiting and laxative abuse are so important in the causation of complications (Beumont et al., 1993), it is important that direct enquiry be made about them. They are likely to be denied, so a tactful approach is necessary. We find it useful to explain that these behaviours are common among young people who are seeking to loose weight (Abraham et al., 1983), but that most patients are ashamed of them and hence unwilling to report their presence. We then ask the mother in front of the patient whether she has any reason to suspect that her child is vomiting or purging. On what is that based? While allowing the patient the opportunity to reply, we do not press to any confrontation about the issue, but return to it later during the interview when the patient is alone with the doctor.

If the patient admits to vomiting, its frequency should be elicited. When did she first use it to control weight? Even if vomiting is denied, it is necessary to discuss it further, perhaps pointing out that, although some young people use vomiting to control weight, it is both ineffective and dangerous. Few patients realize just how dangerous it may be and they should be provided with information about the risks, phrased in language appropriate for their age, education, and clinical status.

Vomiting affects blood chemistry and in particular lowers serum potassium, causing ECG changes and leading to cardiac arrhythmias and decompensation.

Renal damage may also result, due to decreased blood volume, diminished glomerular filtration rate, and acid-base imbalance (Bhanji & Mattingly, 1988). Vomiting is also associated with parotiditis, causing an unsightly swelling at the angle of the jaw; oesophagitis and gastritis with the possibility of oesophageal tears; and erosion of the tooth enamel by the acid in regurgitated gastric contents. Injuries to knuckles (from putting fingers down the throat) or to the mouth and palate (by inserting hard instruments such as toothbrushes) are disfiguring and painful. The use of the emetic drug Ipecac is particularly dangerous because of its cardiotoxic effect.

The issue of laxative or diuretic abuse should also be explored. Specific questions should be asked about so-called herbal laxatives, the use of unprocessed bran (devoid of nutritional content and used for its laxative effects), or drinking large quantities of coffee (a diuretic). Patients often choose to discount the unhealthy nature of these practices. Again, the patient should be educated about the dangers intrinsic to such behaviours. Their effect on weight is entirely the result of dehydration, and they do not influence energy balance as such (Garner et al., 1985). Moreover, they contribute to hypovolemia and hypotension, and to electrolyte disturbances such as hypokalemia and hypocalcemia with their subsequent effects on cardiac rhythm. They also affect bowel function, leading to malabsorption, resulting from abrasion and desquamation of the bowel lining. Inadequate absorption is associated with protein loss and hypoproteinemia and further loss of fluid into the tissues. Explaining these processes to the patient in suitable language may be the crucial step in preventing their occurrence, or in helping the patient to abandon the behaviour if she has previously used it.

## 2.6 Reproductive History

A menstrual history will elicit whether the patient has a primary or secondary amenorrhoea, duration of amenorrhoea, and age at menarche. Menstrual disturbance is almost invariable in young patients who are significantly undernourished (older women appear to be somewhat more resistant). Sometimes the complete cessation of menses is preceded by a phase of irregularity and oligomenorrhoea.

A history of delayed menarche is indicative of long-standing undernutrition prior to the emergence of clinical features of anorexia nervosa. On the other hand, there is an increased frequency of association of anorexia nervosa with Turner's syndrome (Abraham et al., 1981), and this should be borne in mind. A Turner's habitus may be noted, and the diagnosis will be confirmed by karyotyping.

The low oestrogen levels accompanying the amenorrhoea are an important factor in the development of osteoporosis (Rigotti et al., 1991), and this needs to be explained to the patient. Because adequate amounts of bone tissue are not being deposited while she is young, the patient is likely to develop brittle bones and fractures on minimal stress later in life. Low levels of testosterone in male patients retard sexual development, the acquisition of secondary sex characteristics, and the acquisition of mature musculature. They may also affect bone density.

The history of the patient's weight loss should be elicited. Of course, in some children with an insidious onset, it may be more a question of failure to achieve age appropriate weight gain rather than of actual weight loss. It is more common, however, for there to be a clear history of weight loss, which may have been sudden and severe. A rapid loss is more likely to precipitate cardiac problems and is a determinant of the need for urgent hospitalization.

## 2.7 Past Medical and Psychiatric History

The past medical and psychiatric history needs to be carefully evaluated. Prior illnesses such as diabetes, asthma, or cardiac conditions necessitate variations in the approach to therapy. On the other hand, a history of depression or of recent bowel or "malabsorption" problems is likely to be due to the incipient anorexic illness or to the use of laxatives and other agents. In some young patients, anorexia nervosa follows an illness such as glandular fever or gastroenteritis in which appetite and weight are lost. The patient is pleased with the effect and reluctant to resume normal eating and regain weight. This leads to food restriction, perhaps self-induced vomiting, and further weight loss. Thus the illness becomes self-perpetuating. Unfortunately, such patients are sometimes given the inappropriate diagnosis of chronic fatigue syndrome, which leads to much confusion for the parents and reinforces the patients in their assertion that they are not able to eat like other people.

A history of the use of medications is essential, as they may contribute to the physical complications to which these patients are prone. Corticosteroids, which are used in the treatment of asthma, may predispose to infection. Sprays aggravate dry eyes, which are common in anorexia nervosa patients due to the associated vitamin A deficiency. They increase the risk of infection and of corneal injury. Hormone preparations, such as the contraceptive pill, negate the usefulness of the current menstrual history. Even vitamin and mineral supplements may be counterproductive in that they provide patients with further reasons to argue that they do not need to eat normally. Although the predominant nutritional disturbance in anorexia nervosa is energy depletion, deficiencies of protein and of essential nutrients do occur and need to be treated. On the other hand, patients sometimes show ill effects from the excessive use of vitamin supplements, such as gastritis or diarrhoea resulting from massive doses of ascorbic acid (vitamin C).

Perhaps the most troublesome unwanted drug effects in anorexia patients are those resulting from tricyclic antidepressants, inappropriately prescribed for the dysphoria that is often prominent at presentation and is part of the anorexia syndrome. Anticholinergic effects include dry mouth (yet another excuse not to eat), dry eyes, and constipation - which is often already a significant problem, particularly in patients who have chronically abused laxatives. Even more serious are the potential effects on cardiac rhythm in patients whose cardiac function is already compromised by their undernutrition and the electrolytic disturbance consequent on their purging behaviour. The use of tricyclics, particularly in high doses, may precipitate a life-threatening arrhythmia.

## 2.8 Family History

Of particular relevance are conditions in family members that require special dietary management and may have affected family eating patterns, such as a father on a cholesterol-lowering diet. A family history of an eating or dieting disorder in a sibling or a parent may be a further factor preventing full compliance of the family in treatment. A specially difficult problem is that posed by a mother who has herself had an anorexic illness and persists in attitudes and beliefs that are basically inimical to the restoration of a normal eating pattern (Griffiths et al., 1995). On the other hand, obesity in another family member may be a potent precipitant of self-starvation in the child, and one with which the family may well collude.

## 2.9 Exercise

Excessive exercise is frequently part of the anorexic behavioural disturbance, partly as a deliberate means of losing weight and partly as a manifestation of the restless overactivity that has long been known to characterize the anorexia nervosa patient (Beumont et al., 1994). Solitary artistic or athletic pursuits become an important source of self-esteem for a depressed, self-centred youngster, but exercise levels increase paradoxically as weight is lost, contributing to the patient's physical dysfunction. This is particularly dangerous in those whose cardiac function is already compromised. Indicators of loss of control are a history of many hours spent in strenuous activity (e.g., two hours of aerobics every day - and an hour spent running to and from the gymnasium!), solitary exercising, inability to abstain and distress when constrained to do so, and "debting" - i.e., attempting to set energy intake against activity so as always to be in a state of negative energy balance. Although most parents recognize excessive activity as abnormal, there are some who initially condone it on the basis of their own preoccupation with physical fitness. Then there is also the influence of other adults to consider: athletics coaches or ballet teachers who make unreasonable and unhealthy demands of the young people in their care.

The combination of inadequate nutrition with ever-increasing activity eventually leads to a state of utter fatigue with lethargy, dyspnoea, syncope, and depression. Bone pain or stress fractures add to the discomfort, but the patient feels driven to continue to exercise despite the pain. A frank discussion of the obsessive nature of the activity and the impossibility of maintaining high performance or developing strong musculature should be attempted.

## 2.10 Physical Examination: Height and Weight

It is imperative that any patient suspected of having anorexia nervosa is asked to undress so that the doctor can see the extent of the emaciation and the presence of other stigmata of undernutrition, such as lanugo hair (fine, downy hair on the extensor surfaces of the limbs and on the back) and acrocyanosis. Many patients have become adept at hiding the physical effects of their illness under voluminous clothes, and their medical attendants may be deceived into underestimating the severity of their illness.

The patient's height and weight should be recorded and the body mass index (BMI) calculated (weight in kgs divided by the square of height in metres). Patients over 16 should have a BMI of at least 20 (Beumont et al., 1988). However, in younger children the BMI is a less appropriate measure (Bryant-Waugh & Kaminski, 1993). Recourse may be made instead to pediatric tables, setting a weight commensurate to the same percentile as the child's height as a standard of normality. Unfortunately even here there are problems, as longstanding nutritional deprivation may have seriously retarded growth so that a child at the 10th percentile of both weight and height may really be significantly undernourished. To compensate, some authors have suggested that 90% of average weight for age should be set as the absolute minimum for any patient.

## 2.11 General Physical Status

General observations of physical status reveal many of the features of the illness. Anemia may be evident in the pale mucous membranes and an unhealthy pallor of the skin. Previously, it was said to be usually of a normochromic, normocytic type, but with the increasing frequency of vegetarianism among anorexia patients (O'Connor et al., 1987) it is now more likely to be an iron deficiency anemia. In others there is the characteristic orange colouration of carotonemia, especially noticeable on the palms and soles. Its cause remains controversial, attributed variously to the ingestion of massive amounts of carrots and other coloured vegetables, to a enzymatic disturbance, or to a fault in the Krebs cycle (Bhanji & Mattingly, 1988). Patients often show extensive bruising, related to increased capillary wall fragility, low platelet count, and low levels of vitamin K. Nails are brittle and head hair may fall out, leaving areas of alopecia. Yet other patients shamefacedly admit to trichotillomania, the obsessive behavioural disturbance in which hairs are selectively pulled from the scalp. Patients who are severely ill may have significant hypothermia.

## 2.12 Metabolic

Several signs of metabolic disturbance are present. Bradypnoea occurs as a response to the metabolic alkalosis caused by vomiting and purging with loss of $H^+$ and $K^+$ ions. The patient's breath smells acetotic as a result of the breakdown of fat reserves, and ketosis is confirmed by urine testing. Proteinuria is an indicator of renal glomerular damage.

Patients are frequently dehydrated as a result of their purging behaviour and inadequate fluid intake. Oedema, if present, is likely to result from a combination of factors, including increased capillary permeability, hypoproteinuria, congestive cardiac failure, and a lowered glomerular filtration rate associated with hypotension and hypovolemia.

## 2.13 Cardiovascular

The cardiovascular system warrants careful examination (Schocken et al., 1989). Blood pressure should be recorded both standing and lying. Significant hypotension (below 100/60) is cause for caution. Heart rate and rhythm are documented: a pulse rate under 60 per minute is indicative of significant bradycardia. Rates as low as 40 are not uncommon. Because many anorexia patients are hyperactive and exercise excessively, there has been a tendency to attribute the bradycardia to their apparent athleticism. In truth, exercise capacity and oxygen consumption are reduced, and both the heart rate and blood pressure responses to exercise are blunted. These disturbances are probably due to decreased resting catecholamine levels and an attenuated catecholamine response.

Heart size may be dimished, the heart assuming a vertical position in the chest as confirmed by radiography. Auscultation may reveal the characteristic mid systolic click of a mitral valve prolapse. This is an essentially benign complication resulting from a disproportion between the rigid valvular ring and the shrunken left ventricle, and it is accentuated by dehydration. As cardiomyopathy can occur, there may be signs of congestive cardiac failure, especially in instances in which rehydration is pursued too rapidly. The peripheral circulation is affected, with cold, blue extremities and slow venous return.

## 2.14 Gastrointestinal

Examination of the gastrointestinal system includes a careful observation of the mouth, teeth, and gums for evidence of self-induced vomiting such as abrasions caused by the insertion of fingers or hard objects to elicit a gag reflex, erosion of the tooth enamel by gastric contents, or gingivitis. Enlargement of the parotid glands should be noted as it is associated with frequent vomiting. The abdomen is scaphoid but, if constipation is severe, fecal masses may be palpated through the abdominal wall or on rectal examination. Acute gastric dilatation and intestinal obstruction are not uncommon complications early in the refeeding process, a consequence of delayed gastric emptying and hypokalemic paralytic ileus. Various other mechanisms may be involved in the obstruction such as intussusception or a superior mesenteric syndrome. The latter is the result of loss of the retro-peritoneal fat pad, allowing compression of the duodenum between the artery and the spine posteriorly. Fecal impaction may be precipitated by the use of a tricyclic antidepressant such as clomipramine, which causes pronounced constipation. Laxative abuse and its colonic consequences are less likely in the young patient than in adults, but rectal prolapse may result from excessive straining at stool.

## 2.15 Neurological

A mild delirium may be present in patients who are severely undernourished, the symptoms of which may be wrongly attributed to the patient's truculence or lack of co-operation. Myopathy and neuropathy are fairly common, usually associated with hypokalemia, but low Mg, Ca, or PO4 may be involved as well as the toxic effects of Ipecac (an emetic) or of massive amounts of liquorice, used as a purgative. Peripheral nerve compression results from the loss of protective subcutaneous fat. The lateral popliteal nerve is sometimes involved, leading to foot drop (Bhanji & Mattingly, 1988).

Particularly in patients who overexercise, stress fractures are common. They are related to the mechanical stress imposed by an unrealistic exercise schedule together with the inadequate mineralization resulting from the low levels of circulating oestrogen, low dietary intake of calcium, laxative abuse, and a disturbed acid-base balance. A loss of the protein matrix, due to generalized depletion of body nitrogen and protein, may also occur.

## 2.16 Developmental Status

On the basis of the history and physical examination, the physician is able to document the patient's developmental status and consider the likelihood of the illness having caused maturational delay. Of particular importance is the issue of growth retardation. Chronic undernutrition undoubtedly is a major factor in stunting. In a recent study of early onset anorexia nervosa patients, only 10% were found to reach average height at 10 year follow-up and 35% failed to reach even the third percentile for height (G.F.M. Russell, 1985).

Height needs to be carefully recorded at the initial examination so that the patient's progress can be monitored on subsequent visits. However, the decision as to whether any individual patient is growth retarded is often difficult to make because of the wide range in heights that are considered normal. Consideration needs to be given to the influence of genetic factors by measuring parental heights. A patient who is at the 25th percentile, but whose parents are both tall people, may in fact be significantly stunted.

It is important that young children are restored promptly to an adequate state of nutrition, so as to allow for the resumption of growth to offset the retarding effect of the illness. After the age of 13.5 years in girls, or 16 years in boys, few children are able to achieve optimal "catch-up" growth, so the matter is urgent. In deciding on what action to take in these circumstances, it is useful to predict what the patient's adult height should be. Determination of bone age by radiography of the left hand, and of "genetic height", i.e., half the mean height of father and mother, plus or minus 10%, are useful for this purpose. Discussion of the risk of height retardation may help as an inducement to full weight restoration in some patients, particularly boys.

The presence of secondary sexual characteristics is noted, allowing for assessment of the stage of puberty that has been attained, using a system such as that of Tanner (Marshall & Tanner, 1969). Psycho-sexual immaturity is often a striking feature of anorexia nervosa patients, and the consequent low levels of sex steroids are an important factor in the development of osteoporosis.

## 2.17 Special Investigations

There are a few routine tests that should be performed on every patient, but in general the need for laboratory investigations is decided on the basis of the clinical problems posed by the particular patient and should not simply conform to a predetermined list (Beumont et al., 1993). It is relevant to distinguish between those tests that are likely to prove useful in treatment and those undertaken merely to confirm the presence of abnormalities known to occur in anorexia nervosa but which do not require immediate intervention (see Table 1).

Table 1: Laboratory Investigations in Anorexia Nervosa

**Those recommended for all patients**
- Full electrolyte profile, including potassium, magnesium, calcium and phosphates
- Glucose (random)
- Full blood count and ESR (severe sepsis may occur without pyrexia or leucocytosis)
- Full protein, albumin
- Liver function
- Renal function
- Electrocardiogram
- Chest X-ray
- Pelvic ultrasound

**Those indicated for particular patients**
- Further hematological studies, iron, folate, and vitamin B12
- Thiamine and other vitamins
- Bone densitometry (for all with a history of emaciation and amenorrhoea of more than 1 year)
- Abdominal radiographs (for severe bloating)
- Total bowel transit time (for persistent severe constipation)
- Oesophageal sphincter pressure studies (for reflux)
- Lactose deficiency tests (for dairy intolerance)
- Urine and blood osmolality
- Total body nitrogen

**Those of academic interest with expected finding**

| | |
|---|---|
| o LH, FSH | Low (almost invariable) |
| o Oestrogens, testosterone | Low (almost invariable) |
| o Cortisol | Raised (almost invariable) |
| o Thyroid function | Sick euthyroid (likely) |
| o Dexamethasone suppression test | Positive (likely) |
| o Amylase | Raised with vomiting |
| o Brain computed tomography/ magnetic resonance imaging | Pseudoatrophy (likely) |

Patients and their parents, particularly those who have difficulty in accepting a "psychological" cause for the illness, may interpret referral for laboratory testing as an indication that the doctor is unsure of the diagnosis of anorexia nervosa. This may further aggravate difficulties in co-operation. Unless there is a genuine diagnostic difficulty, it is appropriate that the examining doctor explains exactly what tests are being requested and what the reason is for each, relating the physical problem back to the patient's behaviour disturbance.

A full biochemical profile is necessary in all patients and is especially important in those who are suspected of inducing vomiting or abusing laxatives. The characteristic electrolytic disturbance is a hypokalemic, hypochloremic metabolic alkolosis. At least 20% of purging anorexia nervosa patients have significant hypokalemia (Schocken et al., 1989), which may lead to muscular weakness, cardiac arrhythmias, and renal impairment with tubular vacuolation. Potassium supplementation, if required, is best given orally, but even this is not without danger. We have had at least one patient who persistently abused oral K supplements and eventually died of cardiac complications of hyperkalemia.

Once one electrolyte abnormality is discerned, there is a high probability that others will emerge, often during the early phase of refeeding (Hall et al., 1989). Hypomagnesemia is often associated with hypokalemia, as are low values of calcium and phosphate. Sodium levels may also be depressed, normal, or elevated in the presence of dehydration.

Hypoglycemia poses a serious problem (Zalin & Lant, 1984). A random glucose level often reveals significant hypoglycemia in patients whose current energy intake is minimal, or hypoglycemia may be present only early in the morning, indicating how poorly the anorexia patient tolerates the few hours of fasting overnight (Vaisman et al., 1991). This is particularly likely if the diet has been so protein depleted that alanine, which is rate limiting for gluconeogenesis, was in short supply. The resulting low blood sugar levels and their effects on brain function are particularly worrying, as their presence may be obscured by autonomic down-regulation. Easily absorbable sugars should be included in the early refeeding of these patients, together with enough protein to provide alanine for gluconeogenesis. As glucose levels return to normal, phosphate levels may fall, requiring appropriate intervention (Beumont & Large, 1991). Vigorous refeeding without additional phosphate in a patient who is already chronically depleted may drive phosphate intracellularly in muscle and liver, resulting in a dangerous reduction in available phosphate for vital organs such as the heart and brain. Protein and fat supplementation help prevent this development.

Impaired liver function results from starvation induced catabolism, with raised cholesterol and raised enzyme levels. Raised blood urea and serum creatinine levels are commonly found (Mira et al., 1992). High levels of creatinine and uric acid (associated with severe purging) and reduced serum albumin (due to severe and chronic food restriction) are poor prognostic findings (W. Herzog, personal communication, 1993).

Many anorexia nervosa patients nowadays are vegetarian (O'Connor et al., 1987), and this increases the likelihood of significant anemia. Hemoglobin levels may be normal on admission, but drop precipitously on rehydration. Depending on the hematological findings, iron studies may be indicated, or assays of folic acid and vitamin B12. A low white cell count allows bacterial infection to occur without the usual defence mechanisms, and the ESR may be raised only moderately in the presence of an inadequate inflammatory response. Paradoxically, resistance to viral infections appears enhanced, possibly due to elevated cytokines. A lowered platelet count affects clotting and contributes to easy bruising, although increased capillary fragility is more important in this respect.

Some patients present features of specific vitamin deficiencies, requiring assessment of thiamine or other B vitamin levels (Bhanji & Mattingly, 1988).

Because the cardiac complications of anorexia nervosa are potentially so serious, a standard ECG should be part of the routine assessment. Bradycardia is very common, and if severe (below 50/min), warrants further investigation by means of a Holter monitor. Extreme variability in heart rate is an ominous finding, and patients who display it should be under the supervision of a specialist cardiologist, with restricted activity until their nutritional state is improved. Another sign of impending serious arrhythmia is prolongation of the corrected QT interval, presaging the occurrence of a life-threatening arrhythmia (Isner et al., 1985). Other ECG abnormalities that may be found include first degree heart block, ectopic atrial rhythms, modal escape, premature ventricular complexes, ST segment depression, and U waves. A myocardial infarct pattern may accompany severe hypothermia with elevated CPK levels. It reverses with rewarming and refeeding.

Documentation of thyroid status and of the hormonal deficiencies associated with the amenorrhoea and anovulation are of academic interest.

Pelvic ultrasound provides a reliable and nonintrusive means of observing ovarian size and the presence of follicles and it has been proposed as an appropriate means of monitoring the return of normal gonadal functioning during refeeding (Treasure et al., 1988). The determination of bone age has already been discussed in relation to maturational delay. The usual method employs the Greulich and Pyle atlas of radiographs of the left hand and wrist (Greulich & Pyle, 1959).

Osteoporosis is a serious longterm complication of anorexia nervosa (Rigotti et al., 1991). Although its clinical manifestations may only become apparent many years later, osteoporosis is best considered a disease of adolescence and early adult life as inadequate deposition of bone (and possibly of its protein matrix as well) at this time is the prime factor in its aetiology. All patients with a history of secondary amenorrhoea of more than 1 year, or those who still have a primary amenorrhoea at the age of 16, should be investigated by bone densitometry, preferably DEXA (dual energy X-ray absorption). If the results are more than 2 standard deviations below expected values, and if a rapid nutritional restoration to 100% of normal weight for height is not envisaged, the patient should be considered for hormone replacement therapy with low doses of oestrogen and progesterone. The advice and support of an endocrinologist with a specific interest in the area should be canvassed, and the advantages and disadvantages of treatment carefully discussed with the patient and her family.

## 3 Psychological and Family Issues in the Initial Interview, and the Start of Treatment

As anorexia nervosa is a serious illness, effective management must be initiated promptly and must be suitably comprehensive and of sufficient duration to ensure full recovery. Once the diagnosis is made, the need for treatment must be explained to the patient and the family, who individually or collectively may be surprised, hostile, or frankly disbelieving (Touyz & Beumont, 1991). Conflict between parents or between one or both parents and the patient will often emerge and must be explored cautiously and carefully with the aim of promoting parental unity, at least with respect to management decisions.

## 3.1 Establishing the Management Hierarchy

The next objective is to put the adults firmly in charge. This entails establishing a clear therapeutic alliance with the parents, who must be affirmed as figures of authority (empowering the parents) who have engaged the clinician's expert assistance. It is important to be clear at the outset as to the young person's place in the hierarchy of management so as to obviate any attempts at splitting and to disemburse him or her of inappropriate power gained through the illness. This can be achieved, without alienating the patient, by the clinician's demonstration of genuine affirmative interest in his or her opinions, feelings, and observations concerning all other aspects of the illness and its context. At least on one level, most patients see this as acceptable and can be engaged, albeit with apparent reluctance or disdain. Parents should be reassured that children with anorexia nervosa really feel afraid of their own power. By assuming their parental responsibility, they will relieve immense and unspeakable anxiety in their child. Parents must also be encouraged not to be intimidated by their child's angry protestations. This is one battle they must win.

## 3.2 Deciding the Need for Hospitalization

The next step is the decision as to whether hospitalization is indicated. It is mandatory in a number of situations (Lask, 1993):

1. When the nutritional state has deteriorated to a serious level of emaciation;

2. When there is clinical dehydration;

3. When vomiting is persistent, or there is vomiting of blood, abdominal pain, or signs of acute abdomen;

4. When there is cardiovascular compromise – e.g., cardiac failure, ECG changes, severe hypotension and bradycardia, chest pain, dyspnoea, or peripheral oedema;

5. When there is markedly depressed mood or other severe psychiatric or behavioural disturbances. These include delirium, suicidal ideation or gestures, total refusal of oral intake, mutism, self harm, or psychotic phenomena.

Family crisis may warrant admission in a less wasted or otherwise uncomplicated patient, as may significant hypothermia, hypoglycemia, electrolyte disturbances, hypoalbuminemia and oedema, raised creatinine, haematological abnormalities, raised ESR, and surgical complications such as rectal prolapse or suspected pancreatitis. Even in patients who are less obviously ill at first assessment, it is important to warn the family of the possibility of rapid deterioration and to ensure that the medical situation is reviewed frequently and regularly.

### 3.3 Medicolegal Considerations and the Issue of Death

Some form of medicolegal intervention may need to be discussed at the assessment interview, as the parents often feel quite helpless to compel their child to accept the clinician's management recommendations. A reminder of the mortality rate and the parents' responsibility for the preservation of their child's life may assist them in acting decisively and in unison. The issue of death is relevant (J.D. Russell et al., 1991), and enquiry may be made as to who in the family would be most affected if the patient were to succumb (Tranter, 1993). Denial, fear, intellectualization, romanticization or dispassionate acceptance of this possibility may be expressed, and the clinician must be prepared to cut across with a firm statement that an unfortunate outcome can be prevented by effective treatment to which the adults in the situation must make an unswerving commitment. The patient may need to be told firmly that he or she will not be allowed to die.

### 3.4 The Initiation of Outpatient Treatment

If outpatient treatment is deemed appropriate, negotiation with the parents as to eventual hospitalization in the event of poor progress or deterioration must take place early on. If a general practitioner or family doctor is not already involved, the family should be referred to one immediately, and also to a dietitian or nutritionist experienced in the management of eating disorder patients. Prompt contact should be established to discuss treatment goals and conditions. Good communication between the various treating parties is essential, particularly when and if hospitalization needs to be implemented.

## 3.5 The Target Weight Range

Initially, it may be preferable to defer discussion of target weight rather than provoke early confrontation when issues such as dehydration, vomiting, and cardiac compromise are more relevant and demanding of attention. But eventually, the target range must be decided. Reluctance to accept the target weight recommendations must be explored, but ultimately no compromise can be allowed (Touyz & Beumont, 1991).

## 3.6 Refeeding at Home versus Hospital

There will be situations where parents will be keen to implement a refeeding programme at home. With sufficient support and supervision some may be able to do this, thus avoiding the need for hospital admission. Assessment of medical safety, suitability of home milieu, parental motivation, and cohesion is crucial. The medical situation, however, is unstable in young patients and this must be borne in mind (Lask, 1993). Furthermore, even in prepubertal patients, the adolescent task of achieving autonomy and identity may be critically important. It may be manifested either as a wish, a fear, or even a cause for hostility at perceived frustration. The separation dynamic affects both child and parents, and despite initial homesickness, a period of hospitalization in an appropriate setting may provide not only the opportunity for time out but also a mutual "practice separation" in which confiding relationships can be established outside the family. Parental guilt and sense of failure at the need for hospitalization may be assuaged by a simple explanation of these issues.

## 3.7 Choosing the Hospital Setting

Whilst they may agree with the need for hospital treatment, parents not infrequently express concern that their child will learn more dysfunctional and disordered behaviours if exposed to other patients who are older and chronically ill. This is not an unreasonable fear. The hospital setting must be fully discussed with the patient's parents, whose other concerns are likely to relate to the availability of schooling, particularly as anorexia nervosa patients may be perfectionistic in this regard. Requests to allow the patient to continue competitive exercise pursuits such as ballet or athletic training must be firmly resisted during active refeeding, with reassurance that appropriate exercise will be permitted when steady progress is being made (Beumont et al., 1994).

If admission to a specialized eating disorders unit (and one in which the patient will have some suitable peers) is not an option, a paediatric medical setting may be preferable to an adult psychiatric one, provided that the ward personnel have had experience with anorexia nervosa and that there is sufficient supervision along with access to nutritional counselling and consultation-liaison psychiatry services. A relatively brief period of hospitalization to correct medical problems and to initiate and instruct parents in nutritional rehabilitation may be sufficient to permit continuation at home. It is essential, however, to insist on the need for full weight restoration, even if it requires readmission at a more convenient time, possibly during school holidays.

### 3.8 Explaining the Assessment and Treatment Package

The components of treatment need to be fully explained – e.g., correction of medical and acute psychiatric problems, initiation of oral intake, bed rest, the nutritionist's role, cognitive-behavioural therapy, group and individual psychotherapy, exercise, schooling, outings, weekend leave, and the need for regular family meetings. Parent or patient concerns about the use of medication might also be discussed. Anxiety may be allayed by inviting the patient and family to make a conducted tour of the ward and meet some of the staff.

### 3.9 Financial Issues

In the private medical setting, the issue of cost of treatment should be broached early, as this is often an important determinant of treatment setting and compliance. Treatment usually proves to be expensive, and the families of patients with anorexia nervosa can become frankly begrudging, particularly when the patient has relapsed. It is important for the clinician to appreciate the collective sense of being starved and drained and the need to withhold emotional and material supplies. This is as true for the young anorexia patient's experience of the family as for the parents' and siblings' experience of the patient, and it may be projected onto the clinician at first contact. It is important to respond in a warm, generous, and open manner while setting limits (which may entail insisting on the appropriate fees for service or being firm about time allocation). Collaboration with the patient's family in order to formulate the most economical and effective management plan is an essential part of the assessment interview.

## 3.10 Family Therapy and Assessment

Some families and patients are resistant to the notion of family therapy, and the need to include other family members (not necessarily all at once) in the treatment must be stated clearly. Reassurance can be given that the clinician will respect the need to keep some matters private, but this will need to be tempered by clinical judgement. Assessment of family function and dynamics commences with the first meeting, and potential causes for treatment failure and sabotage - such as poor boundaries, parental neediness or disharmony, and parent-child collusion - will often be identified when the issue of treatment is broached (Beumont et al., 1993). Parents may need ongoing assistance in strengthening their dyad if only to co-parent adequately, or one parent may need to be therapeutically "contained" so that the patient's therapy can proceed unhindered.

## 3.11 The Fear of Intrusion

It is important for the clinician to be exquisitely sensitive to the collective fear of intrusion which may prevent adequate assessment or therapeutic engagement. Parents may be guarding family secrets or nursing feelings of shame, failure, guilt, or loss. The patient is terrified of scrutiny of the secret life that is anorexia nervosa, and fearful of being stripped of this last vestige of pride and identity. Furthermore, abusive experiences may render the physical examination a difficult undertaking and one that must be approached with the utmost caution and respect.

## 3.12 Trauma, Grief, and the Pathogenic Secret

The possibility that a child has been the victim of some form of trauma or abuse must be borne in mind, particularly where the patient seems unduly bland and detached, where seemingly adequate treatment has repeatedly failed in the past, and where self-destructive behaviours, psychotic symptoms, and marked mood and sleep disorder characterize the clinical picture. Disclosure is unlikely at first contact, but tactful open-ended enquiry must be followed up when trust and the therapeutic alliance are stronger. Major family psychopathology, particularly mood disorders, eating disorders and alcoholism may be similarly concealed early on. Enquiry is likely to be more fruitful when trauma to the family as a whole is explored. This might include bereavement, separation, divorce, life-threatening or disfiguring illness or accidents, bankruptcy, moving house, or emigration. Any of these might be attended by individual or collective grief for which the patient might be the emissary or to which the patient may be more sensitive than other family members. The patient, when seen alone, may be able to identify a source of private loss, grief, or disappointment (often romantic or academic) of which the family is unaware or dismissive. Grief issues might also be reactivated by projection of parental feelings onto the offspring of an empty or disharmonious marriage. A child in this situation may fear that in growing up he or she will abandon a needy and depressed parent; anorexia nervosa then represents a solution to a painful dilemma. Such issues serve to obstruct acceptance of effective treatment.

### 3.13 Conclusion of the Assessment Interview and Management of Its Aftermath

At the conclusion of the assessment, the patient and accompanying parent(s) should be seen together to discuss the decisions that have been made about treatment. The parents may need to be empowered to manage consequent temper tantrums or running away. Medicolegal options should be explained to the patient if serious resistance is encountered, but this is rarely required if the parents can maintain their resolve. The likely duration of treatment and its components are described in a fashion appropriate to the situation and the age of the child. Again, the seriousness of the illness and the need for long-term treatment must be stressed, as patients and their parents may have inappropriate expectations. Or they may previously have made bargains and compromises with each other that eventually prove to be counter-therapeutic.

### 3.14 Responding to Family Decisions Concerning Management

It is important to reassure patients and their parents that the majority of sufferers will recover with adequate treatment. The family is to be congratulated for seeking treatment, and for recognizing the problem. If treatment is accepted, it is important for the assessment interview to end on an affirmative and cautiously hopeful note. Refusal or failure to make a commitment to treatment must be accepted graciously by the therapist and a suitable treatment alternative suggested, if this can be done without compromising medical safety. Ample opportunity to reconsider, along with the option for further opportunity for questions and discussion, should be provided. Safety is the critical issue, and young patients are in particular danger. The clinician has an obligation to convey this message unequivocally to the patient's parents, while keeping the therapeutic door open.

## References

Abraham, S. F., Beumont, P. J. V., Booth, A., & Smith, A. (1981). Anorexia nervosa, pregnancy and XO/XX mosaicism. *Medical Journal of Australia, 1*, 582-583.

Abraham, S. F., Mira, M., Beumont, P. J. V., Sowerbutts, T., & Llewllyn-Jones, D. (1983). Eating behaviours among young women. *Medical Journal of Australia, 2*, 225-228.

Beumont, P. J. V. (1984a). *Endocrine Function in Magersucht Disorders in the Psychobiology of Anorexia Nervosa* (pp 114-123). K. M. Pirke & D. Ploog (Eds.). Berlin: Springer Verlag.

Beumont, P. J. V. (1984b). A clinician looks at animal models of anorexia nervosa. In N. Bond (Ed), *Animal Models of Psychopathology* (pp 177-210). Sydney: Grune & Stratton.

Beumont, P. J. V. (1986). The dieting disorders: anorexia nervosa and bulimia nervosa. In M. L. Wahlquist & A. S. Truswell (Eds.), *Recent Advances in Clinical Nutrition 2* (pp 293-302). London and Paris: John Libbey.

Beumont, P., Al-Alami, M., & Touyz, S. (1988). Relevance of a standard measure of undernutrition to the diagnosis of anorexia nervosa: use of Quetelet's Body Mass Index (BMI). *International Journal of Eating Disorders, 7*, 399-405.

Beumont, P. J. V., Arthur, B., Russell, J. D., & Touyz, S. W. (1994). Excessive physical activity in dieting disorder patients: proposals for a supervised exercise programme. *International Journal of Eating Disorders, 15*, 21-36.

Beumont, P. J. V., Chambers, T., Rouse, L., & Abraham, S. F. (1981). The diet composition and nutritional knowledge of patients with anorexia nervosa. *Journal of Human Nutrition, 35*, 265-273.

Beumont, P. J. V., & Large, M. (1991). Hypophosphatemia, delirium and cardiac arrythmia in anorexia nervosa. *Medical Journal of Australia, 155*, 519-522.

Beumont, P. J. V., Russell, J. D., & Touyz, S. W. (1993). Treatment of anorexia nervosa. *The Lancet, 341*, 1635-1640.

Bhanji, S., & Mattingly, D. (1988). *Medical Aspects of Anorexia nervosa.* London: Wright.

Bryant-Waugh, R. (1993). Epidemiology. In *Childhood Onset Anorexia Nervosa and related Eating Disorders* (p 61). B. Lask &R. Bryant-Waugh (Eds.). Hove, UK: Lawrence Erlbaum Associates.

Bryant-Waugh, R., & Kaminski, Z. (1993). *Eating disorders in children: an overview, in Childhood Onset Anorexia Nervosa and Related Eating Disorders* (pp 17-30). B Lask & R Bryant-Waugh (Eds.). Hove, UK: Lawrence Erlbaum Associates.

Fichter, M. M., & Pirke, K. M. (1984). Hypothalamic pituitary function in starving healthy subjects. In K. M. Pirke & D. Ploog (Eds.), *The Psychobiology of Anorexia Nervosa* (pp 124-135. Berlin: Springer-Verlag.

Fosson, A., de Bruyn, R., & Thomas, S. (1993). Physical aspects. *In Childhood Onset Anorexia Nervosa and related Eating Disorders* (p 36). B. Lask & R. Bryant-Waugh (Eds.). Hove, UK: Lawrence Erlbaum Associates.

Garner, D. M., Rockert, W., Olmsted, M., Johnson, C., & Coscina, D. V. (1985). Psychoeducational principles in the treatment of bulimia and anorexia nervosa. *In Handbook of Psychotherapy for Anorexia Nervosa and Bulimia* (pp. 513-572). D.M. Garner & P. Garfinkel (Eds.). New York: Guilford Press.

Greulich, W. W., & Pyle, S. I. (1959*). Radiographic atlas of skeletal development of the hand and wrist.* Stanford University, 2nd edition.

Griffiths, R., Beumont, P. J. V., & Touyz, S. W. Anorexie à deux: an ominous feature for treatment. *European Eating Disorders Review*. (In Press)

Hall, R. C. W., Hoffman, R. S., Beresford, T. P., Wooley, B., Hall, A. K., & Kubasak, L. (1989). Physical illness encountered in patients with eating disorders. *Psychosomatics, 30*, 174-191.

Isner, J. M., Roberts, W. C., Heymsfield, S. B., & Yager, J. (1985). Anorexia nervosa and sudden death. *Annals of Internal Medicine, 102*, 49-52.

Lask, B. (1993). Management overview. In B. Lask, R. Bryant-Waugh (Eds.), *Childhood Onset Anorexia Nervosa and Related Eating Disorders* (p. 129). Hove, UK: Erlbaum Associates.

Lucas, A. R., Beard, C. M., O'Fallon, W. M., & Kurland, L. T. (1991). 50-year trends in the incidence of anorexia nervosa in Rochester, Minn.: A population-based study. *American Journal of Psychiatry, 148*, 917-922.

Marshall, W. A., & Tanner, J. M. (1969). Variations in the pattern of pubertal changes in girls. *Archives of Diseases of Childhood, 44*, 291-299.

Mira, M., Stewart, P., Russell, J., & Abraham, S. (1992). Changes in creatinine clearance during treatment of anorexia nervoas and bulimia nervosa. *International Journal of Eating Disorders, 11*, 403-06.

O'Connor, M. A., Touyz, S. W., Dunn, S., & Beumont, P. J. V. (1987). Vegetarianism in anorexia nervosa: a review of 116 consecutive cases. *Medical Journal of Australia, 147*, 540-542.

Pirke, K. M., & Ploog, D. (1987). Biology of human starvation. In P. J. V. Beumont, G. D. Burrows & R. C. Casper (Eds.), *Handbook of Eating Disorders Part 1 Anorexia Nervosa* (pp 79-102). Amsterdam: Elsevier.

Rigotti, N. A., Neer, R. M., Skates, S. J., Herzog, D. B., & Nussbaum, S. R. (1991). The clinical course of osteoporosis in anorexia nervosa: the longitudinal study of cortical bone mass. *Journal of the American Medical Association, 265*, 1133-1138.

Russell, G. F. M. (1985). Premenarchal anorexia nervosa and its sequelae. *Journal of Psychiatric Research, 19*, 363-369.

Russell, J. D., Halasz, G., & Beumont, P. J. V. (1991). Death related themes in anorexia nervosa. *Journal of Adolescence, 13*, 311-326.

Russell, J. D., Mira, M., Allen, B. J., Stewart, P. M., Vizzard, J, Arthur, B, & Beumont, P. J. V. (1994). Protein repletion and treatment in anorexia nervosa. *American Journal of Nutrition, 59*, 98-102.

Schocken, D. D., Holoway, J. D., & Powers, P. S. (1989). Weight loss and the heart: effects of anorexia nervosa and starvation. *Archives of Internal Medicine, 149*, 877-881.

Theander, S. (1985). Outcome and prognosis in anorexia nervosa and bulimia: some results of previous investigations, compared with those of a Swedish longterm study. *Journal of Psychiatric Research, 19*, 493-508.

Touyz, S. W. & Beumont, P. J. V. (1991). The management of anorexia nervosa in adolescents. *Modern Medicine (Australia)*, 86-97.

Tranter, M. (1993). Assessment. In B. Lask & R. Bryant-Waugh (Eds.), *Childhood Onset Anorexia Nervosa and Related Eating Disorders* (p 116). Hove: Erlbaum.

Treasure, J. L., Wheeler, M., King, E. A., Gordon, R. A. L., & Russell, G. F. M. (1988). Weight gain and reproductive function: ultrasonographic and endocrine features of anorexia nervosa. *Clinical Endocrinology, 29*, 607-616.

Vaisman, N., Rossi, M. F., Corey, M., Clarke, R., Goldberg, E., & Pencharz, P. B. (1991). Effect of refeeding on the energy metabolism of adolescent girls who have anorexia nervosa. *European Journal of Clinical Nutrition, 45*, 527-537.

Zalin, A., & Lant, A. (1984). Anorexia nervosa presenting as reversible hypoglycemic coma. *Journal of the Royal Society of Medicine, 77*, 193-195.

# The Inpatient Management of the Adolescent Patient with Anorexia Nervosa

*Stephen W. Touyz, David M. Garner, and Peter J. V. Beumont*

## 1   Introduction

Although it is generally accepted that many anorexia nervosa patients can be treated effectively as outpatients, most clinicians would agree that there is a subgroup of patients who require or greatly benefit from inpatient care (Garner & Sackeyfio, 1993). The main objectives of inpatient management for patients with anorexia nervosa include (1) restoration of body weight or the interruption of acute or insidious weight loss; (2) the interruption of unremitting bingeing, vomiting, or compulsive exercising; (3) the evaluation and treatment of medical complications; (4) the management of associated problems such as severe depression, suicidal behaviour, and substance abuse; (5) addressing the psychological and interpersonal factors that have initiated or maintained the dieting disorder; and (6) occasionally, the disengagement of patients from a social system that both contributes to the maintenance of the disorder and disrupts outpatient treatment. Despite the divergence of opinion regarding the aetiology of eating disorders, there is a general consensus on the parameters that define inpatient treatment (Andersen, 1985; Andersen, Morse, & Santmyer, 1985; Touyz & Beumont, 1985, 1991; Garfinkel & Garner, 1982; Russell, 1970; Strober & Yager, 1985; Vandereycken & Meerman, 1984; Beumont et al., 1993).

Garner and Sackeyfio (1993) have recently stressed that hospitalisation should be regarded as only one facet of what often becomes a lengthy and complex treatment process for the seriously ill patient and does not necessarily lead to a resolution of the eating disorder in the first instance. However, there are times where hospitalisation can result in fairly dramatic improvement in symptomatology, particularly in the younger prepubescent patients. However, in other situations, particularly where there is a therapeutic impasse, inpatient treatment may be a humane alternative to the extraordinary suffering endured by the patient and her family when outpatient treatment has clearly failed because of severe malnutrition or unremitting bingeing, vomiting, and/or compulsive exercising.

In the absence of controlled prospective studies showing clear-cut benefits of any particular type of intervention, it must be concluded that no treatment strategy can be considered definitive at this time. Thus, caution should be exercised in adopting one particular mode of intervention at the expense of others. Rather, one should adopt a broad approach that will suit most patients and follow the first rule of medicine, *primum non nocere* (Andersen, 1985). In cases where there are serious medical or psychological risks, hospitalization may be a desirable and conservative option.

Few clinicians would argue against the notion that anorexia nervosa and the issues surrounding its perpetuation are inextricably tied to developmental concerns (Strober & Yager 1985). It is usually an illness of adolescence and is often triggered by pubertal changes. Any meaningful intervention strategy must take into account the developmental tasks normally achieved during the important teenage years. It is necessary to facilitate the developmental process that usually links adolescent accomplishments with healthy adult adjustments. Strober and Yager (1985) have enunciated some of the important goals to take into consideration when treating the adolescent patient with anorexia nervosa. The clinician should endeavour to:

(a) facilitate the expression of inner feelings; (b) encourage the development of greater tolerance for the uncertainties of change and growth; (c) encourage self-examination, abstract thinking and realistic appraisal of limitations, competencies and potentials; (d) encourage the development of a greater understanding of the issues inhibiting separation and individuation; and (e) encourage the acceptance of a therapeutic relationship that combines dependency with security as a necessary prerequisite for independence.

Finally, it is essential that clinicians involved in the treatment of anorexia nervosa patients familiarise themselves with the physical and psychological consequences of starvation. Starvation has many consequences for both body and mind. Some of these are mechanisms that appear to be both useful and necessary for the body to adapt to the starvation process. Thus, many of the symptoms that have been attributed to the illness are in fact the direct result of the starvation process (Garner et al., 1985). As might be expected, one of the salient aspects of starvation is a pervasive preoccupation with food. The intensity of this preoccupation is such that the patient's whole life becomes devoted to thinking about food, weight, and dieting. Many anorexic patients, whilst adhering tenaciously to their meagre diets, collect recipes, read books on food, and banish others from the kitchen so as to prepare the family meal, which they themselves refuse to eat.

## 2 General Management

### 2.1 Initial Interview

The initial interview is the first step in treatment, engaging both patient and family in the therapeutic endeavour, and it is extremely important that the format and style of the initial or early interviews be aimed at the development of a sense of openness and trust between the patient and the assessing clinician.

Most patients suffering from anorexia nervosa deny the severity of their illness and are brought to treatment by distraught parents, siblings, or friends. Others are terrified that they will be force-fed or placed in solitary confinement on a strict behavioural programme whilst in hospital. They are most apprehensive about the enforced separation from their families. For younger patients this may in fact be the first time that they have been away from their home and families for any length of time. The first major challenge confronting the clinician is to convince the reluctant patient that she is in need of urgent treatment, unlike patients who present with distressing feelings of anxiety or depression and who are actively seeking assistance to alleviate their suffering. Eating disorder patients are often loath to consider relinquishing symptoms such as extreme restrictive dieting, excessive exercise, or self-induced vomiting. Thus, the decision to admit the oppositional patient to hospital often involves the delicate philosophical balance between free will and determinism (Crisp, 1980; Goldner, 1989). Goldner (1989) has provided a summary of recommendations designed to minimise treatment refusal, and they may be paraphrased as follows: seek a voluntary alliance, identify the reasons for treatment refusal, carefully explain the reasons for treatment recommendations, remain flexible, show respect for the patient's belief in the importance of thinness, minimise intrusive interventions, weigh the risks and benefits of active treatment, avoid punitive interventions, involve the family where possible, and consider involuntary treatment only when nonintervention constitutes an immediate or serious danger.

The anorexic patient is often of the opinion that her experiences are idiosyncratic and that no one (especially a clinician who has never suffered from the disorder) could possibly understand the problem as she sees it. It is, therefore, of the utmost importance that the clinician develops a sound understanding of the phenomenology of the illness so as to be able to reassure the patient that her suffering is appreciated and that a firm but compassionate approach to treatment will be undertaken. As a first step, clinicians must familiarise themselves with the physical and psychological consequences of starvation (see Table 1).

Table 1. Physical and Psychological Consequences of Starvation

| Psychological | Physiological |
| --- | --- |
| Anxiety | Amenorrhoea |
| Depression | Dry Skin |
| Lability of mood | Lanugo hair |
| Feelings of inadequacy | Polyuria |
| Irritability | Fatigue |
| Social withdrawal | Paraesthesias |
| Food preoccupation | Hypothermia |
| Poor concentration | Hypotension |
| Hypersensitivity to noise | Disturbed blood chemistry |
| Obsessional thinking and increasing perfectionism | Sinus bradycardia |
|  | Reduced gastric motility |

Most patients are exasperated by their overwhelming preoccupation with thoughts of food and weight and their inability to concentrate on other important issues such as relationships with their peer group. They often respond favourably when told that a reduction in their obsessional rumination and anorexic behaviours and the resumption of a more normal eating pattern would allow better socialisation (Vandereycken & Meermann, 1984). Patients should also be told to expect an improvement in their sleep pattern which may have become fragmented, and to expect to feel both less depressed and less irritable.

By the time they are brought to treatment, anorexic patients usually feel tired and listless, but they express much concern at the prospect of regaining weight, particularly if denied the opportunity to undertake any exercise (Touyz et al.,

1987). They should be reassured that appropriate activity will be permitted, contingent upon their medical status and successful weight gain, and that their energy level and muscle tone will improve with nutritional rehabilitation (Beumont et al., 1994).

Patients may attempt to manipulate the clinician into compromising on the amount of weight to be gained or the varieties of food to be eaten. It is important to be open and honest and not to be trapped into making promises which will have to be broken later. It is a much more productive exercise to focus on the patient's symptoms and the benefits that would accrue as a result of successful intervention than to argue about whether the minimum or target weight should be adjusted down by two or three kilograms to placate the patients' anxieties regarding weight gain. However, the clinician must provide a realistic appraisal about both the length of treatment and what is likely to entail (Touyz & Beumont, 1991).

Most would agree that some patients will need to be admitted to hospital (Touyz & Beumont, 1985; Beumont et al., 1993; Garner & Sackeyfio, 1993). It is an advantage if both the referring doctor or non medical therapist is familiar with the clinical facility which will undertake the treatment so as to be able to allay the patient's fears concerning the specific aspects of therapy. A visit to the unit by the patient and a parent, and a chat with the nursing staff, may facilitate an admission to hospital.

The initial interview thus goes well beyond obtaining a personal, family, medical, and psychiatric history. It should aim at allaying the fears and concerns of both the patient and her family. Furthermore, it should impart realistic expectations concerning the duration of treatment. But the clinician must avoid making any promises that may not be able to be kept at a later date. More specific information pertaining to both the medical assessment and initial interview can be found in the preceeding chapter by Beumont et al. in this volume.

## 2.2 For Whom Outpatient Therapy is Appropriate

In the past, most patients with anorexia nervosa were admitted to hospital for refeeding, as it was generally believed that outpatient intervention would not be successful, especially with an emaciated patient. However, over recent years, we have witnessed a change in the clinical presentation of anorexia nervosa patients, most of whom now present before they have become grossly emaciated. The change may be attributed to the greater awareness of the disorder in the community and by family doctors in particular. In such cases, ambulatory care is clearly preferable to hospitalisation in that it is more economical, reduces the risks of somatization and invalidism, and minimises the likelihood of contamination of patients with a more severe form of the illness (i.e., being exposed to other maladaptive patterns of behaviour that have not yet developed and that may be acquired in a hospital environment). Many patients respond favourably to outpatient therapy thus avoiding an unnecessary hospital admission. Such outpatient treatment usually comprises nutritional counselling by a skilled dietitian (Williams et al., 1985) as well as individual (Beumont et al., 1993, Garner & Sackeyfio, 1993) and family therapy (Stierlin & Weberly, 1987).

A brief trial of outpatient therapy should also be considered with patients who are most skeptical about the benefit of hospitalization, if only to convince them that, despite their assertions to the contrary, they really are unable to change their attitudes or behaviours without the structure that hospital affords. If patients come to realise that they are unable to make satisfactory progress outside of the hospital, they may actually be relieved when presented with a strong recommendation to hospitalise them. Such a trial of outpatient therapy accentuates the patient's inability to modify their irrational beliefs and maladaptive behaviours as outpatients and often facilitates a greater degree of compliance during hospitalisation.

Andersen (1985) has summarised the most common reasons for admitting an anorexia nervosa patient, and they are as follows:

- low body weight (usually a body mass index of 16 or less) or a precipitous loss of weight
- abnormal electrocardiogram, liver function, haematology or biochemistry test results (a low serum potassium level is often evident in patients who induce vomiting and/or use laxatives or diuretics)
- marked dehydration, hypotension (less than 60mm hg. systolic blood pressure) or bradycardia (less than 40 beats per minute) with symptoms of faintness
- depressed mood (e.g., suicidal thoughts or intents)
- a discouraged, demoralised family or the lack of appropriate inpatient facilities.

## 2.3 Hospital Management

The hospital management of patients with anorexia nervosa can be divided into two stages: weight restoration and weight maintenance (Touyz & Beumont, 1985). The effects of starvation must be reversed if the patient is to benefit from other aspects of treatment such as individual, group, or family psychotherapy (Garfinkel & Garner, 1982).

Personal, social, medical and psychiatric histories are confirmed on admission and a comprehensive assessment is made of the dietary history, eating behaviour and level of physical activity of the patient. The ward programme should be clearly explained to both patients and parents to avoid any unnecessary misunderstanding and to minimise the opportunity for a recalcitrant patient to manipulate the staff responsible for the management plan. Once this has been done, parents and siblings should return home, having encouraged the patient to engage in the unit's activities. This also enables the avoidance of a situation in which distraught parents have to endure a barrage of persistent pleas by their child to take him or her home, with unrealistic promises of improved attitudes and behaviours.

## 2.4 Behaviour Modification and the Lenient Flexible Approach

Bachrach, et al. (1965) introduced the concept of using operant techniques in the management of patients admitted to hospital with anorexia nervosa. Most clinicians now incorporate some aspects of behaviour modification in the treatment of emaciated anorexic patients (Touyz et al., 1987). Unfortunately, such programmes are often implemented in a rigid manner without due regard for the contingencies maintaining anorexia nervosa (Garner, 1985). Furthermore, they have tended to be unnecessarily harsh and restrictive, often confining the patient to relative isolation for long periods of time. The programme itself becomes the focus of treatment, and considerable effort is often expended on its strict implementation rather than on the resolution of the patient's psychological conflicts. Patients become resentful, leading to their developing iatrogenic ill-effects that have been well documented (Garner, 1985).

Bruch (1974, 1978) has strongly criticised the use of behaviour modification in the management of anorexia nervosa. She argued that whereas such an approach produces transient weight gain, it ignores the major deficits in the personality development of these patients, namely self-esteem, self-doubt, lack of autonomy, and an inability to lead a self-directed life. Bruch (1974) argued that behaviour modification coerces patients to gain weight under the "pressure of persuasion, force of threats" and that they would literally "...eat their way out of hospital" (p. 1421). Such overeating may, in fact, lead to episode of gorging (bulimia). Traditional operant programmes developed for anorexia nervosa patients during refeeding have tended to be unnecessarily harsh, with the patient kept in isolation and often separated from her peer group and without her possessions. Garner (1985) has also alluded to reports in the literature "... which capture the extraordinary degree of frustration, anger and maltreatment which have prevailed under the guise of behaviour modification" (p. 706). There is no justification whatsoever to implement harsh behavioural regimens to punish patients who have not complied with treatment up to that point in time.

With these criticisms in mind, we have proposed an alternative behavioural programme that allows patients to maintain a greater degree of control over the refeeding process without adversely affecting the rate of weight gain (Touyz et al 1987). Such a lenient, flexible programme was found to have a number of practical advantages in that it is more economical with regard to nursing time, patients are more accessible to psychotherapy, and it is much more acceptable to the patients in general.

At the time of admission, patients are told that they should gain weight at the rate of 1.5 kg/week. Provided they comply with this requirement, they are free to move around the unit or attend outings to a nearby shopping complex. Furthermore, they are permitted to leave the unit on weekends for a few hours with relatives or friends. They understand that if they fail to achieve the weekly target of weight gain, they will be restricted to the unit until they have done so. For example, if a patient only gained 1 kg over the 1-week period, she would be restricted to the unit until she had gained the remaining 0.5 kg. However, if a patient failed to make the weekly target of 1.5 kg over two consecutive weeks, she would be restricted to the unit for an entire week. No further restrictions are imposed and patients have unlimited access to their personal possessions. This programme is even more lenient than the one we reported previously (Touyz et al., 1984). Despite this more humane approach to refeeding, similar results were achieved when compared to other more rigid behavioural programmes in that the patients gained 0.16 kg per day. This approach differs markedly from those that advocate total bed rest for six to eight weeks until the patient reaches the set target weight. It has been our experience that most patients gain weight satisfactorily without being restricted to bed, and they appear to appreciate being able to spend their time more constructively, for example, attending individual and group therapy sessions. Peer pressure within the therapeutic community also contributes to patients attaining their weekly weight gain. However, for the occasional recalcitrant patient who steadfastly refuses to gain weight, a stricter programme may be required for a short period of time.

In conclusion, behavioural programmes used in a responsible manner as an adjunct to refeeding patients with anorexia nervosa are often invaluable in assisting the patient to commence eating appropriately again and in regaining weight. Our lenient, flexible approach provides a humane framework in which this can be achieved.

## 2.5 Nursing Staff

The nursing staff on the unit is responsible for the day-to-day management of the patients and must be well versed in the psychopathology of anorexia nervosa. The importance of the nursing staff in the successful management of these patients cannot be sufficiently emphasised. "The greater burden of responsibility for inpatient treatment should be given to the nurses caring for the patients ... the key to the success of nursing care is the establishment of a relationship of trust [with] those nurses who will have the closest contact with her" (Russell, 1977, p. 281). It is therefore of the utmost importance that the senior nursing staff be comprised of persons who have made a commitment to work on the unit on a regular basis and that the rate of staff turnover is low. The success of any anorexia nervosa unit ultimately rests on the expertise and dedication of the nursing staff.

## 2.6 Minimum or Target Weight

There is no general consensus as to what constitutes an optimal weight for patients with anorexia nervosa, although most clinicians probably use a low average weight for height and sex as a general guideline. This often becomes the most contentious issue in therapy, and clinicians require both the wisdom of Solomon and the patience of Job in addressing it (Touyz & Beumont, 1991).

Fortunately, there are some guidelines to use when coming to a decision that deals with body weight in therapy.

- It is preferable to specify the minimum target weight at the onset of treatment rather than later during the course of an admission.
- The weight should be one that the patient can maintain without continued dieting.
- There should be a range of approximately 2 kg rather than a specific set weight.

Quetelet's body mass index is a useful means of determining target weights. It is derived from the formula where weight (kg) is divided by squared height (m). For those patients aged 16 years or older, a body mass index of 20 should be used as a guide to minimum weight. For those aged between 14 and 15 years, a body mass index of 18.5 - 19.5 appears to be appropriate. However, for patients aged 13 years and under it is best to consult standardised data (see Table 2). There will always be exceptions to any rule, and there is much to be said for using a pragmatic approach. It has been our experience that weighing patients three times per week rather than on a daily basis does not compromise weight gain but reduces the patient's preoccupation with minor fluctuations in their weight (Touyz et al., 1990).

Once patients have reached their target weight they should be "range" weighed. The scale should be set at the lowest acceptable weight and then at a weight 2 or 3 kg higher. This enables the clinician to document whether an individual is maintaining his or her weight within an acceptable range without focusing upon a specific figure, hence avoiding reinforcement of the patient's preoccupation with weight as such.

## 2.7 Tube Feeding

Garfinkel and Garner (1982) have documented concerns regarding the routine application of nasogastric feeding.

- It represents a direct intrusion into the gastrointestinal tract of someone who is already preoccupied and misguided about bodily functions.
- It may be perceived as an assault or an act of hostility, which reinforces the patient's feeling of worthlessness.

- It requires minimal patient cooperation and, as such, leads to increased mistrust.
- There are significant physiological side effects.
- It is almost always unnecessary.

Table 2. Heights, weights and body mass index (BMI) equivalents for girls aged 11 to 18 years

| Age (years) | Height (m) at percentiles ||| Weight (kg) at percentiles ||| BMI at percentiles |||
|---|---|---|---|---|---|---|---|---|---|
| | 25% | 50% | 75% | 25% | 50% | 75% | 25% | 50% | 75% |
| 11 | 1.40 | 1.45 | 1.49 | 31.71 | 35.74 | 40.42 | 16.11 | 17.07 | 18.16 |
| 12 | 1.46 | 1.52 | 1.57 | 35.38 | 39.74 | 44.82 | 16.62 | 17.22 | 18.28 |
| 13 | 1.53 | 1.57 | 1.62 | 40.55 | 44.95 | 50.35 | 17.41 | 18.21 | 19.30 |
| Mean for girls under 14 years |||||||16.79 | 17.58 | 18.64 |
| 14 | 1.56 | 1.60 | 1.64 | 45.27 | 49.17 | 54.29 | 18.58 | 19.30 | 20.26 |
| 15 | 1.58 | 1.61 | 1.65 | 47.67 | 51.48 | 56.20 | 19.17 | 19.84 | 20.67 |
| 16 | 1.59 | 1.62 | 1.66 | 49.17 | 53.07 | 57.70 | 19.55 | 20.17 | 21.02 |
| 17 | 1.59 | 1.63 | 1.66 | 50.08 | 54.02 | 58.79 | 19.81 | 20.46 | 21.31 |
| 18 | 1.59 | 1.63 | 1.66 | 50.44 | 54.39 | 59.33 | 19.95 | 20.60 | 21.50 |

Quoted from Stuart and Stevenson in Documenta Geigy, Scientific Tables, 6th edition, edited by Konrad Diem, Geigy Pharmaceuticals, Manchester 1962.

Nasogastric feeding or parenteral hyperalimentation are very rarely necessary and should be used only as a last resort. It has been our experience that nearly all patients can be persuaded to eat normally, and every endeavour should be made to achieve this, even to the point of feeding the patient with a spoon, if necessary.

If tube feeding is indicated, a transfer to a medical unit is the best option, with an opportunity to return to the anorexia unit once the patient or has resumed eating. This minimises the hostile conflict between patient and therapist when tube feeding has to be enforced. One of our patients described her experience of having been tube fed at another hospital in the following manner (Touyz & Beumont, 1993).

*I didn't know what it was going to involve. I hated pain ... I was afraid, so scared. The tube looked so hard and so long, I began to cry ... the hideous piece of plastic tubing was being forced down my left nostril ... I was screaming... my head thrashed wildly on the bed whilst my body squirmed or moved like a wounded fish out of water.*

*I cried ... Nothing can or will ever remove the memory of that tube.*

*However, this tube was going to save my life... But I decided that I didn't want this tube inside of me nor the fluid flowing into me through the tube. The most sensible thing in my eyes to do was to pull it out. But I didn't want any pain.*

*I gently pulled the tube protruding from my nose and it was sore. I was so afraid and scared of what I could do to myself and also scared of what the staff would do to me ...*

*I lifted my feeble arms and fingers. I placed the tube between my thumb and forefinger and gently yanked it. Something moved inside me. I could now feel the tube inside my stomach. My mind ran amuck. I was so confused. Out came the tube, one hell of a long tube. I hadn't realised how long it actually was. (I later found out that it was 3 feet long).*

This patient even learned how to regurgitate her nasogastric feeds.

*I taught myself how to vomit through the tube... I learnt that by holding my breath and blowing out through my nose, I could regurgitate any fluid that had been passed down through the tube into my stomach (p. 68).*

The above vignette graphically illustrates why tube feeding should only be considered in rare instances in which the patient is in imminent danger and/or completely unresponsive to more conservative methods.

## 2.8 Exercise Counselling

As has been noted in the section on clinical presentation, overactivity and excessive exercise are characteristic features of anorexia nervosa. We have recently described a comprehensive, supervised exercise programme for these patients (Beumont et al., 1994) and a detailed description in booklet form is available from the authors on request. In brief, three general policy statements may be made concerning exercise in patients with anorexia nervosa.

1. Total prohibition of all exercise is not only difficult and time-consuming to enforce but also places the staff, particularly the nurses, in too authoritarian a role. A patient determined or driven to exercise will do so regardless of measures taken to prevent it. Policing activity creates a battle of wills that only serves to distract both patients and staff from the major issues of therapy. The aim of therapy is to facilitate responsibility for self, rather than cause more feelings of loss of control, helplessness, resentment, and dependence.

   However, as with the issue of diet, activity levels cannot be ignored, especially early in treatment. If they are left to themselves, patients are unable to alter many of the behaviors that have necessitated their admission. The staff must adopt at least a supervisory role to expedite the modification of these behaviors, many of which have serious implications for the patients' health.

2. There is a basis of misinformation and misinterpretation underlying much of the patients' behavior. This is particularly true of the beliefs held concerning exercise. Patients usually have little accurate knowledge of matters such as the relatively low level of exercise needed to maintain body shape and tone, the type of exercise most effective in influencing muscle condition, and the deleterious effects of exercise in the presence of undernutrition. False beliefs should be challenged, and accurate information provided.

3. The aim of therapy is to return the patient to as normal a lifestyle as possible. The environment of a psychiatric unit, although designed for maximum therapeutic benefit, is nevertheless artificial. If a patient is discharged from a unit where there is strict supervision of activity, she would have had no help in learning what constitutes a healthy amount of exercise. After discharge the patient has to face the 'real world', where exercise is extolled for its health-promoting effects. A diet that had maintained a normal weight in hospital will be inadequate when the patient resumes normal activity, and another episode of weight loss is likely to ensue.

It seems that a fine balance of supervision and resumption of responsibility is needed. It is particularly patients with unhealthy exercise practices who will need their activity structured, if not restricted, depending on their medical status in the early stages of admission. Once stable within the program, supervision may be withdrawn and a suitable exercise pattern established that will fit into their lifestyle on discharge, without interfering with physical, social, vocational, or psychological well-being.

The principal components of the structured exercise programme include

(a) stretching, (b) posture enhancement, (c) weight training, (d) social sport, and (e) aerobic-style activity.

The inclusion of an exercise programme appears to improve patient compliance and staff satisfaction but does not adversely affect the ability of patients to regain weight (Touyz et al., 1993).

## 2.9 Weight Maintenance

After having regained weight, it is advisable that patients stay a little longer in hospital for a period of weight maintenance. The duration of the weight maintenance period is usually two to three weeks. During this time, the patient reduces his or her kilojoule intake, under the supervision of the dietitian, from approximately 14,650 kilojoules per day to a maintenance level of about 7,500 to 9,200 kilojoules per day.

Patients should be encouraged to spend evenings and weekends at home and to go out with friends and family to eat in restaurants. These should include age-appropriate establishments such as fast food restaurants. Patients often feel safe eating out only when they know they can order foods such as salad and they must be helped to cope in more demanding situations. They should also be permitted to go shopping and be encouraged, if finances permit, to buy a new wardrobe of clothes that will fit comfortably at their recently restored normal weight.

Once patients have successfully reduced their kilojoule intake to a maintenance level, arrangements should be made for them to return to school, university, or work; they may choose to attend work or classes for a week or so prior to discharge. Individual therapy as well as nutritional counselling should continue throughout this period, and a further therapy session should be scheduled at the time of discharge.

Once the maintenance period has been successfully negotiated, patients are discharged from hospital. They should initially attend outpatient appointments on a weekly basis and, dependent on progress, move on to fortnightly and then monthly sessions. Because many patients relapse after treatment, consistent aftercare is most important. If relapse does occur, it is best to arrange prompt readmission rather than wait until the patient is again emaciated and in need of prolonged nutritional rehabilitation.

## 3  Specific Treatment Strategies

### 3.1  Cognitive Therapy

Garner and Bemis (1982; 1985) were the first to develop a coherent model that emphasised the importance of cognitive dysfunction in anorexia nervosa. They applied the cognitive model delineated by Beck (1976) for the treatment of depression and neurotic disorders to anorexia nervosa. Beck had developed a taxonomy of thinking errors, such as dichotomous reasoning and personalisation, he suggested were responsible for the development and maintenance of a variety of neurotic attitudes and beliefs.

Garner and Bemis (1985) have recommended that anorexia nervosa patients become familiar with the cognitive model that encourages them to take cognisance of the following issues:

1. Monitor their thinking or heighten their awareness of their own thinking.
2. Recognise the connection between certain thoughts and maladaptive behaviours and emotions.
3. Examine the evidence for the validity of particular beliefs.
4. Substitute more realistic and appropriate interpretations.
5. Gradually modify the underlying assumptions that are fundamental determinants of more specific beliefs.

More specific techniques include (a) articulation of beliefs — synthesising and condensing vast quantities of information into more manageable ideas or phrases; (b) decentering — evaluating an idea from a different perspective; (c) decatastrophising — dealing with the patient's prediction of calamity in a more realistic fashion; (d) challenging the shoulds — questioning the patient's excessive reliance on words such as "should", "must", and "ought"; (e) challenging beliefs through behavioural exercises, (f) prospective hypothesis testing — generating specific hypotheses based on the patient's belief system to explore their validity in real life situations; and (g) reattribution techniques — providing counter-arguments for some of the patient's most strongly held beliefs.

These cognitive techniques are now undergoing rigorous scientific examination (Butow et al., 1993) and our clinical experience to date suggests that they are a significant adjunct to the treatment of anorexia nervosa and warrant further research.

## 3.2 The Family and Family Therapy

Parental support is vital if an adolescent patient is to be successfully treated (Strober & Yager, 1985). The family needs to be involved in therapy as early as possible, given a full explanation of the illness, and invited to co-operate in treatment.

All family members living in the patient's home are called to attend an initial family therapy session just before or shortly after admission. At this interview, an assessment of family interactional patterns is made and a decision regarding ongoing family therapy is taken. Not all families require regular therapy, and a deliberate decision should be made for each family as to the number of sessions required and the family members who will be asked to attend. For example, if the parents of the index patient have marked marital difficulties, the family therapist may choose to work with the parents alone for a number of sessions before including the patient and siblings. The objectives of family interventions are as follows:

- to enable family members to understand the illness and the goals of treatment
- to bring about a readjustment of family interactional patterns where appropriate
- to encourage participation in post-discharge planning activities - it is often most beneficial for the patient and a parent to meet with the dietitian to discuss the resumption of normal eating behaviour when the patient returns home

Families become increasingly uncertain as to how to relate to children with anorexia nervosa. They are fearful of upsetting them and distressed and bewildered by their behaviour. Because of their own feelings of overwhelming guilt about their alleged role in the development of the disorder, parents experience difficulty in insisting that a child receive professional counselling and treatment when he or she flatly refuses to do so. On the other hand, if the patient has been ill for some time, parents may have depleted their emotional and financial resources and abandoned all responsibility for the child's care. Because of these conflicting forces, there is always a danger of triangulation, with parents seeking the help of professionals and then undermining the treatment offered. It is important that families be approached in a non-blaming way. Andersen (1985) has provided important guidelines when relating to families:

- Do not assume dysfunction exists in a family just because there is an eating problem.
- Assume that families are tired from the stress they have endured.
- Assume families want help.
- Encourage openness and directness in communication within the family.
- Discuss the patient's progress in treatment.
- Encourage the family's interest in becoming knowledgeable about the disorder.

## 3.3 Nutritional Counselling

The dietitian takes a comprehensive nutritional history shortly after admission and is involved in assessment, planning, supervision, and counselling of both inpatients and outpatients. We have stressed that if patients are to return to a healthy, varied diet, they need to learn to eat normal everyday food within some kind of regular meal pattern (Beumont et al., 1987). A daily eating pattern is drawn up to give a weekly weight gain of 1.5 kg This requires between 6,300 KJ and 19000 KJ daily, depending on the stage of weight gain, the size of the patient, the metabolic rate and the level of activity. For example, a patient who has been eating minimally before admission should initially be given a relatively small diet to provide around 6,300 KJ daily. The gastric discomfort of a larger food intake would be hard to tolerate and is unnecessary as long as such patients start to regain weight on a small diet.

Daily menus are written for each patient to ensure that he or she eats a variety of foods and has an adequate energy intake. The prescribed amount of food is gradually increased and, after a few weeks of consistent weight gain, patients are allowed to start selecting their own food. Basically, they are given a nutritionally balanced diet of normal hospital meals, including some high energy foods such as cake, chocolate, and chips. They are not permitted to bring their own food or drink into the hospital. We do not allow patients to hoard food and challenge their belief that they need 'special' food. Commercial dietary products, such as saccharine and low fat milk products, are also forbidden as they are totally counterproductive for weight gain. Specifically, avoidance of red meat is perhaps the most common dietary alteration made by anorexic patients nowadays; we discourage vegetarianism and prohibit it where possible (O'Connor et al., 1987).

Patients with anorexia nervosa usually complain of constipation. Laxative abuse is common, as is the consumption of large amounts of unprocessed bran, which has the added attraction of being a bulky, noncalorific food substitute. Constipation is the result of minimal food residue passing through the digestive system, and a diet providing fibre in the form of wholegrain cereals, fruit, and vegetables will usually regularise bowel habits. For this reason, the use of laxatives is not allowed, except in the most recalcitrant of cases.

Throughout the admission, the dietitian, together with the senior nursing staff and members of the treatment team, have regular meals with patients to provide a model of normal eating in a relaxed setting. This also affords the opportunity to observe the patients' food choices and actual eating behaviour and to correct unhealthy or unusual eating practices. Unusual eating behaviours are identified using our Eating Behaviour Rating Scale (Wilson et al., 1989), which was specifically developed with this purpose in mind. The assumption that patients' eating behaviour improves automatically with weight gain and counselling has not been borne out in clinical practice and special attention needs to be given to correcting disordered eating. Unusual eating behaviours include:

– cutting food into very small portions

– elaborate food preparation procedures, often involving an excessive handling of food

– precise measurement of portions

- leaving the table frequently during a meal
- the excessive use of condiments
- restricting choice to a rigid pattern of very few foods
- agonising over the choice of what to eat
- paying undue attention to what others are eating
- avoiding conversation and social contact whilst eating

We have found that videotaping a meal and then playing it back to the patient after the meal is completed, in the presence of a senior nurse or dietitian, may actually improve eating behaviour (Touyz et al., 1994). This avenue of exploration warrants further attention in the research literature.

## 3.4 Psychoeducational Principles

Anorexia nervosa is a complex psychosomatic disorder that is caused and then maintained by a multitude of social, psychological, and biological factors. It is often of great benefit to patients to familiarise themselves with the relevant scientific literature relating to semi-starvation, weight regulation, dieting, obesity, and the cultural milieu and with how these factors not only contribute to the development of their disorder but to the maintenance of their symptomatology. Garner, et al., (1985) have produced a comprehensive manual that exhorts patients to alter their eating patterns and attitudes towards food, weight, and their bodies in the context of meaningful scientific findings. Such psychoeducational material should not be a substitute for psychotherapy but rather used as an adjunct to it.

The consequences of starvation of body and mind is of particular importance to patients with anorexia nervosa. Some of these are mechanisms that appear to be both useful and necessary for the body to adapt to the starvation process. As might be expected, one of the salient aspects of starvation is a pervasive preoccupation with food. The intensity of this preoccupation is such that the patient's whole life is devoted to thinking about food, weight, and dieting. Patients are often surprised to discover that many of the symptoms that they have attributed to their illness are in fact the direct result of the starvation process (Table 1).

## 3.5 Self-Help Groups

There has been a dramatic increase in the popularity of self-help groups worldwide. Many of these groups were established by individuals who had become increasingly frustrated at the lack of adequate treatment methods and facilities and often felt despondent at the lack of understanding of their particular problem by the professional community (Touyz, 1988). United by a common affliction, they turned to one another for mutual support in the form of self-help groups. Stunkard (1982) has summarised this phenomenon rather well.

> In the early days of our nation, Alex de Tocqueville described the proclivity of Americans to organise in informal groups to achieve ends that are the responsibility of government in other societies. Nowhere is this proclivity more impressively expressed than in the organisation of patients to cope with their illness. Although the origins of the self-help movement can be traced to nineteenth century England and beyond, the pioneering American motivation was Alcoholics Anonymous, and many of the current self-help groups have been modelled on it (p. 563).

Despite the apparent success of self-help/support groups, a great deal of confusion exists as to what such groups do and to what extent they differ from conventional counselling and psychotherapy groups. Baker Enright et al. (1985) have stressed the importance of distinguishing between self-help and support groups. Although they both refer to peer networks addressing a common affliction, support groups often have professional affiliations whereas self-help groups usually do not. Alcoholics Anonymous has been particularly successful, and its success is due in no small way to the universal and often unquestioned acceptance of its charter. Unfortunately, there is no such consensus when it comes to the treatment of anorexia nervosa. Because of this, there is always the real danger that a recalcitrant anorexia nervosa patient establishes a self-help group and then either conveys inappropriate information to an impressionable patient or information that could be potentially dangerous or harmful to that individual. It is our opinion that support groups for patients with anorexia nervosa that compliment traditional treatment approaches or avail themselves to the professional community are preferable to self-help groups that are run independently by the patients themselves. The effectiveness of support groups have yet to be determined, but their future seems assured in that they will not only open the door to more comprehensive services but will pay a vital role in stimulating community awareness about this frustrating disorder.

## 3.6 Day Hospital Treatment and Community Houses

Day patient programmes are gaining increasing recognition as an alternate form of treatment (Piran et al., 1989a, 1989b). They have clinical and financial advantages over the more traditional inpatient programme. However, a major difference between the day program and inpatient setting is the degree of containment offered to the patient and control over the patients behaviour, restricting their use to less severe cases (Piran et al., 1989b). Most of the psychological treatment is conducted in a group setting using a multidisciplinary approach. Piran et al. (1989b) have also alluded to the possible pitfalls in the use of day hospital programmes including staff burnout, pathological group processes, higher risk of patients engaging in impulsive behaviour, and poor clinical outcome in those patients who are poorly motivated.

We have recently begun to explore the rather novel approach of treating the more chronic patients on a longer term basis in community houses. This avenue of exploration warrants further investigation to evaluate its efficacy in the treatment of such patients.

## 4 Conclusions

It is now generally regarded that the majority of eating-disordered patients can be managed effectively as outpatients (Garner & Sackeyfio, 1993). However, this chapter has focussed on those patients who either require or benefit greatly from an admission to an inpatient facility. The inpatient treatment of the adolescent with anorexia nervosa is a complex task involving both the patient and her family. Furthermore, an illness that commences in adolescence, and which often has a chronic course requiring repeated admissions, imposes a substantial financial burden on the community (Beumont, Russell & Touyz, 1993). In the United States of America, insurance companies are now challenging the need of hospital care for patients with anorexia nervosa. They are seeking to limit reimbursement for treatment (McManus & Comerci, 1986), although the need for hospital care is well documented (Silver, Delaney & Samuels, 1989). Such managed care approaches aim to provide cheap and effective treatments in the short-term but these may ultimately turn out to be counterproductive and lead to increased rates of relapse, disability and social handicap (Wooley, 1993).

The onus of care ultimately falls on the individual clinicians, both medical and non medical. It is important to bear in mind that anorexia nervosa is often a chronic, relapsing illness. Even those patients who ultimately recover may take several years to do so, sometimes requiring several admissions. Others are likely to remain severely handicapped. It is so important to maintain realistic expectations regarding treatment outcome. While relapses in chronic schizophrenia are accepted as being outside the patient's own control, relapse in a chronic anorexic patient is often met by anger and frustration. Clinicians treating patients with anorexia nervosa who acknowledge that the difficulties that such patients face are just as real as those of any other sick person will find the treatment of anorexia nervosa patients both interesting and rewarding.

## References

Andersen, A. E. (1985). *Practical comprehensive treatment of anorexia nervosa and bulimia.* Baltimore: Edward Arnold.
Andersen, A. E., Morse, C., & Santmyer, K. (1985). Inpatient treatment for anorexia nervosa. In D. M. Garner & P. E. Garfinkel (Eds.). *Handbook of Psychotherapy for Anorexia Nervosa and Bulimia* (pp. 311-343). New York: Guildford Press.
Bachrach, A. J., Erwin, W. J., & Mohr, J. P. (1965). The control of eating behaviour in an anorexic by operant conditioning techniques. In L. P Ullman, & L. Kranser (Eds.). *Case Studies in Behaviour Modification* (pp. 153-163). New York: Holt Rinehart & Winston.
Baker Enright, A., Butterfield, P., & Berkowitz, B. (1985). Self-help and support groups in the management of eating disorders. In D. M. Garner, & P. E. Garfinkel (Eds.). *Handbook of Psychotherapy for Anorexia Nervosa and Bulimia.* (pp. 491-512). New York: The Guilford Press.
Beck, A. T. (1976). *Cognitive therapy and emotional disorders.* New York: International Universities Press.
Beumont, P. J. V., Arthur, B., Russell J. D., & Touyz, S. W. (1994). Excessive physical activity in dieting disordered patients: Proposals for a supervised exercise program. *International Journal of Eating Disorders*, 15(1).
Beumont, P. J. V., Lowinger, K., & Russell, J. D. (1995). Medical assessment and the initial interview in the management of young patients with anorexia nervosa. In *Eating Disorders in Adolescence.* In H.-C. Steinhausen (Ed.)
Beumont, P. J. V., O'Connor, M., Touyz, S. W., & William, H. (1987). Nutritional counselling in the treatment of anorexia and bulimia nervosa. In P. J. V. Beumont, G. D. Burrows & R. Casper (Eds.). *Handbook of Eating Disorders.* Volume 1, Anorexia and Bulimia. (pp. 351-361). Amsterdam: Elsevier Biomedical Press.
Beumont, P. J. V., Russell, J. & Touyz, S. W. (1993). Treatment of anorexia nervosa. *The Lancet*, 341, 8861, 1635-164.
Bruch, H. (1974). Perils of behaviour modification in the treatment of anorexia nervosa. *Journal of the American Medical Association*, 23, 1419-1422.
Bruch, H. (1978). Dangers of behaviour modification in the treatment of anorexia nervosa. In J. P. Brady & H. K. H. Brodie (Eds.), *Controversy in Psychiatry* (pp. 645-654). Philadelphia: W. B. Sanders.

Butow, P., Beumont, P. J. V., & Touyz, S. W. (1993). Cognitive processes in dieting disorders. *International Journal of Eating Disorders, 14, 3*, 319-329.

Crisp, A. H. (1980). *Anorexia nervosa*. New York: Grune and Stratton.

Garfinkel, P. E., & Garner, D. M. (1982). *Anorexia nervosa: a multidimensional perspective*. New York: Brunner/Mazel.

Garner, D. M. (1985). Iatrogenesis in anorexia nervosa and bulimia nervosa. *International Journal of Eating Disorders, 4*, 71-726.

Garner, D. M. & Bemis, K. M. (1982). A cognitive-behavioral approach to anorexia nervosa. *Cognitive Therapy and Research, 6*, 123-15.

Garner, D. M., & Bemis, K. M. (1985). Cognitive therapy for anorexia nervosa. In D. M. Garner, & P. E. Garfinkel (Eds.), *Handbook of Psychotherapy for Anorexia Nervosa and Bulimia*. (pp. 17-146). New York: The Guilford Press.

Garner, D. M., & Sackeyfio, A. H. (1993). Eating Disorders. In A. S. Bellack & M. Hersen (Eds.). *Handbook of Behavior Therapy in the Psychiatric Setting*. (pp. 477-497). New York: Plenum Press.

Garner, D. M., Rockert, W., Olmsted, M., Johnson, C., & Cosina, D. V. (1985). Psychoeducational principles in the treatment of bulimia and anorexia nervosa. In D. M. Garner, & P. E. Garfinkel (Eds.), *Handbook of Psychotherapy for Anorexia Nervosa and Bulimia*. (pp. 513-572). New York: The Guilford Press.

Goldner, E. (1989). Treatment refusal in anorexia nervosa. *International Journal of Eating Disorders, 8*, 297-36.

Macmanus, M., & Comerci, G.D. (1986). Financial barriers in the care of adolescents with anorexia nervosa and bulimia. *Seminars in Adolescent Medicine, 2*, 89-92.

O'Connor, M. A., Touyz, S. W., Dunn, S., & Beumont, P. J. V. (1987). Vegetarianism in anorexia nervosa? A review of 116 consecutive cases. *The Medical Journal of Australia, 147*, 54-542.

Piran, N., Kaplan, A., Kerr, A., Shenker-Wolfson, L., Winocur, J., Gold, E., & Garfinkel, P. E. (1989a). A day hospital program for anorexia nervosa and bulimia. *International Journal of Eating Disorders, 8(5)*, 511-521.

Piran, N., Langdon, L., Kaplan, A., & Garfinkel, P. E. (1989b). Evaluation of a day hospital program for eating disorders. *International Journal of Eating Disorders, 8(5)*, 523-532.

Russell, G. (1970). Anorexia nervosa: Its identity as an illness and its treatment. In J. H. Price (Ed). *Modern Trends in Psychological Medicine*. Vol. 2 (pp. 131-164). London: Butterworth's.

Russell, G. F. M. (1977). The present status of anorexia nervosa (editorial). *Psychological Medicine, 7*, 363-367.

Silver T.H., Delaney, D., & Samuels, D. (1989). Anorexia nervosa: hospitalization in adolescent medicine units and third party payments. *Journal of Adolescent Health Care, 10*, 122-125.

Stierlin, H., & Weberly. (1987). Anorexia nervosa: Family dynamics and family therapy. In P. J. V. Beumont, G. D. Burrows & R. C. Casper (Eds.), *Handbook of Eating Disorders: Part 1. Anorexia and Bulimia Nervosa*. (pp. 319-347). Amsterdam: Elsevier.

Strober, M., & Yager, J. A. (1985). A development perspective on the treatment of anorexia nervosa in adolescents. In D. M. Garner, P. E., Garfinkel (Eds.), *Handbook of Psychotherapy for Anorexia Nervosa and Bulimia*. (pp. 363-369). New York: The Guilford Press.

Stunkard, A. J. (1982). Obesity. In A. S. Bellack, M. Hersen, & A. E. Kazdin (Eds.), *International Handbook of Behaviour Modification and Therapy*. (pp. 535-573). New York: Plenum Press.

Touyz, S. W. (1988). Self-help groups. In G. D. Burrows, P. J. V. Beumont & R. C. Casper (Eds.), *Handbook of Eating Disorders: Part 2: Obesity*. (pp. 261-268). Amsterdam: Elsevier.

Touyz, S. W., & Beumont, P. J. V. (1985). A comprehensive, multidisciplinary approach for the management of patients with anorexia nervosa. In S. W. Touyz & P. J. V. Beumont (Eds.). *Eating Disorders: Prevalence and Treatment*. (pp. 11-22). Sydney: Williams and Wilkins/Adis.

Touyz, S. W., & Beumont, P. J. V. (1991). The management of anorexia nervosa in adolescence. *Medical Journal of Australia, 34(11)*, 86-97.

Touyz, S. W., & Beumont, P. J. V. (1993). Overcoming anorexia nervosa. In S. Schwartz (Ed), *Case Studies in Abnormal Psychology*. (pp. 53-72). Brisbane: John Wiley and Sons.

Touyz, S. W., Beumont, P. J. V., & Dunn, S. M. (1987). Behaviour therapy in the management of patients with anorexia nervosa: A lenient, flexible approach. *Psychotherapy and Psychosomatics, 48*, 151-156.

Touyz, S. W., Beumont, P. J. V., Glaun, D., Philips, T., & Cowie, I. (1984). Comparison of lenient and strict operant conditioning programmes in refeeding patients with anorexia nervosa. *British Journal of Psychiatry, 144*, 512-52.

Touyz, S. W., Lennerts, W., Arthur, B., & Beumont, P. J. V. (1993). Anaerobic exercise as an adjunct to refeeding patients with anorexia nervosa. Does it compromise weight gain? *European Eating Disorder Review, 1(3)*, 177-182.

Touyz, S. W., Lennerts, W., Freeman, R. J., & Beumont, P. J. V. (1990). To weigh or no to weigh: Frequency of weighing and rate of weight gain in patients with anorexia nervosa. *British Journal of Psychiatry, 157*, 752-754.

Touyz, S. W., Williams, H., Marden, K., Kopec-Schrader, E., & Beumont, P. J. V. (1994). Videotape feedback of eating behaviour in patients with anorexia nervosa: does it normalise eating behaviour? *Australian Journal of Nutrition and Dietetics, 51(2)*, 79-82.

Vandereycken, W. & Meermann, R. (1984). *Anorexia nervosa: A clinician's guide to treatment.* Berlin: Walter de Gruyter.

Williams, H., Touyz, S. W., & Beumont, P. J. V. (1985). Nutritional counselling in anorexia nervosa. In S. W. Touyz. & P. J. V. Beumont (Eds.), *Eating Disorders: Prevalence and Treatment.* (pp. 23-31). Sydney: William and Wilkins/Adis.

Wilson, A. J., Touyz, S. W., & Beumont, P. J. V. (1989). The Eating Behaviour Rating Scale (EBRS). A measure of eating pathology in anorexia nervosa. *International Journal of Eating Disorders, 8(5)*, 583-592.

Wooley, S.C. (1993). Manage care and mental health: The silencing of a profession. *International Journal of Eating disorders, 14 (4)*, 387-401.

# Psychopharmacology in Adolescents with Eating Disorders

*Denise M. Heebink and Katherine A. Halmi*

## 1 Introduction

The onset of anorexia nervosa (AN) and bulimia nervosa (BN) typically occurs during the adolescent years. Given this, the potential role for pharmacotherapy in the treatment of eating disorders in adolescents needs to be critically examined. After a thorough search of the literature, we found neither a controlled study of psychotropic drugs performed exclusively in adolescents with eating disorders, nor one comparing their response to that of adults. For purposes of the search and this chapter, an adolescent was defined as anyone 12 to 19 years old. Case reports in adolescents and controlled trials in primarily adult populations will be described and their potential application to the treatment of eating disorders in adolescents discussed.

Eating disorders symptomatology will be divided into three categories: (1) anorexia nervosa, restricting subtype (AN-R); (2) anorexia nervosa, with concurrent bingeing and/or purging (AN-B); (3) bulimia nervosa (BN); (American Psychiatric Association, 1994).

## 2 Neuroleptics

Neuroleptics were among the first medications used in the treatment of patients with AN. Barry and Klawans (1976) have hypothesized that increased dopaminergic activity may account for the major symptoms of anorexia nervosa (AN) and suggested treatment with selective dopamine-blocking agents. Others have noted that some patients with eating disorders display transient psychotic symptoms during the course of their illness (Grounds 1982; Hudson et al., 1984). Clinicians have also been puzzled by the fact that the body image distortion in AN can assume delusional proportions. Theoretical lines of reasoning and clinical observations have led to the use of the dopamine-blocking neuroleptics in AN.

The earliest trials of neuroleptics in patients with AN included adolescents (Dally & Sargant, 1960; 1966). In these open trials, patients received the phenothiazine chlorpromazine in high dosage combined in some cases with insulin to induce hunger and weight gain. Control patients, like the experimental ones, received nursing care and psychological intervention but no chlorpromazine. Treatment with chlorpromazine and insulin led to more rapid weight gain and earlier discharge from the hospital. The treatment was not without complications - 17% developed seizures and 45% at follow-up had developed bulimia, whereas 12% of the control group became bulimic. Overall, no long-term benefit of neuroleptic treatment was shown.

Crisp (1984) who initially advocated chlorpromazine in patients with AN, has largely abandoned its use. The drug appears to have very little effect on appetite or ingestion but rather renders patients more compliant and less active. Our experience has been that in selected patients the anxiety-reducing effect of phenothiazines can help the patient overcome fears of eating and gaining weight; the sedating effect may decrease restlessness, and the known side effect of weight gain may benefit some. The disadvantages of these drugs must also be considered. Chlorpromazine has been reported to have induced hemolytic anemia in a 15-year-old girl with AN (How & Davidson, 1977). Phenothiazines are also known to decrease blood pressure, cause agranulocytosis and hyperprolactinemia, aggravate leukopenia, and alter fluid balance. These problems can be especially troublesome in the emaciated patient, and a careful assessment of risks and benefits should made before using phenothiazine medications in patients with AN.

Plantey (1977) reported dramatic improvement in a 17-year-old anorectic male treated with the dopamine-blocking drug pimozide. Within three weeks on pimozide, he gained 20 pounds, his body image disturbance diminished, and his overactivity decreased. Hoes (1980) reported improvement in 10 anorectic adolescent girls treated with pimozide. Vandereycken and Pierloot (1982) treated 18 inpatients with pimozide and a placebo in a crossover design study and found a trend towards greater daily weight gain in those receiving the drug. Ratings of activity level and characteristic anorectic attitudes did not show a consistent advantage for medication.

Vandereycken (1984) also studied the a antipsychotic agent sulpiride - which is known to stimulate appetite and weight gain - in a double-blind, placebo-controlled trial of anorectic females that included adolescents. Weight gain during the first three weeks was greater in the patients receiving sulpiride, but overall, this effect did not reach statistical significance. No significant changes in behavioral or attitudinal characteristics were noted in drug-treated patients.

Munford (1980) described a single-subject experimental analysis to assess the effects of haloperidol and behavioral treatment in a 17-year-old anorectic female. Although the study attempted to evaluate the separate effects of medication and behavioral therapy, no firm conclusions regarding the contributions of either could be drawn. No serious side effects of haloperidol in this adolescent were reported.

In summary, the evidence does not support clear efficacy of neuroleptic medication in the treatment of the adolescent with an AN or BN. Given the untoward side effects associated with these drugs, they should be used with caution. However, in patients with AN in which cognitive-behavioral and supportive nursing care are inadequate, a trial of neuroleptic medication may be warranted after a careful analysis of risks and benefits has been made.

## 3  Antidepressants

Antidepressants are frequently used in the treatment of eating disorders, and the literature suggests that these disorders have features in common with depression (Pope et al., 1983; Herzog, 1984). A current or past history of depression and some neuroendocrine changes similar to those in depression are seen in eating disorder patients. These patients also seem to have a familial aggregation and genetic predisposition to affective disorders. Hudson and coworkers (1983) have reported that 88% of patients with eating disorders have a history of affective disorder.

### 3.1  Tricyclic Antidepressants

### 3.1.1  Anorexia Nervosa

White and Schnaultz (1977) have reported the successful treatment of AN in two depressed adolescents - one a 15-year-old female, the other a 16-year-old male - using imipramine 150-175 mg/day. Others have reported successful treatment of

AN in six adolescents, five female patients age 11-17 and one male patient age 16, using amytriptyline in doses ranging from 75-150 mg for 1-3 months (Needleman & Waber, 1977). All gained weight and seemed to have diminution of depressive symptoms and abnormal eating patterns while on medication. Hudson and coworkers (1985) reported no improvement in anorectic symptoms in a 17-year-old female patient treated with both imipramine and desipramine.

The first placebo-controlled trial of amitriptyline in AN was done in a mixed group of in- and outpatients (Biederman et al., 1985). After five weeks on amytriptyline, no evidence was found that it was significantly better than the placebo in increasing the rate of weight gain or improving depressive and eating disorder symptomatology. A larger, placebo-controlled trial was conducted in two centers by Halmi and others in which the serotonin antagonist cyproheptadine was compared to amytriptyline in hospitalized patients with AN (Halmi et al., 1986). They found that overall amytriptyline had no significant advantage over placebo in promoting weight gain or improving mood.

The few studies that do exist do not support a major role for the use of tricyclic antidepressants (TCA) in the treatment of adolescents with AN. In addition, side effects of these medications can include orthostatic hypotension and cardiac arrhythmia, both of which can worsen the clinical condition of an emaciated patient with AN.

### 3.1.2 Bulimia Nervosa

Pharmacologic trials of TCA's in BN were prompted by the clinical observation that mood disturbances appeared to be widespread in bulimic patients. The relation between depression and BN remains unclear, but the results of these trials have been much more hopeful than those in the AN trials.

Of the eight controlled studies of tricyclic antidepressants in BN, virtually all have shown that medication is superior to placebo in reducing binge eating episodes in adult females (Pope et al., 1983; Mitchell & Groat, 1984; Hughes et al., 1986; Agras et al., 1987; Barlow et al., 1988; Blouin et al., 1988; Mitchell et al., 1990; Walsh et al., 1991). The dosages used in these studies were similar to those used in treating depression. No trials have been done exclusively in adolescents with BN but several did include 18 and 19 year olds.

Double-blind, placebo-controlled studies of the antidepressant mianserin have been done and included bulimic patients as young as 16 (Sabine et al., 1983). No improvement in anxiety, depression, or eating disorder symptoms was found with mianserin.

The presence of depression has not been shown to be a good predictor of response to antidepressants in BN (Hughes et al., 1986; Agras et al., 1987). Both depressed and nondepressed patients appear to have similar reductions in bulimic symptoms with TCA's. This is surprising in view of the original rationale for using these medications in bulimic patients.

Work has also begun with comparing psychopharmacologic and psychotherapeutic interventions in the treatment of BN. Recently, Mitchell and colleagues (1990) found that intensive group therapy was superior to imipramine. A later study compared response to individual cognitive-behavioral treatment, desipramine, and a combination of both in bulimic women. Cognitive-behavioral therapy was superior to medication alone and overall, a combination of both was superior in decreasing bingeing and purging episodes and reducing hunger and dietary preoccupations (Agras et al., 1992).

Results of placebo-controlled studies of TCA's in depressed adolescents are mixed and have yet to clearly show their efficacy (Ryan, 1992). This may be because clinical improvement in adolescents treated with TCAs is not as robust as that in adults or that certain subgroups of depressed adolescents are nonresponders. For these same reasons, caution must be exercised in applying findings in adult patients with BN to the adolescent with BN, but current studies would suggest that a trial of a TCA may be helpful to some.

## 3.2 Serotonin-Reuptake Inhibitors

### 3.2.1 Anorexia Nervosa

The selective serotonin-reuptake inhibitor (SSRI) medications have been used in the treatment of depression in both adolescents and adults, and more recently, for obsessive-compulsive disorder. Hudson and coworkers (1983) reported that 81% of patients with AN-R and 92% of those with AN-B have had a history of affective disorder. A high prevalence of obsessive compulsive symptoms in patients with

AN has also been reported (Solyom, et al., 1982; Hudson, et al., 1983), and disturbances in the serotonin system have been implicated (Zohar & Insel, 1987). Patients with AN have also been shown to have disturbances in serotonergic activity that persist after long-term weight restoration (Kaye et al., 1991a). These lines of evidence suggest that SSRI medications may be helpful in the treatment of AN in adolescents.

Two case reports describe the successful treatment of two 16-year-old females with AN-B with the SSRI fluoxetine (Lyles et al., 1990; Inacu et al., 1992). In the patient described by Inacu and colleagues, hyperprolactinemia and galactorrhea developed on fluoxetine 60 mg/day but remitted on 40 mg/day.

Kaye and coworkers reported an open trial of fluoxetine in patients with anorexia nervosa admitted to out- and inpatient eating disorder programs (Kaye et al., 1991b). No particular regimen of psychotherapy was prescribed. In this study, 21 of the 31 patients reported were adolescents. A good outcome with fluoxetine was reported when a patient had unimpaired daily functioning and improvement in three areas: (1) reduction of depression, anxiety, and obsessive-compulsive symptoms; (2) reduction in pathological eating behavior and maintenance of weight above 85% of normal body weight; (3) abstinance from bingeing and purging behaviors. A poor response was judged when there was continued symptomatology in these areas, and a partial response was intermediate between good and poor.

Of the 10 patients in this study with a good response to fluoxetine, nine were adolescents. Eight of the nine had AN-R, the other AN-B. All adolescents with a good response were treated with 20-40 mg/day of fluoxetine. In the partial response group, 10 of the 17 patients were adolescents; two had AN-R, three AN-B, and five had AN-R and also began bingeing while on fluoxetine. All adolescents with a partial response were treated with fluoxetine 10-60 mg/day. Two of the four with a poor response were adolescents with AN-R who had been treated with 60-80 mg/day of fluoxetine.

These investigators found that significantly more patients with AN-R were in the good response group and significantly more with AN-B were in the fair and poor response group. They found that no patient reported increased difficulty in eating while in the study, and also concluded that fluoxetine seemed to be particularly effective in helping those with AN-R to maintain a healthy weight. This is a noteworthy finding considering that a well-known side effect of fluoxetine is diminished appetite. Kaye and colleagues (1984) have also reported that patients with AN-R may have increased serotonin turnover in comparison to those with AN-B. Clearly, there is evidence that fluoxetine may be helpful in weight restoration and improving affective symptoms in adolescents with anorexia nervosa, particulary AN-R, but controlled trials are still needed before definitive treatment recommendations can be made.

Clomipramine, a tricyclic antidepressant with strong serotonergic action, has been studied in patients with AN (Lacey & Crisp, 1980). In a placebo-controlled trial of low-dose clomipramine (50mg/day) these investigators found no significant increase in rate of weight gain in the drug-treated group. Although clomipramine has theoretical efficacy in the treatment of AN, further studies using standard dosages need to be done.

### 3.2.2 Bulimia Nervosa

The serotonin system in the medial hypothalamus appears to be an important component of satiety mechanisms (Liebowitz et al., 1985), and manipulations that increase serotonergic neurotransmission have been shown to decrease food consumption (Blundell & Hill, 1987). These findings suggest that the SSRI medications could be useful in decreasing the unrestrained bingeing patterns in patients with BN.

The SSRI fluoxetine has been studied and shown to be effective in reducing bingeing and purging behaviors in persons with BN but has not been systematically studied in adolescents. Double-blind, placebo-controlled studies have shown that fluoxetine is more effective than placebo in reducing bingeing and purging behaviors in BN (Fichter et al., 1991; Fluoxetine collaborative study group, 1992). The fluoxetine collaborative study performed in 13 centers is the largest controlled trial to date. Fluoxetine at doses of 60 mg/day proved superior to placebo in decreasing the frequency of bingeing and purging in bulimic women. Improvement in patients on 20 mg/day was intermediate between 60 mg/day and placebo. Depression, carbohydrate craving, and pathological eating attitudes also showed more robust improvement on 60 mg/day than 20 mg/day. The mean age of the study participants was about 27 years and separate data analysis was not performed on adolescents (Fluoxetine bulimia nervosa collaborative study group, 1992).

Other serotonin agonists such as fenfluramine and fluvoxamine have also been shown to be helpful in reducing abnormal eating behaviors (Robinson et al., 1985; Blouin et al., 1988; Gardiner et al., 1992).

Although the response of bulimic adolescents to medications can not be predicted from adult studies, our clinical impression is that fluoxetine has been well tolerated and helpful to adolescents in decreasing their bingeing and purging behaviors, but again, controlled studies of the SSRI's in adolescents are needed.

### 3.3 Monoamine Oxidase Inhibitors

The monoamine oxidase inhibitor (MAOI) medications have been used in the treatment of depression for over three decades. The high prevalence of mood disorder symptoms in eating disorder patients has led to investigations to examine their utility in AN and BN.

#### 3.3.1 Anorexia Nervosa

Kennedy and Walsh (1987) compared the effects of the MAOI isocarboxazid and placebo in an open trial of five patients with AN-R. They saw no trend towards improvement in weight gain or abnormal eating attitudes while patients were on isocarboxazid. Hudson and coworkers (1985) have reported on one adolescent with AN who received phenelzine and showed no appreciable clinical improvement. These modest findings suggest a negligible role for MAOI's in the treatment of AN.

#### 3.3.2 Bulimia Nervosa

Kennedy and others (1988) have performed a double-blind, placebo-controlled study of isocarboxazid in 18 bulimic women and found a significant reduction in bingeing and vomiting. There was only one adolescent in this study, and specific information about her response was not reported. Walsh and colleagues (1985) performed a controlled trial of phenelzine and placebo and reported a reduction in bingeing in bulimic women with phenelzine. Others also reported improvement in bingeing in a case series of bulimic women treated with phenelzine (Jonas et al., 1983). Overall, given the danger of hypertensive crisis with the ingestion of tyramine-rich foods in patients on MAOI's and the impulse control problems of bulimic patients, MAOI's appear to be of limited value in adolescents with BN.

## 4 Anxiolytic Medication

Anxiety about body size and shape plays a major role in the genesis of eating disorders, and the anxiety relief provided by food restriction and purging behavior may be reinforcing and ultimately maintain these symptoms. No controlled studies have been done examining the use of benzodiazepenes in eating disorder patients. Anderson (1987) has advocated the judicious use of small doses of lorazepam before meals in very anxious patients with AN. Because of their addictive potential, caution must be exercised in the use of benzodiazepenes in eating disorders patients and should be avoided in those with a history of substance abuse.

## 5 Lithium

Lithium carbonate has been used for over two decades for mood stabilization in bipolar disorder and augmentation of antidepressants in unipolar depression. These mood stabilizing properties and the well-known side effect of weight gain have led some investigators to use lithium in eating disorder patients.

### 5.1 Anorexia Nervosa

Stein and others (1982) have reported on a 16-year-old girl with a 5-year history of AN who was successfully treated with lithium after several trials of neuroleptics, TCA's, and behavioral management had failed. Their impression was that lithium did not influence her AN but rather stabilized her moods and so enabled her to be more responsive to nursing care and psychotherapy. In a double-blind, placebo-controlled trial of lithium carbonate in patients also receiving behavioral therapy, the lithium group showed greater weight gain at the third and fourth weeks of treatment than those in the placebo group (Gross et al., 1981). The lithium-treated patients also showed improvement in the denial or minimization of illness item on the Psychiatric Rating Scale. Patients in this study were age 12-32, but no separate analysis of the adolescents was conducted. The physiological explanation for these findings is uncertain. Lithium has been shown to increase glucose uptake in muscle, suggesting an insulin-like effect (Plenge et al., 1970). Untreated patients with AN have an increased sensitivity to glucose, which has been explained by increased insulin binding resulting from an increased number of receptors without change in receptor affinity (Wachslicht-Rodbard, 1979). An insulin-like effect of lithium may promote weight gain in AN, and further study may be warranted. Nevertheless, lithium is not widely used in the treatment of AN because of its potential toxicity in emaciated or dehydrated patients.

## 5.2 Bulimia Nervosa

In an open trial of lithium and cognitive behavioral treatment in 14 bulimic women, three adolescents were included (Hsu, 1984). Two of the adolescent subjects showed marked improvement and one moderate improvement in depressive and eating disorder symptoms at 8-14 month follow-up. All adolescents received lithium for at least four weeks but had stopped the drug at follow-up. The significance of this finding is unclear, but lithium is generally not used in bulimic patients. The potential toxicity of lithium in patients who are vomiting, abusing laxatives and diuretics, or reducing fluid intake is very dangerous. The use of lithium as a first line drug in adolescents with BN is not warranted.

## 6 Cyproheptadine

Cyproheptadine, an antihistamine and a serotonin antagonist, has been widely used to stimulate appetite and promote weight gain. Benady (1970) described the successful use of cyproheptadine in a 14-year-old female with refractory anorexia nervosa. In the first double-blind, placebo-controlled trial of cyproheptadine, Vigersky and Loriaux (1972) reported that 12 mg/day of cyproheptadine was not significantly more effective than placebo in promoting weight gain in patients with AN.

More extensive studies of cyproheptadine in AN have since been done by Halmi and colleagues. In their first report of 81 patients, they showed that cyproheptadine had a significant effect on weight gain in patients with a history of birth complications, severe emaciation, and several failures of outpatient treatment (Goldberg et al., 1979). Doses of up to 32 mg/day were used and virtually no side effects were reported. In a follow-up study of 105 patients, improvements were also found in the characteristic attitudinal and behavioral features of AN (Goldberg et al., 1980). A later study showed that cyproheptadine at doses of 32 mg/day promotes weight gain and decreases depressive symptoms (Halmi et al., 1983). Motor activity has also been shown to be suppressed in patients with AN during the first two weeks of treatment with cyproheptadine - a finding that may in part explain the weight increase (Falk et al, 1985).

In a placebo-controlled trial of cyproheptadine and amytriptyline in hospitalized patients with AN, cyproheptadine was shown to have a marginal effect on decreasing the number of days necessary for achieving normal weight (Halmi et al., 1986). Cyproheptadine was also not shown to affect anorectic attitudes and behaviors. There was, however, a differential drug effect found in AN-B and AN-R subtypes. Efficiency of weight gain was significantly increased in patients with AN-R and decreased in those with AN-B who received cyproheptadine. Also, in the early stages of treatment, cyproheptadine was found to have an antidepressant effect. No significant side effects from cyproheptadine were reported. These findings suggest that cyproheptadine can be useful for increasing the rate of weight gain and reducing depression in patients with AN-R, but it should be avoided in patients with AN-B.

After a re-analysis of the data in the study described above (Halmi et al., 1986), we found that, although anorectic adolescent patients who received cyproheptadine did not respond differently from adults with respect to weight gain, they did show significantly greater improvement in depressive, obsessive compulsive, and anxiety symptoms than did the adolescents who received placebo (Data submitted for publication).

## 7 Conclusions

In the absence of controlled trials of medication in adolescents with eating disorders, definitive treatment recommendations are impossible. Great caution must be exercised in extrapolating the results of experimental work done primarily in adults to the clinical treatment of adolescents. When choosing a medication for an adolescent with an eating disorder, a careful assessment of eating disorder symptomatology and medical and psychiatric comorbidity must be made. General principles for prescribing medications in adolescents with eating disorders might include the following:

1. Neuroleptics have a limited role except in carefully selected patients with AN in whom cognitive-behavioral techniques and supportive nursing care have failed.

2. The SSRI fluoxetine may be useful in patients with AN-R in improving affective symptoms and weight restoration but carefully controlled studies remain to be done. Fluoxetine has been shown to be effective in reducing bingeing and vomiting in adult bulimic women.

3. TCA's have not been shown to be effective in AN but have been shown to reduce bulimic symptoms in adult women, particularly when combined with cognitive-behavioral or group therapies.

4. Benzodiazepenes and MAOI's are of limited value in treating eating disorder patients.

5. Lithium is probably of negligible value in the treatment of adolescents with AN or BN.

6. Cyproheptadine is a safe drug that promotes weight gain and improves mood in adolescents with AN-R but should be avoided in patients with AN-B.

**References**

Agras, W.S., Dorian, B., Kirkley, B.G., Arnow, B., & Bachman, J. (1987). Imipramine in the treatment of bulimia: A double-blind controlled study. *International Journal of Eating Disorders, 6*, 29-38.

Agras, W.S., Rossiter, E.M., Arnow, B., Schneider, J.A., Telch, C.F., Raeburn, S.D., Bruce, B., Perl, M., & Koran, L.M. (1992). A comparison study of antidepressants and structured intensive group psychotherapy in the treatment of bulimia nervosa. *American Journal of Psychiatry, 149*, 82-87.

American Psychiatric Association.(1994). *Diagnostic and Statistical Manual*, 4th Ed. Washington D.C.:American Psychiatric Press.

Andersen, A.E. (1987). Uses and potential misuses of antianxiety agents in the treatment of anorexia nervosa and bulimia nervosa. In Garfinkel, P.E., & Garner, D.M. (Eds.), *The Role of Drug Treatments for Eating Disorders* (pp. 59-73). New York: Brunner/Mazel.

Barlow, J., Blouin, J., Blouin, A., & Perez, E (1988). Treatment of bulimia with desipramine: A double-blind crossover study. *Canadian Journal of Psychiatry, 33*, 129-133.

Barry, V.C., & Kawans, H.L. On the role of dopamine in the pathophysiology of anorexia nervosa (1976). *Journal of Neuron Transmission, 38*, 107-122.

Benady, D.R. Cyproheptadine hydrochloride (Periactin) and anorexia nervosa: A case report (1970). *British Journal of Psychiatry, 117*, 681-682.

Biederman, J., Herzog, D.B., Rivinus, T.M., Harper, G.P., Ferber, R.A., Rosenbaum, J.F., Harmatz, J.S., Tondorf, R., Orsulak, P.J., & Shildkraut, J.J. (1985). Amytriptyline in the treatment of anorexia nervosa: A double-blind, placebo-controlled study. *Journal of Clinical Psychopharmacology, 5*, 10-16.

Blouin, A.G., Blouin, J.H., Perez, E.L., Bushnik, T., Zuro, C., & Mulder, E. (1988). Treatment of bulimia with fenfluramine and desipramine. *Journal of Clinical Psychopharmacology, 8*, 261-269.

Blundell, J.E., & Hill, A.H. (1987). Serotonergic modulation of the pattern of eating and the profile of hunger-satiety in humans. *International Journal of Obesity, 11* (Suppl 3), 141-155.

Crisp, A.H. (1984). Treatment of anorexia nervosa: What can be the role of psychopharmacological agents? In Pirke, K.M., Ploog, D. (Eds.), *The Psychobiology of Anorexia Nervosa* (pp. 148-160). Berlin-New York:Springer-Verlag.

Dally, P.J., & Sargant, W. (1960). A new treatment of anorexia nervosa. *British Medical Journal, 1*, 1770-1773.

Dally, P.J., & Sargant, W. (1966). Treatment and outcome of anorexia nervosa. *British Medical Journal, 2*, 793-795.

Falk, J.R., Halmi, K.A., & Tyron, W.W. (1985). Activity measures in anorexia nervosa. *Archives of General Psychiatry, 42*, 811-814.

Fichter, M.M., Leibl, K., Rief, W., Brunner, E., Schmidt-Auberger, S, & Engel, R.R. (1991). Fluoxetine versus placebo: A double-blind study with bulimic inpatients undergoing intensive psychotherapy. *Pharmacopsychiatry, 24*,1-7.

Fluoxetine bulimia nervosa collaborative study group. (1992). Fluoxetine in the treatment of bulimia nervosa. A multicenter, placebo-controlled, double-blind trial. *Archives of General Psychiatry, 49*, 139-147.

Gardiner, H.M., Freeman, C.P.L, Jesinger, D.K., & Collins, S.A. (1993). Fluvoxamine: An open pilot study in moderately obese female patient suffering from atypical eating disorders and episodes of bingeing. *International Journal of Obesity, 17*, 301-305.

Goldberg, S.C., Halmi, K.A., Eckert, E.D., Casper, R.C., & Davis, J.M. (1979). Cyproheptadine in anorexia nervosa. *British Journal of Psychiatry, 134*, 67-70.

Goldberg, S.C., Eckert, E.D., Halmi, K.A., Casper, R.C., Davis, J.M., & Roper, M. (1980). Effects of cyproheptadine on symptoms and attitudes in anorexia nervosa. *Archives of General Psychiatry, 37*, 1083.

Gross, H.A., Ebert, M.H., Faden, V.B., Goldberg, S.C., Nee, L.E., & Kaye, W.H. (1981). A double-blind controlled trial of lithium carbonate in primary anorexia nervosa. *Journal of Clinical Psychopharmacology, 1*, 376-381.

Grounds A. (1982). Transient psychoses in anorexia nervosa: A report of 7 cases. *Psychological Medicine, 12*, 107-113.

Halmi, K.A., Eckert, E.D., & Falk, J.R. (1983). Cyproheptadine, an antidepressant and weight-inducing drug for anorexia nervosa. *Psychopharmacology Bulletin, 1*, 103-105.

Halmi, K.A., Eckert, E., LaDu, T.J., & Cohen, J. (1986). Anorexia nervosa. Treatment efficacy of cyproheptadine and amytriptyline. *Archives of General Psychiatry, 43*, 177-181.

Herzog D.B. Are anorexic and bulimic patients depressed? (1984). *American Journal of Psychiatry, 141*, 1594-1597.

Hoes, M.J.A. (1980). Copper sulfate and pimozide in anorexia nervosa. *Journal of Orthomolecular Psychiatry, 9*, 49-51.

How, J., & Davidson, R.J.L. (1977). Chlorpromazine-induced haemolytic anaemia in anorexia nervosa. *Postgraduate Medical Journal, 53*, 278-279.

Hsu, L.K.G. (1984). Treatment of Bulimia with lithium. *American Journal of Psychiatry, 141*, 1260-1262.

Hudson, J.I., Pope, H.G., & Jonas, J.M. (1984). Psychosis in anorexia nervosa and bulima. *British Journal of Psychiatry, 145*, 420-423.

Hudson, J.I., Pope, H.G., Jonas, J.M., & Yurgelun-Todd, D. (1983). Phenomenologic relationship of eating disorders to major affective disorders. *Psychiatry Research, 9*, 345-354.

Hudson, J.I., Pope, H.G., Jonas, J.M., & Yurgelun-Todd, D. (1985). Treatment of Anorexia nervosa with antidepressants. *Journal of Clinical Psychopharmacology, 5*, 17-23.

Hughes, P.L., Wells, L.A., Cunningham, C.J., & Ilstrup, D.M. (1986) Treating bulimia with desipramine. *Archives of General Psychiatry, 43*, 182-186.

Iancu, I., Ratzoni, G., Weitzman, A., & Apter, A. (1992). More fluoxetine experience (Letter). *Journal of the American Academy of Child and Adolescent Psychiatry, 31*, 755-756.

Jonas, J.M., Hudson, J.I., & Pope, H.G. (1983). Responses to "The Psychiatrist as Mind Sweeper": Eating Disorders and Antidepressants (Letter). *Journal of Clinical Psychopharmacology, 3*, 59-60.

Kaye, W.H., Ebert, M.H., Gwirtsman, H.E., & Weiss, S.R. (1984). Differences in brain sertonergic metabolism between nonbulimic and bulimic patients with anorexia nervosa. *American Journal of Psychiatry, 141*, 1598-1601.

Kaye, W.H., Gwirtsman, H.E., George, D.T., & Ebert, M.H. (1991a) Altered serotonin activity in anorexia nervosa after long-term weight restoration: Does elevated CSF 5-HIAA correlate with rigid and obsessive behavior? *Archives of General Psychiatry, 48*, 556-562.

Kaye, W.H., Weltzin, T.E., Hsu, L.K.G., & Bulik, C.M. (1991b). An open trial of fluoxetine in patients with anorexia nervosa. *Journal of Clinical Psychiatry, 52*, 464-471.

Kennedy, S., & Walsh, B.T. (1987). Drug therapies for eating disorders: Monoamine oxidase inhibitors. In Garfinkel, P.E., & Garner, D.M. (Eds.), *The Role of Drug Treatments for Eating Disorders* (pp. 3-35). New York: Brunner Mazel.

Kennedy, S.H., Piran, N., Warsh, J.J., Prendergast, P., Mainprize, E., Whynot, C., & Garfinkel, P.E. (1988). A trial of isocarboxazid in the treatment of bulimia nervosa. *Journal of Clinical Psychopharmacology, 8*, 391-396.

Lacey, J.H., & Crisp, A.H. (1980). Hunger, food intake and weight: The impact of clomipramine on a refeeding anorexia nervosa population. *Postgraduate Medical Journal, 56* (suppl 1), 79-85.

Liebowitz, S.F., Weiss, G.F., & Shor-Posner, G. (1985) Medial hypothalamic serotonin in the control of eating behavior. *International Journal of Obesity, 11* (suppl 3), 110-123.

Lyles, B., Sarkis, E., & Kemph, J.P. (1990). Fluoxetine and anorexia (Letter). *Journal of the American Academy of Child and Adolescent Psychiatry, 29*, 984-985.

Mitchell, J.E., & Groat, R. (1984). A placebo-controlled, double-blind crossover trial of amitriptyline in bulimia. *Journal of Clinical Psychopharmacology, 4*, 186-193.

Mitchell, J.E., Pyle, R.L., Eckert, E.D., Hatsukami, D., Pomeroy, C., & Zimmerman, R. A. (1990). A comparison study of antidepressants and structured group psychotherapy in the treatment of bulimia nervosa. *Archives of General Psychiatry, 47*, 149-157.

Munford, P.R. (1980). Haloperidol and contingency management in a case of anorexia nervosa. *Journal of Behavior Therapy and Experimental Psychiatry, 11*, 67-71.

Needleman, H., & Waber, D. (1976). Amytriptyline therapy in patients with anorexia nervosa (Letter). *Lancet, 2*, 580.

Plantey, F. (1977). Pimozide in treatment of anorexia nervosa (Letter). Lancet, 1, 1105.

Plenge, P., Mellerup, E.T., & Rafaelsen, O.J. (1970). Lithium effect on glycogen synthesis in rat brain, liver, and diaphragm. *Journal of Psychiatric Research, 8*, 29-36.

Pope, H.G., Hudson, J.I., Jonas, J.M., & Yurgelun-Todd, D. (1983). Bulimia treated with imipramine: A placebo-controlled, double-blind study. *American Journal of Psychiatry, 140*, 554-558.

Robinson, P.H., Checkley, S.A., & Russell, G.F.M. (1985). Suppression of eating by fenfluramine in patients with bulimia nervosa. *British Journal of Psychiatry, 146*, 169-176.

Ryan, N.D. Pharmacological treatment of major depression. (1992). In Shafii, M., Shafii, S.L. (Eds). *Clinical Guide to Depression in Children and Adolescents* (pp. 210-232). Washington, D.C.: American Psychiatric Press.

Sabine, E.J., Yonace, A., Farrington, A.J., Barratt, K.H., & Wakeling, A. (1983). Bulimia nervosa: A placebo controlled double-blind therapeutic trial of mianserin. *British Journal of Pharmacology, 15*, 195s-202s.

Solyom, L.S., Freeman, R.J., & Miles, J.E. (1982) A comparative psychometric study of anorexia nervosa and obsessive neurosis. Canadian Journal of Psychiatry, 27, 282-286.

Stein, G.S., Hartshorn, J., Jones, J., & Steinberg, D. (1982) Lithium in a case of severe anorexia nervosa. *British Journal of Psychiatry, 140*, 526-528.

Vandereycken, W. (1984). Neuroleptics in the short-term treatment of anorexia nervosa. A double-blind, placebo-controlled study with sulpiride. *British Journal of Psychiatry, 144*, 288-292.

Vandereycken W., & Pierloot R. (1982). Pimozide combined with behavior therapy in the short-term treatment of anorexia nervosa. A double-blind placebo-controlled crossover study. *Acta Psychiatrica Scandanavia, 66*, 445-450.

Vigersky, R.A., & Loriaux, D.L. (1977). The effect of cyproheptadine in anorexia nervosa: A double-blind trial. In Vigersky, R.A. (Ed.), *Anorexia Nervosa* (pp. 349-356). New York: Raven Press. 1977.

Wachlicht-Rodbard, H., Gross, H.A., Rodbard, D., Ebert, M.H., & Roth, J. (1979). Increased insulin binding erthythrocytes in anorexia nervosa. *New England Journal of Medicine, 300*, 882-887.

Walsh, B.T., Hadigan, C.M., Devlin, M.J., Gladis, M., & Roose, S.P. (1991). Long-term treatment outcome of antidepressant treatment for bulimia nervosa. *American Journal of Psychiatry, 148*, 1206-1212.

Walsh, B.T., Stewart, J.W., Roose, S.P., Gladis, M., & Glassman, A.H. (1985). A double-blind trial of phenelzine in bulimia. *Journal of Psychiatric Research, 19*, 485-489.

White, J.H., & Schnaultz, N.L. (1977). Successful treatment of anorexia nervosa with imipramine. *Diseases of the Nervous System, 38*, 567-568.

Zohar, J., & Insel, T.R. (1987). Obsessive-compulsive disorder: Psychobiological approaches to diagnosis, treatment, and pathophysiology. *Biological Psychiatry, 22*, 667-687.

# The Place of Family Therapy in the Treatment of Eating Disorders

*Walter Vandereycken*

## 1 Introduction

Through the influence of family systems theories eating disorders have been relabeled as interpersonal problems within a dysfunctional family context. The logical consequence of this view, the application of family therapy, is critically questioned in this chapter. After a discussion of the empirical evidence, our personal and rather pragmatic viewpoint is presented, situating family therapy within a multidimensional and eclectic approach to eating disorders.

## 2 Treating the Disordered Family?

For about a century since its introduction in the medical nosology, anorexia nervosa was considered to be an intrapersonal matter with the implicit belief that faulty parenting could cause or aggravate the disorder. It is no wonder, then, that traditional treatment often implied a form of "parentectomy": as a pathogenic influence, the parents had to be separated from the patient (Vandereycken, Kog, & Vanderlinden, 1989). In the 1970s, a radical change took place through the rapidly growing field of systems theory and family therapy. Minuchin and coworkers (1978) stated that the family structure and interactions should be the focus of treatment; anorexia nervosa could only be understood "in context". Around the same time, the Italian family therapist, Selvini Palazzoli (1974), called this a shift "from an intrapsychic to a transpersonal approach". Food refusal was seen as an interpersonal problem: being a "symptom" of pathological family interactions, it would refer to the adaptive reaction - be it in the form of protest or escape - of a vulnerable child to a given type of family dysfunctioning.

A logical consequence of the family systems view on eating disorders was to make family interactions the main target of the treatment. But this was more a question of ideology than of an empirically derived viewpoint (Vandereycken, 1987). In the meantime, various family characteristics have been investigated in eating disorders: genetic, physiological, cognitive, behavioral, emotional, and interactional. All the findings, however, are correlational in nature and should be interpreted with caution for the following reasons (Vandereycken, Kog, & Vanderlinden, 1989).

*First*, no family theory can explain the mechanisms whereby so-called typical family patterns are translated into the many psychological and physiological features of eating disorders. *Second*, it remains to be substantiated that specific interactions occur in families of eating disorder patients and that they are causally related to the development of this disorder. *Third*, even if one can identify a particular family factor as having played a specific role in the development of the eating disorder, it does not automatically imply that an alteration of this factor — if this were possible — would be necessary for a beneficial change of the eating disorder itself.

The latter issue applies in particular to the conclusion of long-term follow-up studies with respect to the prognostic significance of certain family features: a "disturbed" parent-child relationship was found to be associated with poor outcome of anorexia nervosa (Herzog, Rathner, & Vandereycken, 1992; Steinhausen, Rauss-Mason, & Seidel, 1991). Should one interpret this finding as an argument in favor of family therapy? The disturbed family interaction might have been a sign or epiphenomenon of the severity of the eating disorder itself, indicating that the family was not able to cope with a serious or disruptive disorder such as anorexia nervosa. In this case family therapy is coming "too late" or its impact can only be limited. Similarly, should we suppose the disturbed relationship was an important causal factor, then we might assume that the "damage" is irreparable or the interaction "untreatable". In that case, the best therapeutic measure might be to separate the patient from the family as a form of tertiary prevention.

We will now try to judge the value of family therapy in eating disorders by referring to two sources of information: the opinions of clinicians and patients, and the existing research data.

## 3 Opinions on the Use of Family Therapy

In 1978, a survey on the opinions and practices of British physicians with respect to anorexia nervosa patients showed that 48% of the responding psychiatrists (N = 60) had often used family therapy in these cases, usually combined with individual psychotherapy (Bhanji, 1979). In a similar survey in 1980, US-American psychiatrists (N = 90) and psychologists (N = 94) responded that family therapy was their preferred treatment for anorexia nervosa (very often in combination with individual psychotherapy) in respectively 94% and 87% of the respondents (Whyte & Kaczkowski, 1983). Participants of the 1988 and 1990 International Conference on Eating Disorders in New York were asked to complete a questionnaire on which type of treatment they endorsed in their most recent case of anorexia nervosa or bulimia nervosa. The responding physicians (N = 125; the majority probably being psychiatrists) and psychologists (N = 99) answered that they preferred or had prescribed a form of family therapy in about 60% of the cases of restricting anorexics versus 45% in bingeing anorexics and 26% in patients with bulimia nervosa. Family therapy was practically always combined with some form of individual psychotherapy or group therapy (Herzog, Keller, Strober, Yeh , & Pai, 1992).

Because of the many differences in the samples surveyed in these three studies, a comparison of the results should be made with great caution. Moreover, the form and content of what was meant by "family therapy" probably varied considerably within and between the samples surveyed. Nevertheless, an interesting trend emerges from these figures. At the end of the 1980s, about 90% of the American clinicians treating anorexia nervosa were endorsing the use of family therapy. A decade later its popularity dropped to about half of this percentage, and a distinction is made according to the subtype of eating disorder: the more "bulimic" a patient, the less likely is family therapy the treatment of choice!

Due to mass media coverage, eating disorders have become more widely known to the general public. Lay people seem to hold elaborate and consensual beliefs about the nature of anorexia and/or bulimia nervosa. In a study on attitudes and knowledge about eating disorders, more than 50 % of US-American high school and college students rate "influence of family" as an important causal factor and family therapy as an effective treatment (Smith, Pruitt, McLaughlin Mann , & Thelen, 1986). In a more recent US-American study about lay theories of anorexia nervosa, respondents ascribed a causal role to family factors, but they do not consider the family to be important in the treatment (Furnham & Hume-Wright, 1992). However, a British study comparing the opinions of lay persons and eating disorder experts found that both groups look at family therapy as an important component in the management of eating disorders. Both groups were asked what they thought about the following statement: "The successful management of anorexia nervosa in the future will depend on more effective forms of family therapy". In general, the experts were quite unsure about this issue, whereas lay people were more inclined to agree with it (Slade, Butler, & Newton, 1988).

Strikingly little attention has been paid to the opinions of the most important parties involved in family therapy: *the patients and the family members themselves*. To our knowledge, no systematic study has been carried out on this issue. An impression of the patients' opinions about family therapy can be made from the following five survey studies in which patients were asked to evaluate the therapies they had undergone.

1. In a US-American study, intensive interviewing of 25 recovered anorexics revealed that many perceived their problems as a function of their family's difficulties, but that only five received family therapy, which was usually valued rather positively. Many participants ascribed the ineffectiveness of their therapy to the lack of family involvement in treatment (Maine, 1985).

2. A study of the treatment experiences of Dutch anorexia nervosa patients (N = 78) in the mid 1980s showed that only a fifth of the patients had been in family therapy, an experience they evaluated as moderately positive (Noordenbos, 1989).

3. In a pilot study of 13 US-American women who considered themselves as being recovered from anorexia nervosa, all subjects attributed the eating disorder to "deeply engrained family conflicts and the roles played in the family". Only a third of the group had been exposed to family therapy, usually during inpatient treatment, and this experience received a very mixed review - from "invaluable" to "harmful" (Beresin, Gordon, & Herzog, 1989).

4. At least one year after discharge from the inpatient program at the Eating Disorder Center of Toronto General Hospital, patients (N = 47) were asked to evaluate the treatment. Although family therapy received a slightly positive

satisfaction score, on the average its rating was clearly lower than all other forms of therapy (Kennedy & Garfinkel, 1989).

5.  At the time of discharge from an inpatient treatment program for eating disorders at St. Luke's Medical Center in Phoenix (Arizona), 28 patients completed an anonymous opinion survey. The treatment components focusing on the family ("family education", "multiple family group therapy") were on the average rated as "somewhat helpful", although 25% of the patients considered it "least helpful" (Lemberg & May, 1991).

Regardless of the scarcity of specific data and the lack of comparability between these surveys, the least one can say is that family therapy seems to evoke very divergent reactions in the patients concerned. Unfortunately, we do not know the opinions of other family members, parents in particular.

## 4  Testing the Outcome of Family Therapy

Instead of relying on clinical opinions and therapists' preferences, the application of family therapy should be evaluated on the basis of well-designed research. The frequently-cited outcome study of Minuchin and coworkers (1978) focused on the effect of structural family therapy in anorexia nervosa. They studied 53 restricting anorexics after an average of five months treatment (predominantly outpatient family therapy), and after a follow-up period ranging from 1.5 to 7 years (80% of the sample was followed-up after at least two years). The outcome criteria included both the medical aspects of anorexia nervosa (mainly weight restoration) and psychosocial functioning in relation to home, school, and peers. The results after treatment and at follow-up revealed that 86% of the cases were considered to be "recovered". This unusually high success rate should be regarded, however, with great caution (Vandereycken, Kog, & Vanderlinden, 1989). *First*, a selected bias existed in the patient sample of this study: it concerned young adolescents, with a short duration of food restriction, and all coming from intact families. Each of these selection features have been shown to be prognostically favorable factors. *Second*, outcome evaluations were performed by members of the clinical team and not by neutral assessors. *Third*, no specific assessment of family functioning was carried out, which is a remarkable omission for a team emphasizing a family model. *Finally*, this study did not use a control group or comparison with another form of therapy.

Another research project involving family therapy was carried out at St. George's Hospital in London. In the first part of the project (Hall & Crisp, 1987), 30 single, female outpatients aged 13-27 with anorexia nervosa (mean duration of 27 months) were randomly allocated to either twelve sessions of dietary advice or twelve sessions of combined individual and family psychotherapy. At one year follow-up, both groups showed significant overall improvement, but with some differences. Four patients in the psychotherapy group were considered as being recovered and the remaining eleven patients attended the recommended further therapy. All fifteen patients of the dietary advice group were felt to require further treatment, but only eight followed this recommendation. From these findings it is difficult, however, to evaluate the impact of family therapy because families were also seen occasionally in the dietary advice group, and a mixture of family and individual therapy was used in the other group.

In a subsequent and larger study at St. George's (Crisp, Norton, Gowers, Halek, Bowyer, Yeldham, Levett , & Bhat, 1991), 90 female anorexia nervosa patients (mean age 22 years, mean length of illness 39 months) were randomly allocated to one of the four options: (1) inpatient treatment, (2) outpatient individual and family psychotherapy plus separate dietary counseling, (3) outpatient group psychotherapy (patients and parents in separate groups), (4) no further treatment. All three treatment regimes were significantly effective at one year in terms of weight gain, return of menstruation, and aspects of social and sexual adjustment. Again, the combination of treatment forms in this study does not allow judgment of the differential effect of family interventions. In our own investigation of the influence of a family-oriented inpatient treatment program, we were faced with a similar problem (Vanderlinden & Vandereycken, 1987).

Up to now the best controlled study of family therapy in eating disorders was carried out at the Institute of Psychiatry in London (Russell, Szmukler, Dare , & Eisler, 1987). After inpatient treatment (average duration 10.4 weeks), 80 eating disorder patients (57 anorexics, 23 bulimics; 7 males; mean age 17.9 years; mean length of illness 3.8 years) were randomly allocated for further outpatient treatment to a series of one hour sessions during one year of either family therapy or individual supportive therapy. At the end of the treatment, i.e., one year after discharge from the hospital, the outcome was in general poorer in bulimia nervosa patients. For anorexia nervosa, outcome differed according to the age of onset (more or less than 18 years) and the duration of illness (more or less than 3 years).

Family therapy was found to be more effective than individual therapy in younger, non-chronic patients. Older patients tended to respond better to individual therapy.

A most interesting part of this research project is the analysis of the considerable number of drop-outs: 15 out of 41 family therapy patients, and 13 of 39 individual therapy patients. Again, an age factor seemed to be related to the premature termination of treatment: patients over 18 years of age more often tended to remain engaged in individual therapy, whereas among younger patients family therapy appeared to be the more acceptable treatment. An important finding was that high levels of "*Expressed Emotion*" (EE), especially critical comments, in the mothers were associated with dropping out of family therapy - an association that was more pronounced in bulimia nervosa. If the predictive ability of EE is as good as it was found to be for relapse in schizophrenia, it may be a most valuable finding, and even more so should the critical attitude of parents be amenable to change through directed therapeutic interventions (Szmukler, Eisler, Russell, & Dare, 1985).

The same group of researchers undertook a second study evaluating two forms of outpatient family therapy for families with an anorexic child. The classic form of conjoint family therapy, in which the therapist sees the entire family together in the treatment sessions, was compared to *family counseling*, in which the therapist sees the parents together and advices them about the best way to manage their child's eating problem. In the latter case, the same therapist also sees the patient in individual sessions to provide support and counseling. We currently only have data from a pilot study (Le Grange, Eisler, Dare, & Russell, 1992) that included 18 anorexia nervosa patients (16 girls and 2 boys; mean age 15.3 years; mean duration of illness 13.7 months). Over a period of six months, the patients and families received an average of 8.6 sessions of family therapy as compared to a mean of 9.3 sessions in the family counseling group. At the 32 week assessment, both treatment forms appeared to bring about similar improvements in symptomatic and psychosocial functioning.

Because their previous study showed EE to be related to drop-out from treatment, the researchers now paid special attention to this issue (Le Grange, Eisler, Dare, & Hodes, 1992). It was found that parental criticism, if present at the beginning of therapy, rendered the treatment less effective when evaluated after six months. Moreover, if the anorexia nervosa had not improved at this point, family criticism was likely to have increased in comparison with the initial assessment. This emphasizes once more the importance of a treatment strategy being capable of tackling high levels of intrafamilial criticism and dissatisfaction. Although the results of this investigation are still preliminary (small groups, no follow-up data), it showed that conjoint family therapy may be too confrontational in some cases and carry the risk of negative influence on family interactions!

## 5  A Pragmatic, Eclectic Viewpoint

The question of in which cases family therapy may be indicated in patients with eating disorders is a misleading one, because family therapy can have many different meanings in form and content. This might, for instance, explain the divergent opinions on the usefulness of family therapy as perceived by the patients. Nevertheless, the absence of a clearly positive judgment and of unequivocal research findings can be seen as arguments for a nuanced and cautious evaluation. In this respect we propose the following situations as *relative contra-indications* for conjoint family therapy:

* When the parents are divorced or separated, otherwise one might reinforce the idea of re-uniting the family (a fantasy or wish often found in anorexics).

* When a parent displays severe psychopathology (e.g. manic depressive psychosis), necessitating some protection of the parent's individual vulnerability.

* When a parent has physically and/or sexually abused the partner or a child - a situation that demands protection of the victim and avoidance of loyalty dilemmas.

* When family interactions are highly negative or destructive, increasing the risk that direct confrontations in the presence of an "important other" (the therapist) might lead to more disruption.

Of course, the previous situations do not exclude the use of family therapy if it is conducted by experienced therapists and/or counterbalanced by other therapeutic measures. In fact, in most specialized centers for the treatment of eating disorders, family therapy is seen as just one component in a multidimensional approach (Vandereycken, Kog, & Vanderlinden, 1989). As such, the issue of family therapy is probably much more a question of therapeutic attitude than of therapeutic technique. We, therefore, plead for a *constructive and flexible family approach* to eating disorders. Its concrete form may range from parent counseling groups to classical family therapy, from some informal meetings to marital therapy of the parents, depending on the functional analysis of the eating disorder within the family context and the willingness of family members to engage in therapy.

More important than the therapeutic methods are the following principles or guidelines of a family-oriented approach (Vandereycken, 1987; Vanderlinden & Vandereycken, 1991):

* A family *crisis* does not mean family pathology; start from the assumption that the parents did their best, but were lacking essential problem-solving capacities.

* All kinds of family problems or disturbed interactions can be both *cause and consequence* of the eating disorder; hence, consider the patient to be at the same time "victim" and "architect" of the situation.

* Do not consider parents to be "guilty" but *co-responsible* for the development of the eating disorder, implying that their cooperation is quite valuable in the treatment.

* Involve brothers and sisters in the treatment, not just because they may be neglected "co-patients", but also because *siblings* can act as reliable "consultants" and excellent "co-therapists" (Vandereycken & Van Vreckem, 1992).

In adolescent anorexics or bulimics, the most difficult, if not critical, point in the course of the treatment arises when one attempts to deal with the separation-individuation issue, which practically always lies at the heart of the eating disorder. In a sense, one may look at anorexia or bulimia nervosa as a maladaptive reaction to, or an escape from, a critical phase in the evolving family life cycle. The fact that the eating disorder itself can be the stagnating factor in the developmental process of the adolescent implies indirectly that it hampers the healthy evolution in the family life cycle. Hence, the treatment of an anorexic or bulimic adolescent cannot but affect the family in one sense or another. Often the parents fear the "loss" of their child, while overlooking that they already have "lost" contact due to the disorder. The inevitable crisis during therapy will be overcome when everyone realizes that at the end of treatment all parties involved will gain from it.

## References

Beresin, E.V., Gordon, C., & Herzog, D.B. (1989). The process of recovering from anorexia nervosa. *Journal of the American Academy of Psychoanalysis, 17*, 103-130.
Bhanji, S. (1979). Anorexia nervosa: Physicians' and psychiatrists' opinions and practices. *Journal of Psychosomatic Research, 23*, 7-11.
Crisp, A.H., Norton, K., Gowers, S., Halek, C., Bowyer, C., Yeldham, D., Levett, G., & Bhat, A. (1991). A controlled study of the effect of therapies aimed at adolescent and family psychopathology in anorexia nervosa. *British Journal of Psychiatry, 159*, 325-333.
Furnham, A., & Hume-Wright, A. (1992). Lay theories of anorexia nervosa. *Journal of Clinical Psychology, 48*, 20-36.
Hall, A., & Crisp, A.H. (1987). Brief psychotherapy in the treatment of anorexia nervosa: Outcome at one year. *British Journal of Psychiatry, 151*, 185-191.
Herzog, D.B., Keller, M.B., Strober, M., Yeh, C., & Pai, S.Y. (1992). The current status of treatment for anorexia nervosa and bulimia nervosa. *International Journal of Eating Disorders, 12*, 215-220.
Herzog, W., Rathner, G., & Vandereycken, W. (1992). Long-term course of anorexia nervosa: A review of the literature. In W. Herzog, H.C. Deter & W. Vandereycken (Eds.), *The course of eating disorders* (pp. 15-29). Berlin-New York: Springer Verlag.
Kennedy, S.H., & Garfinkel, P.E. (1989). Patients admitted to hospital with anorexia nervosa and bulimia nervosa: Psychopathology, weight gain, and attitudes toward treatment. *International Journal of Eating Disorders, 8*, 181-190.
Le Grange, D., Eisler, I., Dare, C., & Hodes, M. (1992). Family criticism and self-starvation: A study of expressed emotion. *Journal of Family Therapy, 14*, 177-192.
Le Grange, D., Eisler, I., Dare, C., & Russell, G.F.M. (1992). Evaluation of family treatments in adolescent anorexia nervosa: A pilot study. *International Journal of Eating Disorders, 12*, 347-357.
Lemberg, R., & May, M. (1991). What works in in-patient treatment of eating disorders: The patient's point of view. *British Review of Bulimia and Anorexia Nervosa, 5*, 29-38.
Maine, M. (1985). Effective treatment of anorexia nervosa: The recovered patient's view. *Transactional Analysis Journal, 15*, 48-54.
Minuchin, S., Rosman, B., & Baker, L. (1978). *Psychosomatic families: Anorexia nervosa in context*. Cambridge, MA: Harvard University Press.
Noordenbos, G. (1989). Improving the process of recovery of patients with anorexia nervosa. *British Review of Bulimia and Anorexia Nervosa, 4*, 17-32.
Russell, G.F.M., Szmukler, G.I., Dare, C., & Eisler, I. (1987). An evaluation of family therapy in anorexia nervosa and bulimia nervosa. *Archives of General Psychiatry, 44*, 1047-1056.
Selvini-Palazzoli, M. (1974). *Self-starvation: From the intrapsychic to the transpersonal approach to anorexia nervosa*. London: Human Context Books/Chaucer. American edition: *Self-starvation: From individual to family therapy in the treatment of anorexia nervosa*. New York: Jason Aronson, 1978.
Slade, P., Butler, N., & Newton, T. (1988). Attitudes towards anorexia nervosa and bulimic disorders: Expert versus lay opinion. In D. Hardoff & E. Chigier (Eds.), *Eating disorders in adolescents and young adults* (pp. 1-13). London: Freund Publishers.
Smith, M.C., Pruitt, J.A., McLaughlin Mann, L., & Thelen, M.H. (1986). Attitudes and knowledge regarding bulimia and anorexia nervosa. *International Journal of Eating Disorders, 5*, 545-553.
Steinhausen, H.C., Rauss-Mason, C., & Seidel, R. (1991). Follow-up studies of anorexia nervosa: A review of four decades of outcome research. *Psychological Medicine, 21*, 447-454.
Szmukler, G.I., Eisler, I., Russell, G.F.M., & Dare, C. (1985). Anorexia nervosa, parental "expressed emotion" and dropping out of treatment. *British Journal of Psychiatry, 147*, 265-271.
Vandereycken, W. (1987). The constructive family approach to eating disorders: Critical remarks on the use of family therapy in anorexia nervosa and bulimia. *International Journal of Eating Disorders, 6*, 455-467.
Vandereycken, W., Kog, E., & Vanderlinden, J. (1989). *The family approach to eating disorders: Assessment and treatment of anorexia nervosa and bulimia*. Costa Mesa, (CA)-London: PMA Publishing.

Vandereycken, W., & Van Vreckem, E. (1992). Siblings as co-patients and co-therapists in the treatment of eating disorders. In F. Boer & J. Dunn (Eds.), *Children's sibling relationships: Developmental and clinical issues* (pp. 109-123). Hillsdale (NJ): Lawrence Erlbaum Associates.

Vanderlinden, J., & Vandereycken, W. (1987). The effect of a residential treatment program on eating disorder patients and their families. In W. Huber (Ed.), *Progress in psychotherapy research* (pp. 407-420). Louvain-la-Neuve: Presses Universitaires de Louvain.

Vanderlinden, J., & Vandereycken, W. (1991). Guidelines for the family therapeutic approach to eating disorders. *Psychotherapy and Psychosomatics, 56,* 36-42.

Whyte, B.L., & Kaczkowski, H. (1983). Anorexia nervosa: A study of psychiatrists' and psychologists' opinions and practices. *International Journal of Eating Disorders, 2(3),* 87-92.

# Part IV

# Course and Outcome

# Comparative Studies on the Course of Eating Disorders in Adolescents and Adults. Is Age at Onset a Predictor of Outcome?

*Manfred M. Fichter and Norbert Quadflieg*

## 1 Introduction

Over the past decades quite a bit of data and knowledge has accumulated about the course of *anorexia nervosa* (see review by Steinhausen & Glanville, 1983; Steinhausen et al., 1991). The findings about age at onset of anorexia nervosa as a predictor are, however, inconclusive and contradictory. Whereas some earlier studies have concluded that early onset anorexia has a more favourable course than late onset anorexia, more recent studies have not confirmed this finding, and in a few other studies the contrary was reported. A methodological problem is that age is often confounded with other variables. In those samples early onset anorexics also have a shorter duration of illness (less chronicity), which appears to be a strong predictor for the course of illness. On the other hand, it could be argued that patients who develop a mental illness at an early age are more likely to have a chronic course, especially when additional environmental factors (familiy climate, etc.) are present in the history of a child or young adolescent with increased biological vulnerability.

In contrast to anorexia nervosa, there is very little literature about the course of *bulimia nervosa*. Some major studies on the course of bulimia nervosa have been published by Mitchell and Pyle (1992), Lacey et al. (1991), Herzog et al. (1991), Fallon et al. (1991) and Fichter et al. (1992). Few of these studies have commented on the association between age at onset and course of illness. In a study on outcome of anorexia nervosa and prognostic factors Ratnasuriya et al. (1991) found that after 20 years, patients with an onset at younger age had a better long-term prognosis. On the other hand, Swift (1982) has argued that the evidence that an onset before the age of 15 years is an indicator of good prognosis is inconclusive. Other authors, such as Bryant-Waugh et al. (1988), found that prepubertal onset was even associated with poor prognosis. However, Bryant-Waugh et al. defined early onset as onset before the age of eleven. Frequent *methodological problems* in studies addressing the issue of differential effects of age at onset on the course of an anorexic or bulimic eating disorder are a limited variation concerning age at presentation or age at onset in the samples assessed in each single study and a low sample size. Thus, in the sample studied by Ratnasuriya et al. (1991) there were only two patients who developed anorexia nervosa before their menarchy.

Recent *long-term follow-up* studies on *anorexia nervosa* over an intervall of ten or more years (Halmi, 1988; Theander, 1985; Ratnasuriya et al., 1991) showed further improvement in many patients but also high mortality rates. Willi et al. (1989) and Theander (1970, 1985) assessed anorexics treated as inpatients in a geographically circumscript area (in Switzerland and Sweden respectively). According to the 10-year follow-up of Willi et al., 11% were free of symptoms, 71% were improved, 14% were unchanged and in a bad health status, and one patient (4%) had died as a consequence of anorexia nervosa. The mortality rate by the end of 20 years of follow-up was 15% in the British study by Ratnasuriya et al. (1991). In the Swedish study by Theander (1985), which covered a course of 24 years, it was even a bit higher. On the other hand, fairly low longer-term mortality rates have been reported for young patients treated in child and adolescent psychiatry (Tolstrup et al., 1985; Steinhausen & Seidel, 1993). Do these findings imply that anorexia nervosa patients with early onset have a more favourable prognosis? Further data on the course of anorexia nervosa and other eating disorders have recently been published in a book edited by Herzog, Deter and Vandereycken (1992).

The age at onset of anorexia nervosa may vary considerably although most patients have the first episode before, during, or shortly after puberty. Although the authors of this chapter have personally never come across a case of very late onset that did not include a clear or abortive episode of anorexia nervosa during adolescence or young adulthood, a few such cases have been described in the literature. Hsu and Zimmer (1988) reported five cases with very late onset, one of which appeared to be the first onset; Rammell and Brown (1988) described another case of anorexia nervosa that revealed no previous evidence of an eating disorder before a post-menopausal onset. Recently, Gowers and Crisp (1990) described a case of an eighty-year-old woman who experienced a brief episode of anorexia nervosa at the age of 15 and a relapse of the eating disorder at the age of 80. On the other hand, onset of anorexia nervosa has been reported in young girls several years before puberty, but it is questionable whether such cases should be classified as anorexia nervosa.

Far fewer studies have been carried out concerning the *course* and characteristics of *bulimia nervosa*. One study in particular (Schmidt et al., 1992) proposed — in analogy to Alzheimer-type dementia and coronary heart disease — that an early onset of bulimia nervosa constitutes an indicator of unfavourable course. They compared 23 cases with early onset bulimia nervosa (< 15 years) and 23 matched cases with later onset bulimia (onset age 17 to 21 years). Although they found no differences over time concerning the eating symptomatology, early onset bulimics showed more acts of deliberate self-harm, a trend for more depression among their relatives, and inadequate parental control (whereas other indicators of intra-familial disturbance did not differ between the two groups).

Bulimia nervosa usually starts in adolescence or early adulthood; the peak age of onset is around age 18 (Mitchell et al., 1987). Other reports show that bulimia nervosa may also start at an earlier age (Remschmidt & Herpertz-Dahlmann, 1990). Maloney et al. (1989) and Collins (1991) have suggested that dieting and concerns about body shape and weight are increasingly affecting cohorts of younger children and adolescents. Because dieting has been shown to be associated with an increased risk for developing an eating disorder (Patton et al., 1990), these findings concerning dieting habits may have an impact on the age at onset of anorexia and bulimia nervosa in future years.

Even if carried out properly, longitudinal studies in eating disorders encounter many *methodological short comings*. First of all, almost all anorexia nervosa samples published are samples that consist of *treated* patients. The mechanisms of patient selection between studies can differ highly and the selection criteria are usually unknown. Further potential short comings of longitudinal studies include selective attrition over the course of the study, reliability and validity of the assessments, and problems in retrospective recall.

In the context of the contradictory findings concerning the relevance of early or late onset for the course of anorexia nervosa and the fact that only very little research has been conducted concerning the issue of early vs. late onset in bulimia nervosa, in the present chapter we review the literature on outcome of eating disorders in general and the prediction of outcome on the basis of age at onset in particular. Several reviews on the course of eating disorders exist (Steinhausen & Glanville, 1983; Steinhausen, Rauss-Mason, & Seidel, 1991; and Herzog, Keller, & Lavori, 1988). In order to obtain an understanding of more recent developments concerning research on the course of eating disorders, we have reviewed several studies not covered in these reviews. Most studies date from 1989 and later.

In addition, we have analyzed the data of the *"German Anorexia and Bulimia Nervosa Study" (GABS)* in order to address the issue of age at onset of the disease. The study is exceptional for several reasons: (a) A very large sample size of inpatients with eating disorders was studied, and (b) the patients were assessed four times over a six-year period with a high completion rate. The findings are, however, restricted to patients treated at age 16 or older. The present paper describes the two year course. The *German Anorexia and Bulimia Nervosa Study* is a longitudinal prospective study of 635 consecutively admitted eating disordered inpatients treated in the Roseneck Hospital for Behavioural Medicine, Prien (Germany) between May 1985 and June 1988. Only patients who, at admission, met DSM-IV criteria for a major eating disorder (American Psychiatric Association [APA], 1994) were included in the final analyses concerning outcome and course of anorexia and bulimia nervosa. Of the total sample, 102 female patients were diagnosed as having anorexia nervosa and 196 female patients as having bulimia nervosa (purging type).

For analysis of age at onset, patients were grouped according to whether onset occured at or before age 16 (early onset) or after age 16 (late onset). In bulimia nervosa patients, duration of illness did not differ between early and late onset. In anorectics the early onset group showed longer duration of illness.

## 2   Diagnosis

Although in most outcome studies an eating disorder diagnosis is stated, it is often less clear on what grounds the diagnosis was made. Many studies use their own diagnostic criteria for anorexia nervosa, generally based on some variation of the criterion "being underweight". In this regard, however, the Diagnostic and Statistical Manual, 3rd Edition (DSM-III, APA, 1980) and 3rd Revised Edition

(DSM-III-R, APA, 1987) have brought about marked changes. In their reviews Steinhausen et al. (1983, 1991) noted a trend towards the use of standardized criteria (usually Feighner et al., 1972). In more recent studies DSM-III or DSM-III-R clearly begin to dominate. Tables 1, 2, and 3 illuminate these problems of differing sample definitions.

The diagnosis of bulimia nervosa was first defined and described by Russell as late as 1979 and it was introduced into the DSM-criteria in 1980. Almost all studies on bulimia nervosa since then have used the relatively stringent criteria according to Russell or the DSM-III (APA, 1980) (Herzog, Keller, & Lavori, 1988). The development in the past two decades of operationalized diagnostic criteria is — among other things — helpful in increasing comparability in longitudinal outcome studies.

## 3  Psychiatric Comorbidity at the First Assessment During a Longitudinal Study

Only rarely are additional psychiatric disorders reported at first assessment in longitudinal studies on eating disorders. Even when data on comorbidity are reported, expressions like "depressive syndrome" or "psychotic symptoms" are frequently used and the severity of illness and diagnosis remain unclear. Similarily, the formulation "x percent had no comorbidity" is equivocal and does not specify which diagnoses were considered.

Taking into account the sparse information about psychiatric comorbidity at first assessment, mood disorders are clearly the most frequently reported comorbid diagnostic categories in eating disorders. The comorbidity of major depression in bulimia nervosa varied considerably between studies. Whereas Mitchell et al. (1991) reported a lifetime comorbidity rate of 34%, Fallon et al. (1991), using the SCID-Interview of DSM-III-R-diagnoses, found 73.9% of 52 female patients having a major depression in addition to the eating disorder. The assessment in this study was, however, retrospective. For anorexia nervosa, high rates of depression have been reported, too. In the more recent studies concerning anorexia nervosa, little information on comorbidity can be found.

Another comorbid disorder that is frequent in bulimia nervosa is substance abuse. Fallon et al. (1991) reported 30.4% alcohol abuse, Mitchell et al. (1989) 10%

lifetime alcohol/drug abuse, and Swift et al. (1987) reported 37% lifetime drug abuse and 20% alcohol abuse in bulimia nervosa patients.

Information on comorbid anxiety disorders as well as personality disorders is scarce. Suicide attempts (lifetime) have been found in 34.8% (Fallon et al., 1991) and 30% (Swift et al., 1987) of bulimia nervosa patients.

In the *German Anorexia and Bulimia Nervosa Study (GABS)*, on admission we found a rate of 23% for affective disorders (clinical diagnoses according to DSM-III) in female patients with bulimia nervosa (purging type) and a rate of about 10% in patients with anorexia nervosa. Dysthymia (DSM-III: 300.40) was by far the most frequent depressive disturbance. Substance abuse was found in 11.2% of purging bulimia nervosa and in 5.3% to 6.5% of anorexia nervosa. Personality disorders were quite frequent in purging bulimia nervosa female patients as well as in bulimic-type anorexia nervosa patients (21.1%). In contrast, restricting anorexia nervosa patients had a lower rate of personality disorders (8.7%) than bulimics. The rate of anxiety disorders in bulimia nervosa was 3.6%; in bulimic anorexia nervosa the rate was 12.3%; in anorexia nervosa without full bulimia nervosa it was 18.4% and in restricting anorexia nervosa it was 4.3%. Comorbidity rates in the *German Anorexia and Bulimia Nervosa Study (GABS)* were not different between patients with an early onset eating disorder (before or at age 16) and patients with a late onset eating disorder (onset after age 16). Anxiety disorders appeared to be more pronounced in bulimia nervosa patients with an early onset.

Generally, eating disordered patients showed relatively high rates of psychiatric comorbidity (especially affective disorders and personality disorders in bulimia nervosa). Data indicate lower comorbidity rates of anxiety disorders and personality disorders in restricting as compared to bulimic anorexia nervosa patients. Age at onset appeared of little relevance concerning comorbidity.

## 4 Treatment

Information about duration and type of treatment for more recent studies are listed in Tables 1 (anorexia nervosa), 2 (bulimia nervosa), and 3 (combined studies).

Table 1. Characteristics of Outcome Studies of Anorexia Nervosa

| First author (year) | Med./Psych. services for[x] | Design Retro-(R)/Prospective (P) | N | Sex F=female M=male | Age at first assessment (yrs) Range | Age at first assessment Mean ±SD | Age at onset Range | Age at onset Mean ±SD | Diagnosis | Diagnost. criteria | Type of therapy | N | In-(I)/Outpatient (O) treatment I/O | Duration of therapy in weeks |
|---|---|---|---|---|---|---|---|---|---|---|---|---|---|---|
| Arroyo 1985 | C | R | 27 / 1 | F / M | | 15[a] / 17.5[a] | | 14* / 16** | AN | part. DSM-III | n.r | 20 / 8 | I / O | n.r. |
| Calvo 1989 | A | R | 40 / 1 | F / M | | 18.6 ±5 | 11-25 | 15.9±3 | AN | DSM-III | PT | 19 | I | 43-156 |
| Crisp 1992 | A | R | 105 / 63 | F / F | | 20.8±6 / 21.1[a] | | 16.8±4 / 19.1±5 | AN | DSM-III-R Crisp 1977 | PT/MT | unclear | I or O | n.r. |
| Deter 1989/92 | A | R | 91 / 12 | F / M | 12-48 | 20.8 ±6 | 12-38 | 18.0±5 | AN | DSM-III-R | PT | 86 | I | 12 |
| Greenfeld 1991 | A | R | 40 | F | 13-21 | 16.3 ±2 | | n.r. | AN | DSM-III-R | n.r. | | I | 9 |
| Halmi 1991 | A | R | 76 | F | 12-36 | 20.1 ±5 | | 17[b] | AN | DSM-III-R | PT/MT | | I | 5 |
| Higgs 1989 | C | R | 19 / 8 | F / M | | n.r. / n.r. | 8-16 | 12 | AN | Russell | MT | | I | n.r. |

Table 1. continued

| First author (year) | Med./ Psych. services for$^x$ | Design Retro-(R)/ Prospec- tive (P) | N | Sex F=female M=male | Age at first assess- ment (yrs) Range Mean ±SD | | Age at onset Range | Mean ±SD | Dia- gno- sis | Dia- gnost. criteria | Type of the- rapy | In- (I)/Out- patient (O) treatment N I/O | | Duration of therapy in weeks |
|---|---|---|---|---|---|---|---|---|---|---|---|---|---|---|
| Jenkins 1987 | C | P | 21 | F | | 15.0 ±1 | 12 -17 | 14.1±1 | AN | Weight | MT | I | | 27 |
| Kreipe 1989 | C | R | 62 | F | 9 -22 | 16.0 | n.r. | n.r. | AN | un- clear | PT /MT | un- clear | I or O | >2 |
| Ratnasuriya 1991 | A | R | 38 3 | F M | | 21.5 ±9 | | 18.0±7 | AN | Russell 1970 | PT | I | | 4-26 |
| Remschmidt 1990 | C | R | 99 4 | F M | | 14.5 | 9 -19 | 13.3 | AN | DSM -III ICD-9 Feighner | PT /MT | I | | 20 |
| Rosenvinge 1990 | — | R | 39 2 | F M | 15 -51 | 24.5 ±9 | | 21.5$^b$ | AN | DSM -III Feighner | n.r. | I | | n.r. |
| Santonas- taso 1991 | A | P | 49 1 | F M | | 20.9 ±8 | | 17.7±5 | AN | DSM -III | MT | I | | n.r. |
| Steiner 1990 | C | P | 41 | F/M | | 14.8 ±2 | | 13.0±2 | AN | DSM -III | PT | un- clear | I O | 6-70 |

Table 1 continued

| First author (year) | Med./ Psych. services for[x] | Design Retro-(R)/ Prospec- tive (P) | N | Sex F=female M=male | Age at first assess- ment (yrs) Range | Age at first assess- ment (yrs) Mean ±SD | Age at onset Range | Age at onset Mean ±SD | Dia- gno- sis | Dia- gnost. criteria | Type of the- rapy | In- (I)/Out- patient (O) treatment N I/O | Duration of therapy in weeks |
|---|---|---|---|---|---|---|---|---|---|---|---|---|---|
| Steinhausen 1992-94 | C | P | 57 3 | F M | 15.7 ±2 | | 12 -17 | 14.7 | AN/ BN[c] | Feighner ICD-10 | PT | I+O | 4-60 13.9 |
| Walford 1991 | C | R | 12 3 | F M | 9 -15 | 12.4 | 8 -14 | 11.9 | AN | Bryant- Waugh | PT | I | 6-65 18 (mean) |

- n.r = not reported
- AN = Anorexia nervosa, BN = Bulimia nervosa
- PT = Psychotherapy, MT = Medical Treatment
- * = restricters, ** = bulimics
- a = Computed from mean age at onset and mean duration of illness
- b = Computed from mean age at first assessment and mean duration of illness
- c = At follow-up 48 AN, 6 AN bulimic type, 5 BN, 1 partial AN
- x = Adults (A), Children (C)

Table 2. Characteristics of Outcome Studies of Bulimia Nervosa

| First author (year) | Design Retro-(R)/ Prospec- tive (P) | N | Sex F=female M=male | Age at first assess- ment (yrs) Range | Age at first assess- ment (yrs) Mean ± SD | Age at onset (yrs) Range | Age at onset (yrs) Mean ± SD | Dia- gno- sis | Dia- gnost. criteria | Type of the- rapy | In- (I)/Out- patient (O) treatment I/O | Duration of therapy in weeks |
|---|---|---|---|---|---|---|---|---|---|---|---|---|
| Abraham 1983 | R | 51 | | | 23[a] | | 17 ± 4 | BN | DSM -III | PT | O | n.r. |
| Baell 1992 | P | 21 | F | | 26.3 ± 6 | | 20.2[b] | BN | DSM -III-R | PT | O | 16 |
| Brotman 1988 | R | 14 | F | 19 -35 | 24.3 | | 20.8[b] | BN | DSM -III-R | PT /PhT | O | 13-260 |
| Johnson- Sabine 1992 Collings 1994 | P | 49 1 | F M | 14 -40 | 23.5 ± 5 | 10 -36 | 19.0 ± 4 | BN | Russell DSM-III | PhT | O | n.r. |
| Fahy 1993 | P | 43 | F | 18 -45 | 23.8 ± 5 | | 18.8 ± 2[c] 21.1 ± 6[d] | BN | DSM -III-R | PT /MT | O | 8 |
| Fairburn 1987/91/93 | P | 75 | F | | 24.2 | | 19.8[b] | BN | DSM -III-R 88 % | PT | O | 18 |

Table 2. continued

| First author (year) | Design Retro-(R)/ Prospec- tive (P) | N | Sex F=female M=male | Age at first assess- ment (yrs) Range | Age at first assess- ment (yrs) Mean ± SD | Age at onset (yrs) Range | Age at onset (yrs) Mean ± SD | Dia- gno- sis | Dia- gnost. criteria | Type of the- rapy | In- (I)/Out- patient (O) treatment I/O | Duration of therapy in weeks |
|---|---|---|---|---|---|---|---|---|---|---|---|---|
| Fallon 1991 | R | 52 | F | 17-50 | 24.4 ±7 | | 16.2[b] | BN | DSM -III-R | PT /PhT | I | n.r. |
| Herzog, 1988, 1991, 1993 | P | 47 | F | | 23.9 | | 18.9[b] | BN | DSM -III | PT /PhT | O | n.r. |
| Herzog/ Hartmann, 1991 | P | 42 | F | 17-35 | 23.7 ±3 | | 17.7[b] | BN | DSM -III-R | PT | O | 104 |
| Hsu 1986/89 | P | 56 | F | 16-36 | 26.6 ±5 | | 22.2[b] | BN | Russell | PT | O | 8-16 |
| Johnson 1990 | P | 55 | F | | 25 ±5 | | 16.7 | BN | DSM -III-R | PT | O | n.r. |
| Lacey 1992 | P | 250 | F | 16-40 | 24.8 ±5 | 13-33 | 20.3 | BN | DSM -III-(R) | PT | O | 10 |
| Maddocks 1992 | P | 86 | F | | 24.9 ±7 | | 17.3 ±5 | BN | DSM -III-R | PT | O | 11.4 (mean) |

Table 2. continued

| First author (year) | Design Retro-(R)/ Prospective (P) | N | Sex F=female M=male | Age at first assessment (yrs) Range | Age at first assessment (yrs) Mean ±SD | Age at onset (yrs) Range | Age at onset (yrs) Mean ±SD | Diagnosis | Diagnost. criteria | Type of therapy | In- (I)/Out-patient (O) treatment I/O | Duration of therapy in weeks |
|---|---|---|---|---|---|---|---|---|---|---|---|---|
| Mitchell 1989 | P | 100 | F | 17-44 | 22 (med.) | 11-27 | 17 (med.) | BN | DSM-III-(R) | PT | O | 10 |
| Norman 1986 | R | 27 | F | 19-48 | 28.0 | | 21.4[b] | BN | DSM-III | PT/PhT | O | n.r. |
| Pope/Hudson 1985 | P | 20 | F | 17-43 | 28.7 | | 21.2[b] | BN | DSM-III | PhT | O | 6 |
| Pyle 1990 | P | 68 | F | 18-40 | n.r. | | n.r. | BN | DSM-III | PT/PhT | O | 12 |
| Swift 1987 | R | 38 | F | 14-25 | 19.3 | | 16.4[b] | BN | DSM-III | PT | I | 3.5 (mean) |

- n.r. = not reported
- BN = Bulimia nervosa
- PT = Psychotherapy, PhT = Pharmacotherapy, MT = Medical Treatment
- med. = median
- a = Computed from mean age at follow-up and mean follow-up interval
- b = Computed from mean age at first assessment and mean duration of illness
- c = Good outcome group
- d = Poor outcome group

Table 3. Characteristics of Outcome Studies of Mixed Groups of Anorexia and Bulimia Nervosa

| First author (year) | Design Retro-(R)/ Prospec-tive (P) | N | Sex F=female M=male | Age at first assess-ment (yrs) Mean ± SD | Age at onset (yrs) Mean ± SD | Dia-gno-sis | Dia-gnost. criteria rapy | Type of the-rapy | In- (I)/Out-patient (O) treatment | Duration of therapy in weeks |
|---|---|---|---|---|---|---|---|---|---|---|
| Fichter (GABS) | | | | | | | | | I/O | |
| early onset = before or at age 16 | P | 96 | F | 22.9±4 | 14.4±2 | BN pur-ging type early onset | DSM-IV | PT /PhT | I | 14.4 |
| late onset = after age 16 | | 100 | F | 28.2±8 | 20.6±5 | BN pur-ging type late onset | | | | 12.8 |
| | | 52 | F | 22.0±5 | 1.4±2 | AN early onset | | | | 17.1 |
| | | 50 | F | 27.9±7 | 22.8±7 | AN late onset | | | | 17.0 |
| Herzog/Sacks 1993 | P | 41 | F | 24.9±6 | 19.2±6 | AN | DSM-III-R | n.r. | n.r. | n.r. |
| | | 98 | F | 22.8±7 | 18.8±4 | BN | | | | |
| | | 90 | F | 26.1±7 | 17.5±5 | AN+BN | | | | |
| Vandereycken 1992 | R | 92 Σ309 F 115 Σ 6 M | | 20.1±6 23.8±6 | 16.6[a] 18.4[a] | AN rest. AN bul. | DSM-III-R | PT | I/O | up to 26 |
| | | 78 | | 23.7±5 | 17.3[a] | BN | | | | |
| | | 30 | | 25.8±8 | 21.0[a] | EDNOS | | | | |

n.r. = not reported; AN= Anorexia nervosa, BN = Bulimia nervosa, EDNOS = Eating Disorder Not Otherwise Specified restr.= restrictors, bul. = bulimics; PT= Psychotherapy, PhT = Pharmacotherapy;
a= Computed from mean age at first assessment and mean duration of illness

In most studies patients received some kind of psychotherapy. Several striking differences between studies of anorexia nervosa and studies of bulimia nervosa can be derived from Tables 1 to 3:

1) While there are many reports on the treatment of anorexia nervosa in general, quite a few studies on the course of anorexia nervosa give very little information about the type of therapy (e.g., somatic treatment, psychotherapy) and details of the therapy that the patients received.

2) It appears that inpatient treatment is more common in anorexia nervosa than in bulimia nervosa patients. This makes comparison of the duration of therapy difficult. Conclusive findings are not possible as information is not given in some of these studies. However, it seems that treatment of anorexia nervosa patients in hospitals specializing in child and adolescent psychiatry (Jenkins, 1987; Kreipe et al., 1989; Remschmidt et al., 1990; Steiner et al., 1990; Steinhausen & Seidel, 1992; 1993a, b;1994a, b; Walford & McCune, 1991) is of rather long duration.

Patients with early and late onset did not differ significantly from patients with late onset concerning the duration of inpatient treatment in the *German Anorexia and Bulimia Nervosa Study (GABS)*.

## 5  Methodological Issues of Longitudinal Research

The *length of the follow-up interval* differs greatly between longitudinal studies. Another source of variation in reported outcome is the length of individual follow-up intervals within the same study, amounting to an extreme of follow-up intervals ranging between 4 and 43 years in one single study (Bassoe & Eskeland, 1982, cited in Herzog et al., 1988). However, the average duration of the follow-up interval is only of limited value. For example, the study of Fallon et al. (1991) gives a mean interval of 4 1/2 years, thus meeting Morgan and Russell's (1975) criteria of at least 4 years of follow-up. The individual follow-up period in the Fallon et al. study, however, varies from 2 years to 9 years.

In addition, *drop-out rates* vary considerably, amounting to as high as three-quarters of the original sample (Steinhausen & Glanville, 1983). In some studies the drop-out rate remains unclear because the original sample size has not been reported. In some studies like that of Maddocks et al. (1992) the sample itself was defined retrospectively. Of 86 females, for whom treatment was finished more than two years earlier, only 43 were actually eligible (based on retrospective report) for the follow-up. For purposes of evaluating outcome, this was considered the original sample. On the other hand, sample characteristics were given for all 86 patients in therapy. This example illustrates the problems of outcome studies arising from imprecise information. In the two-year follow-up of the *"German Anorexia and Bulimia Nervosa Study" (GABS)* only two bulimia nervosa patients dropped out. None of the anorexia nervosa patients dropped out. In follow-up, questionnaires as well as interview methods were used.

## 6 Outcome of Eating Disorder

Documentation of outcome varies considerably. Many studies of anorexia nervosa give detailed results concerning body weight or menstrual status. In many studies percentages of distinct eating-related behaviour — such as binging, dieting, or vomiting and laxative abuse — are given. Most studies derive a general score of outcome either by rating several scales comprising special areas of outcome (e.g., General Outcome Assessment Scale, Morgan & Russell, 1975) or by integrating this information into one outcome score (e.g., Psychiatric Status Rating Scale for Bulimia Nervosa [PSRSB], Herzog et al., 1990). Generally, the frequency of disturbed eating behaviours or the restrictions caused by eating symptoms are criteria for outcome categories. An alternative approach is the use of standardized self- or expert-rating scales (e.g., Eating Attitude Test [EAT], Garner & Garfinkel, 1979) with a sum score and cut-off scores for good or bad outcome.

In their review of 45 follow-up studies on the course of anorexia nervosa Steinhausen and Glanville (1983) conclude that "long-term improvements of 20 - 50% emerge from most follow-up reports ...". Steinhausen et al. (1991) see this conclusion confirmed in their up-date covering another 10 years of long-term studies. A similar pattern of results can be found in more recent studies summarized in Table 4. Herzog et al. (1988) include in their review some studies on bulimia nervosa; no deaths were reported in the reviewed studies on bulimia nervosa patients. As shown in Table 5, the mortality rate for bulimia (nervosa) in

Table 4. Results of Follow-up Studies of Anorexia Nervosa

| First author (year) | FU N | FU % | Dropout N | Dropout % | Mortality rate N | Mortality rate % | Interval in months range | Interval in months average | Method | Outcome good N | good % | intermed. N | intermed. % | poor N | poor % | Comorbidity |
|---|---|---|---|---|---|---|---|---|---|---|---|---|---|---|---|---|
| Arroyo 1985 | 25 | 89 | 2 | 7 | 1 | 4 | 3-70 | | Q | 0 | 0 | 14 | 56 | 11 | 44 | |
| Calvo 1989 | 35 | 85 | 6 | 15 | 0 | 0 | 60-108 | | I | 27 | 77 | 2 | 5 | 6 | 17 | 8.6% Body shape delusions |
| Crisp 1992 | 97 | 92 | 4 | 4 | 4 | 4 | | 262 | Q,I | Mortality Study | | | | | | |
| | 53 | 84 | 2 | 3 | 8 | 13 | | 265 | | | | | | | | |
| Deter 1989/92 | 86 | 83 | 1 | 1 | 16 | 16 | 108-228 | 151 | Q,I | 54 | 44 | 23 | 26 | 10 | 13 | 22% Pers.dis., 14% Subst. abuse, 12% Phobia, 8% Major depression |
| Greenfeld 1991 | 30 | 75 | 10 | 25 | 0 | 0 | 14-120 | 55 | I | 6 | 20 | 9 | 30 | 15 9 AN, 6 BN | 60 | 13 Major Depression, 6 Dysthymia, 11 anxiety dis., 4 Phobias, 3 obs.-comp. dis. |
| Halmi 1991 | 71 | 93 | 0 | 0 | 5 | 7 | 96-120 | 115 | I | 18 | 24 | 44 | 58 | 9 | 12 | |
| Higgs 1989 | 23 | 85 | 4 | 15 | 0 | 0 | 12-312 | 62 | I | 7 | 30 | 7 | 30 | 9 | 40 | |
| Jenkins 1987 | 21 | 100 | 0 | 0 | 0 | 0 | | 36 | Q,I | 10 | 48 | 4 | 19 | 5 | 24 | 1 Bipolar Dis., 1 BN |
| Kreipe 1989 | 49 | 79 | 12 | 19 | 1 | 2 | 48-150 | 80 | I | 27 | 55 | 15 | 31 | 7 | 14 | 41% health problems |
| Ratnasuriya 1991 | 34 | 83 | 0 | 0 | 7 | 17 | | 242 | Q,I | 12 | 30 | 13 | 32 | 15 incl. deaths | 37 | 3 alcohol abuse, 15 depressive |
| Remschmidt 1990 | 81 | 79 | 19 | 18 | 3 | 3 | | 141 | Q,I | 58 | 72 | 9 | 11 | 14 | 17 | 4 subst. abuse, 15 depressive sympt. |

Table 4. continued

| First author (year) | FU N | % | Dropout N | % | Mortality rate N | % | Interval in months range | average | Method | Outcome good N | % | intermed. N | % | poor N | % | Comorbidity |
|---|---|---|---|---|---|---|---|---|---|---|---|---|---|---|---|---|
| Rosenvinge 1990 | 30 | 73 | 7 | 17 | 4 | 10 | 72-324 | 172 | Q,I | 11 | 37 | 0 | 0 | 19 | 63 | 23% Major Depresion 13% Ob.-comp., 23% Borderline Pers.Dis 20% Histrionic Pers.Dis. 13% Passive-dep. Pers.Dis. |
| Santonastaso 1991 | 28 | 56 | 19 | 38 | 3 | 6 | | 91 | Q,I | 17 | 61 | 6 | 21 | 5 | 18 | 7 Major Depression, 1 Dysth., 4 Pers. Dis. |
| Steiner 1990 | 41 | 100 | 0 | 0 | 0 | 0 | 12-72 | 32 | Q,I | 15 | 37 | 14 | 34 | 12 | 29 | 10 Major Depression |
| Steinhausen 1992-94 | 50 | 83 | 6 | 10 | 4 | 7 | | 58 | Q,I | 34 | 68 | 9 | 18 | 7 | 14 | n.r. |
| Walford 1991 | 14 | 93 | 0 | 0 | 1 | 7 | 36-172 | 64 | notes, I | 10 | 71 | 3 | 21 | 1 | 8 | 1 Schizophr., 1 neurotic depression |

- Q = Questionnaire
- I = Interview
- AN = Anorexia nervosa, BN = Bulimia nervosa

Table 5. Results of Follow-up Studies of Bulimia Nervosa

| First author (year) | FU N | % | Dropout N | % | Mortality rate N | % | Interval in months range | average | Method | Outcome good N | % | intermed. N | % | poor N | % | Comorbidity |
|---|---|---|---|---|---|---|---|---|---|---|---|---|---|---|---|---|
| Abraham 1983 | 43 | 84 | 8 | 16 | 0 | 0 | 14 - 72 | | Q,I I only: | (29-40) 17 | 40 | (17-49) 13 | 31 | (21-55) 12 | 29 | |
| Baell 1992 | 20 | 95 | 1 | 5 | 0 | 0 | | 3 | Q | n.r. | | | | | | n.r. |
| Brotman 1988 | 14 | 100 | 0 | 0 | 0 | 0 | 12 - 60 | | Q | 8 | 57 | 4 | 28 | 2 | 14 | 2 depressed |
| Johnson-Sabine 1992/ Collings 1994 | 44 | 88 | 5 | 10 | 1 | 2 | 93-161 | 117 | Q,I | 23 | 52 | 13 | 30 | 8 | 18 | 12 Depressive dis., 1 Substance abuse, 1 Simple phobia |
| Fahy 1993 | 39 | 91 | 4 | 9 | 0 | 0 | | 12 | Q | 21 | 54 | | | 16 | 41 | |
| Fairburn 1987/ 1991/93 | 50 | 66 | 25 | 34 | 0 | 0 | | 12 | Q,I | 22 | 44 | | | | | |
| Fallon 1991 | 46 | 88 | 5 | 10 | 1 | 2 | 24-108 | 54 | Q,I | 18 | 39 | 9 | 20 | 19 | 41 | 1 AN |
| Herzog 1988, 1991, 1993 | 30 | 64 | 17 | 36 | 0 | 0 | 6 - 18 | | I | 17 | 57 | 0 | 0 | 13 | 43 | 10 of 17 recovered from aff. disorder |
| Herzog/Hartmann 1991 | 42 | 100 | 0 | 0 | 0 | 0 | | 12 | Q | marked improvement | | | | | | |
| Hsu 1986/89 | 35 | 63 | 21 | 37 | 0 | 0 | 48 - 72 | | I | 21 | 60 | 0 | 0 | 14 | 40 | 7 Maj. Depr., 8 Dysthymia |
| Johnson 1990 | 40 | 73 | 15 | 27 | 0 | 0 | | 12 | Q | 11 | 28 | 18 | 44 | 11 | 28 | |

Table 5. continued

| First author (year) | FU N | FU % | Dropout N | Dropout % | Mortality rate N | Mortality rate % | Interval in months range | Interval in months average | Method | Outcome good N | Outcome good % | intermed. N | intermed. % | poor N | poor % | Comorbidity |
|---|---|---|---|---|---|---|---|---|---|---|---|---|---|---|---|---|
| Lacey 1992 | 232 | 93 | 18 | 7 | 0 | 0 | | 18 | Q,I | 161 | 63 | 60 | 24 | | 5 | |
| Maddocks 1992 | 35 | 81 | 7 | 16 | 1 | 3a | | 24 | Q | 16 | 46 | 9 | 26 | 10 | 28 | |
| Mitchell 1989 | 91 | 91 | 8 | 8 | 1 | 1 | 20 - 60 | 42 | I | 60 | 66 | 8 | 9 | 23 | 25 | |
| Norman 1986 | 18 | 66 | 9 | 34 | 0 | 0 | 34 - 36 | | Q | about 50 % improved | | | | | | |
| Pope/Hudson 1985 | 20 | 100 | 0 | 0 | 0 | 0 | 2 - 28 | | I | 10 | 50 | 9 | 45 | 1 | 5 | |
| Pyle 1990 | 61 | 91 | 6 | 9 | 0 | 0 | | 6 | I | 31 | 51 | 8 | 13 | 22 | 36 | |
| Swift 1987 | 30 | 79 | 8 | 21 | 0 | 0 | 25 - 50 | 40 | Q,I | 8 | 27 | 12 | 40 | 10 | 33 | |

[a] „eligible for follow-up" N = 43
– Q = Questionnaire
– I = Interview

Table 6. Results of Follow-up Studies of Mixed Groups of Anorexia and Bulimia Nervosa

| First author (year) | FU N | % | Dropout N | % | Mortality rate N | % | Interval in months: average | Method | Outcome good N | % | intermed. N | % | poor N | % | Comorbidity |
|---|---|---|---|---|---|---|---|---|---|---|---|---|---|---|---|
| Fichter (GABS) 1993 | 96 | 100 | 0 | 0 | 0 | 0 | 24 | Q,I | 21 | 22 | 36 | 38 | 37 | 39 | 37 % Affective Dis. 11 % Anxiety Dis. 26 % Substance Abuse 5 % Borderline Pers. Dis. |
|  | 98 | 98 | 2 | 2 | 0 | 0 | 24 |  | 26 | 28 | 28 | 30 | 40 | 43 | 23 % Affective Dis. 15 % Anxiety Dis. 22 % Substance Abuse, 5 % Borderline Pers. Dis. |
|  | 49 | 94 | 0 | 0 | 3 | 6 | 29 |  | 6 | 12 | 12 | 25 | 31 | 63 | 37 % Affective Dis. 17 % Anxiety Dis. 37 % Substance Abuse 12 % Borderline Pers. Dis. |
|  | 48 | 96 | 0 | 0 | 2 | 4 | 31 |  | 14 | 29 | 15 | 31 | 19 | 40 | 28 % Affective Dis. 25 % Anxiety Dis., 19 % Substance Abuse 8 % Borderline Pers. Dis. |

Table 6. continued

| First author (year) | FU N | FU % | Dropout N | Dropout % | Mortality rate N | Mortality rate % | Interval months average | Method | Outcome good N | Outcome good % | intermed. N | intermed. % | poor N | poor % | Comorbidity |
|---|---|---|---|---|---|---|---|---|---|---|---|---|---|---|---|
| Herzog/Sacks 1993 | 41 | 100 | 0 | 0 | 0 | 0 | 12 | I | 4 | 10 | 13 | 32 | 24 | 58 | |
| | 96 | 98 | 2 | 2 | 0 | 0 | | | 53 | 56 | 15 | 16 | 28 | 28 | |
| | 88 | 98 | 2 | 2 | 0 | 0 | | | 16 | 18 | 36 | 41 | 36 | 41 | |
| Vandereycken 1992 | 61 | 66 | 31 | 34 | 0 | 0 | 60 | Q,I | 34 | 56 | 23 | 38 | 4 | 7 | |
| | 54 | 47 | 61 | 53 | 0 | 0 | | | 17 | 32 | 24 | 44 | 13 | 24 | |
| | 45 | 58 | 28 | 36 | 5 | 6 | | | 15 | 33 | 17 | 38 | 13 | 29 | |
| | 14 | 47 | 16 | 53 | 0 | 0 | | | 3 | 21 | 8 | 57 | 3 | 21 | |

– Q = Questionnaire
– I = Interview

more recent studies with longer follow-up intervals was lower than had been reported for anorexia nervosa. Only 3 deaths altogether were reported in 20 follow-up studies of bulimia nervosa. In the two year course of the *GABS* we did not observe any deaths in the bulimia nervosa sample (purging type). It seems that mortality over the course of time is higher in anorexia than in bulimia nervosa. In the GABS (Table 6), the general outcome was assessed at two-year follow-up by the Psychiatric Status Rating Scale for Bulimia nervosa (Herzog et al., 1990). In the bulimia nervosa (purging type) subsample 22.3% of the early onset group and 27.7% of the late onset group showed a good outcome, 38.3% and 29.8% (early and late onset, respectively) had an intermediate outcome, and 39.4% of the early onset group and 42.6% of the late onset group showed poor two-year outcome. The two-year outcome rates for patients treated for anorexia nervosa with early onset and those with late onset, respectively, are: (a) good outcome — 12.2% and 29.2%; (b) intermediate outcome — 24.5% and 31.3%; and (c) poor outcome — 63.3% and 39.6%.

At the two-year follow-up 1% of the *patients treated for bulimia nervosa* (purging type) with early onset had anorexia nervosa and 40.6% fulfilled the criteria for bulimia nervosa. At the two-year follow-up of those patients with late onset 1% had anorexia nervosa only, 1% had both anorexia nervosa and bulimia nervosa, 40.8% had bulimia nervosa only, and 4.1% had an eating disorder not otherwise specified (NOS). All diagnoses were made according to DSM-III-R. In the *patients treated for anorexia nervosa* the rates of DSM-III-R-diagnoses at the two-year follow-up were for early and late onset, respectively: 28.8% (early onset) and 18.0% (late onset) respectively met criteria for anorexia nervosa, 13.5% and 12.0% respectively had both anorexia nervosa and bulimia nervosa, 17.3% and 6.0% respectively had bulimia nervosa only, and 1.9% and 2.0% respectively had an eating disorder not otherwise specified (NOS). Several conclusions can be drawn from these data:

1) The two-year outcome appears to be worse for anorexia nervosa than for bulimia nervosa. Both groups had received intensive psychotherapy during the same time period and in the same hospital.

2) In anorexia nervosa, patients with early onset (before age 16) tended to have more severe eating disturbances over time than those with later onset.

3) Although patients with bulimia nervosa very seldom developed anorexia nervosa, a considerable proportion (18%) of the patients with anorexia nervosa had bulimia nervosa at the two-year follow-up. This occured more frequently in patients with early onset than in those with late onset. In the section on predictors, this issue will be discussed further.

## 7   Psychiatric Comorbidity of Eating Disorders at Follow-up

In most studies psychiatric comorbidity is better documented at follow-up; it is also better documented for anorexia than for bulimia nervosa (see Tables 4 and 5). In the *GABS*, affective disorders, anxiety disorders, personality disorders, and substance abuse were the most frequent concomitant disorders. In anorexia nervosa overall about one quarter of the patients showed major depression at two-year follow-up. The two other studies of bulimia nervosa giving information on comorbidity (Herzog et al., 1988; Hsu et al., 1986, 1989) confirm this rate for bulimia nervosa.

The documentation of comorbidity at follow-up in patients treated for bulimia nervosa is unsatisfactory. Few of the existing studies addressed this issue. From the data available there is no indication that early or late onset eating disorders differ with respect to psychiatric comorbidity. In the *GABS*, comorbidity at two-year follow-up was assessed according to the DSM-III-R for affective and anxiety disorders, substance abuse/dependence, and borderline personality disorder.

In patients treated for bulimia nervosa (purging type) 37.0% of those with early onset and 22.8% of those with late onset had an affective disorder at follow-up (chi$^2$ = 4.38; p < 0.05). Anxiety disorders were found in 10.9% and 15.2% (early and late onset, respectively). Alcohol or drug abuse occurred in 26.1% (early onset) of the former patients and 21.7% (late onset) and 5.4% in each group had a borderline personality disorder.

In the patients treated for anorexia nervosa, rates for affective disorders at follow-up were 37.5% and 27.8%; anxiety disorders were found in 17.5% and 25.0%, substance abuse in 37.5% and 19.4%, and a borderline personality disorder in 12.5% and 8.3% (early and late onset, respectively). Thus, affective disorders were more frequent in patients with an early onset of eating disorder (before or at age

16). In anorexia nervosa, early onset was associated with more substance abuse. This may be attributed to the longer duration of the illness in these patients.

## 8   Psychosocial Adaption

Results concerning psychosocial adaption and sexuality are very heterogeneous in published studies and clear-cut categories are frequently lacking. Apparently, the age at onset is not associated with the psychosocial adaptation at a later point of time. This negative finding may result from heterogeneous follow-up intervals within samples. In the GABS 39.3% and 32.6% of the bulimia nervosa patients and 55.6% and 47.5% of the anorexia nervosa patients were without a partner at the two-year follow-up (early and late onset, respectively).

## 9   Prognostic Factors

In studies on the course of eating disorders (mainly anorexia nervosa) a large number of predictors of the course and outcome has been evaluated. In the following, a brief summary of the relevance of prognostic factors will be given separately for anorexia and bulimia nervosa.

### 9.1   Prognostic Factors for Anorexia Nervosa

In their review Steinhausen et al. (1983, 1991) identified a longer duration of illness as a predictor of poor outcome of anorexia nervosa. This finding is supported by Herzog et al. (1988), as well as by several more recent studies (cf. Table 7). Steinhausen et al. also reported a good parent-child relationship to be a predictor of good outcome. This is supported by Herzog et al. (1988a), who found a disturbed parent-child relationship a predictor of negative outcome. Histrionic personality disorder, too, has been reported to predict a better outcome of eating disorder (Steinhausen et al., 1983, 1991).

The findings concerning the predictive value of duration of inpatient treatment, socioeconomic status, type of anorexia nervosa, and comorbidity are inconclusive. Duration of inpatient treatment and higher socioeconomic status have been reported as an indicator of better outcome in some but not in all other studies (cf.

Table 7. Predictor of Outcome of Anorexia Nervosa

| First author and year | Positive predictor | Negative predictor | No predictor |
|---|---|---|---|
| Arroyo 1985 Calvo 1989 Crisp 1992 Deter 1989/92 Greenfeld 1991 | - Comprehensive Treatment | - Duration of Illness, Low serum albumin - Greater height | - Social class, weight, age at onset serum phosphate, hemoglobin - Age at onset, weight, depression previous treatment |
| Halmi 1991 | | - Higher age at onset, alcohol abuse, vomiting, lax. abuse | |
| Higgs 1989 Jenkins 1987 Kreipe 1989 Ratnasuriya 1991 | - Earlier follow-up | - Vomiting, binge eating - Later age at onset, personality disorder, longer duration of illness | |
| Remschmidt 1990 | - Early age at onset (< 12.7 yrs.) | | - Weight loss, duration of illness previous treatment, duration of treatment, weight at discharge, IQ, social class, personality structure, length of FU-interval, artificial nourishment |
| Rosenvinge 1990 | - Histrionic Pers. Dis. | - Long duration of illness, sleeping difficulties, Borderline Pers. Dis., depression | |
| Santonastaso 1991 | | - Greater number of hospitalizations unsatisfactory school/work adjustment | - Social class, marital status, age at first menstruation, age at onset, duration of illness, duration of FU, weight loss, vomiting, bulimia, lax. abuse, family relationship, sexual relationship |
| Steiner 1990 Steinhausen 1992-94 | | - Depression, bulimia - Low body weight | - Age at onset, duration of illness duration of treatment, depression socioeconomic status |
| Walford 1991 | | | - Social class, weight, sex, duration of illness |

Steinhausen et al., 1983, 1991). The same is true for comorbidity (Herzog et al., 1988).

Results concerning the predictive value of the type of anorexia nervosa (restricting vs. nonrestricting) also appear to be inconclusive. There are, however, several studies that indicate that bulimic symptoms are associated with a poorer outcome (cf. Steinhausen et al., 1991; Herzog et al., 1988).

## 9.2 Prognostic Factors for Bulimia Nervosa

In a review of the limited literature on the issue, Herzog et al. (1988) concluded that a history of alcohol abuse, a history of suicide attempts, and depression were predictors of poor outcome in bulimia nervosa. Duration of illness, age at first presentation to a physician, past history of anorexia nervosa, and frequency of bulimic episodes were found to be unrelated to outcome of bulimia nervosa. These findings were partly confirmed by newer studies listed in Table 8. More recently, the presence of a borderline syndrome has been shown to be associated with a negative outcome.

In the GABS, psychiatric comorbidity emerged as a predictor for an unfavourable two year outcome. Scales measuring depression showed inconclusive results concerning their predictive value. Higher body weight at the beginning of inpatient treatment was found to be a predictor of positive outcome of the eating disturbance. No predictive value was found for the drive for thinness and laxative abuse (Fichter, Quadflieg, & Rief, 1992).

## 10 Does the Age at the Onset of the Eating Disorder Have a Predictive Value?

Tolstrup (1965) studied 24 female and 4 male patients over a follow-up period ranging from half a year to 12 years and found no essential differences in symptoms between the youngest and the oldest patients, nor were there any differences concerning the course of illness. Remschmidt et al. (1990) reported on the course of 103 anorexia nervosa inpatients treated in a department of child psychiatry. Reliable information was obtained on 81 living subjects, whereas three patients had died and for nineteen patients insufficient or no information was obtained. Predictors of unfavourable course of illness were premorbid eating disorder, late age at onset of the eating disorder, and some weight parameters during inpatient treatment. The finding of a positive association between a relatively low age at onset of the eating disorder and a good or at least intermediate outcome was in accordance with several earlier studies (Frazier, 1965; Theander, 1970; Halmi et al., 1973, 1976; Morgan & Russell, 1975; Willi & Hagemann, 1976; Sturzenberger et al., 1977; Hsu, Crisp, & Harding, 1979).

Steinhausen et al. (1991) analyzed 22 more recent studies on the course of anorexia nervosa and compared them to 45 follow-up studies published between 1953 and 1981. Concerning age at onset and course of illness they concluded that "three of the more recent studies (Steinhausen & Glanville, 1983; Hawley, 1985; Nussbaum et al., 1985) found age at onset to be insignificant with regard to outcome. Despite the considerable variation of data among the samples, there is, however, still some evidence — especially in the older studies — that an early onset of the disease is associated with favourable prognosis." According to Steinhausen and Glanville (1983, p. 246): "most workers associate an early onset (of anorexia nervosa) with a favourable prognosis (Lesser et al., 1960; Frazier, 1965; Theander, 1970; Halmi et al., 1973, 1976; Morgan & Russell, 1975; Pierloot et al., 1975; Willi & Hagemann, 1976; Sturzenberger et al., 1977; Hsu et al., 1979). A few authors (Tolstrup, 1965; Warren, 1968; Browning & Miller, 1968; Garfinkel et al., 1977), on the other hand, report no prognostic distinction between illnesses of early and of late onset. Seidensticker and Tzagournis (1968) regard an onset up to the age of 30 as prognostically favourable and Dally (1969) even claims that the prognosis of anorexia nervosa commencing before the age of 14 is unfavourable." Thus, there is some evidence for each hypothesis: age at onset predicts poor outcome; age at onset predicts good outcome; age at onset is no predictor at all.

This evaluation by Steinhausen and Glanville (1983) was later slightly revised by Steinhausen et al. (1991), and the predictive value of age at onset for poor outcome was not supported by studies of the eighties. This situation is well illustrated by Herzog et al. (1988 — see Table 8). The controversy continues, as Tables 7, 8, and 9 show. However, the direction of the association seems to indicate that early age at onset of anorexia nervosa is associated with positive outcome and later age at onset is associated with negative outcome (e.g., Crisp et al., 1977) — if age at onset is connected with outcome at all. In bulimia nervosa no predictive value can be attributed to age at onset (see Tables 8 and 9, Fairburn et al., 1987, 1991, 1993; Fallon et al., 1991; Herzog et al., 1993; and Fichter et al., 1992).

The relatively large samples of the GABS make it possible to study homogeneous diagnostic groups (anorexia nervosa, bulimia nervosa) and to subdivide the samples into groups with early and late onset, and to compare outcome between these groups at two-year follow-up. Psychiatric comorbidity rates at admission did not differ between early and late onset groups of anorexia nervosa and bulimia nervosa, as did the duration of inpatient therapy.

In a previous section we stated that poor outcome according to the PSRSB was more often found in anorexia nervosa patients with early onset. This is reflected in the means and standard deviations of the PSRSB scores (range from 1 (= "usual self") to 6 (= "severe AN") at follow-up. The average scores for bulimia nervosa were 3.74 (± 1.50) and 3.71 (± 1.56) and for anorexia nervosa 4.39 (± 1.35) and 3.65 (± 1.55) (early and late onset, respectively). The anorexia nervosa subgroups differed significantly from each other ($t = 2.51$; $p < 0.05$). In order to check possible interactions between diagnosis and age at onset, further analyses were conducted; these revealed no significant differences. The eating disorder diagnoses at follow-up did not differ between age at onset groups. Comorbidity rates at follow-up were the same in both of the age at onset groups, with the exception of affective disorders in bulimia nervosa patients, where early onset patients showed a higher rate than their later onset counterparts. Thus, our results question the hypothesis that in anorexia nervosa early onset is associated with a more favourable outcome (Steinhausen et al., 1991).

In a study on mortality Patton (1988) found about equal mortality rates in anorexia nervosa (3.3%) and bulimia nervosa (3.1%). Deter et al. (1989, 1992), Ratnasuriya et al. (1991) and Crisp et al. (1992) found mortality rates above 10% in anorexia nervosa in long-term follow-ups (cf. Table 4). Long-term studies on the 10 to 20 year course of bulimia nervosa have not yet been carried out. Shorter-term (two-year) results of the *GABS* point to higher mortality rates in anorexia as compared to bulimia nervosa.

Concerning age at onset and mortality, it seems that early onset is not a risk factor for death. Studies such as those by Remschmidt et al. (1990) and by Collings and King (1994) support this statement; so does the *GABS* for bulimia nervosa. For anorexia nervosa the *GABS* found late onset to be a predictor of positive outcome,

Table 8. Predictors of Outcome of Bulimia Nervosa

| First author and year | Positive predictor | Negative predictor | No predictor |
|---|---|---|---|
| Abraham 1983 | - Age at onset before age 16 | - Suicide attempts | - Duration of illness, age at presentation history of AN |
| Baell 1992 | | - Low self-esteem | - Duration of illness |
| Brotman 1988 | | | |
| Johnson-Sabine 1992/ Collings 1994 | - Younger age at onset higher social class family history of alcohol abuse | | - History of AN |
| Fahy 1993 | | - Personality disorder, longer duration of illness | - Impulsivity, history of AN or substance abuse, family history of depression |
| Fairburn 1987/ 1991/93 | - High self-esteem | - Personality disorder, level of attitudinal disturbance | - Age at onset, duration of illness, history of AN, depression |
| Fallon 1991 | - Shorter duration of BN, long FU-interval, history of laxative abuse | | - Age at onset, history of substance abuse, AN at admission |
| Herzog 1988, 1991, 1993 | | - High EDI-Bulimia score | - Depression |
| Herzog/Hartmann 1991 | | - Borderline Symptoms (BSI) | - History of AN, depression, abuse of alcohol |
| Hsu 1986/89 | | - Long duration of illness, treatment response, family history of depression and alcohol abuse | - Age at presentation, history of AN or obesity, weight, frequency of bulimic episodes |
| Johnson 1990 | | - Borderline symptoms | |
| Lacey 1992 | | - Alcohol abuse | |
| Maddocks 1992 | | | |
| Mitchell 1989 | | | |
| Norman 1986 | | | - Age, weight, bulimic behaviour, marital status, social class |
| Pope/Hudson 1985 | | | |
| Pyle 1990 | | | - Duration of illness |
| Swift 1987 | | | - Frequency of bulimic episodes |

Table 9. Predictors of Outcome of Mixed Groups of Anorexia and Bulimia Nervosa

| First author and year | Positive predictor | Negative Predictor | No predictor |
|---|---|---|---|
| Fichter (GABS) | - AN: late age at onset | | - BN: age at onset |
| Herzog/Sacks 1993 | | - Low weight, diagnosis of AN, duration of illness | - Age at onset, age at admission |
| Vandereycken 1992 | | - Binge eating, vomiting, lax. abuse | |

which is, however, not supported by the other studies cited above. All three studies which report mortality rates above 10% were performed in institutions for adult psychiatry. Evidently anorexia nervosa is the more life-threatening illness, especially when onset occurs at age 18 or later.

There are several studies that follow-up different diagnostic groups separately but simultaneously, such as the *GABS*. Two of these studies (Herzog, Sacks et al., 1993; Vandereycken & Pieters, 1992) are listed in Tables 3, 6, and 9. The studies of Herzog, Hopkins et al. (1993), of Sohlberg, Norring, and co-authors (Norring & Sohlberg, 1993; Sohlberg et al., 1989, 1992) and of Yager et al. (1987/1988) are not listed because they give important data (e.g., age at first assessment or age at onset) for the complete sample only and do not differentiate diagnostic groups.

The study of Vandereycken and Pieters (1992) is in accordance with several other studies concerning the more positive outcome in early onset anorexia nervosa. The best outcome is found in the diagnostic group with the lowest age at onset (anorexia nervosa, restricting type). This finding is not supported by Herzog, Sacks et al. (1993), the worst outcome being in the youngest age at onset group (bulimic anorexia nervosa), which, however, has a later age at onset than the youngest group of Vandereycken and Pieters. Age at onset may not be a good predictor of the course of the eating disorder as it appears to be confounded with the type of eating disorder. Anorectic patients acquire bulimic symptoms during the course of illness and may then have a poorer prognosis in the long run.

## 11 Conclusions

The evaluation of age at onset as predictor in anorexia nervosa remains inconclusive. The *GABS* contributes additional data on this issue in large homogeneous samples. Nevertheless, the issue remains unsettled. The findings by Schmidt et al. (1992) that early onset bulimics had the worse prognosis was not confirmed in our study. As we have seen, there are severe difficulties with the definitions of outcome. Several types of outcome measures were discussed. The lack of standardized outcome measures makes comparison between studies difficult. Therefore other studies have to be conducted to confirm or disconfirm our findings. Especially, there is a lack of appropriate prospective studies that compare longitudinal outcome data in different age-at-onset groups. Longer follow-up intervals are also needed, at least for bulimia nervosa.

Another problem is the definition of early and late onset. What is an early onset? In the GABS we arbitrarily dichotomized the sample at the median. Finding the most appropriate definition of early or late onset remains an empirical issue for future studies. With the increase of treated cases of eating disorders, our understanding concerning the association between age of onset and course of illness in anorexia and bulimia nervosa will certainly increase in the coming years. What is needed are studies with large samples and with a wide age distribution, which will follow patients over a long period of time with appropriate methodology.

A number of intervening variables may help us understand the controversy concerning the significance of age at onset on course of illness. Quite a few other factors are directly or indirectly related to age. In younger patients the illness is usually less chronic (shorter duration of illness). Except for cases of severe family enmeshment, the family is highly motivated to assist in inducing change in their anorectic child. This includes that harsher therapeutic procedures, such as (possibly compulsory) tube feeding are more easily accepted. A child may be less likely to win a power struggle concerning its health status than an adult patient on whom the parent's influence is minimal. On the other hand, it would appear plausible that the occurence of severe psychopathology in earlier age is indicative of a high degree of family disturbances and/or biological vulnerability for a mental disorder and, thus, be a predictor of unfavourable course of illness. It may also be possible that the relationship between age at onset and course of illness is not linear but curvilinear, but further data are necessary.

A methodological problem of prediction of outcome is the varying statistical analysis of prediction. One could use tests from the ANOVA family, regression analysis, discriminant analysis, or several others. Each method gives its own results without guarantee that another method derives the same conclusions from the same data. For a correct interpretation one must know what statistical analysis was used and we must know how many and which predictors were used. The predictive value of one variable may vary depending on which combination of variable interactions are considered.

For eating disorders other than anorexia and bulimia nervosa — such as the recently proposed and defined binge eating disorder (Spitzer et al., 1992) or recurrent overeating — no data whatsoever is available yet concerning possible associations between age at onset and course of illness.

## References

Abraham, S. F., Mira, M., & Llewellyn-Jones, D. (1983). Bulimia: A study of outcome. *International Journal of Eating Disorders, 2*, 175-180.
American Psychiatric Association (APA). (1980). *Diagnostic and statistical manual of mental disorders (3rd ed.): DSM-III.* Washington DC: American Psychiatric Association.
American Psychiatric Association (APA). (1987). *Diagnostic and statistical manual of mental disorders (3rd ed.) Revised: DSM-III-R.* Washington DC: American Psychiatric Association.
American Psychiatric Association (APA). (1994). *Diagnostic and statistical manual of mental disorders (4th ed.): DSM-IV.* Washington, DC: American Psychiatric Association.
Arroyo, D., & Tonkin, R. (1985). Adolescents with bulimic and nonbulimic eating disorders. *Journal of Adolescent Health Care, 6*, 21-24.
Baell, W. K., & Wertheim, E. H. (1992). Predictors of outcome in the treatment of bulimia nervosa. *British Journal of Clinical Psychology, 31*, 330-332.
Brotman, A. W., Herzog, D. B., & Hamburg, P. (1988). Long-term course in 14 bulimic patients treated with psychotherapy. *Journal of Clinical Psychiatry, 49*, 157-160.
Browning, C. H., & Miller, S. I. (1968). Anorexia nervosa: A study in prognosis and management. *American Journal of Psychiatry, 124*, 1128-1132.
Bryant-Waugh, R., Knibbs, J., Fosson, A., Kaminski, Z., & Lask, B. (1988). Long-term follow-up of patients with early onset anorexia nervosa. *Archives of Disease in Childhood, 63*, 5-9.
Calvo Sagardoy, R., Fernandez Ashton, A., Ayuso Mateos, J. L., Bayon Perez, C., & Santo-Domingo Carrasco, J. (1989). Between 5 and 9 years' follow-up in the treatment of anorexia nervosa. *Psychotherapy and Psychosomatics, 52*, 133-139.
Casper, R. C. (1990). Personality features of women with good outcome from restricting anorexia nervosa. *Psychosomatic Medicine, 52*, 156-170.
Collings, S., & King, M. (1994). Ten-year follow-up of 50 patients with bulimia nervosa. *British Journal of Psychiatry, 164*, 80-87.
Collins, M. E. (1991). Body figure perceptions and preferences among preadolescent children. *International Journal of Eating Disorders, 10*, 199-208.
Crisp, A. H., Callender, J. S., Halek, C., & Hsu, L. K. G. (1992). Long-term mortality in anorexia nervosa. A 20-year follow-up of the St. George's and Aberdeen cohorts. *British Journal of Psychiatry, 161*, 104-107.
Crisp, A. H., Kalucy, R. S., Lacey, J. H., & Harding, B. (1977). The long-term prognosis in anorexia nervosa: Some factors predictive of outcome. In R.A. Vigersky (Ed.), *Anorexia nervosa* (pp. 55-65). New York: Raven Press.
Dally, P. J. (1969). *Anorexia nervosa.* London: Heinemann Medical Books.
Deter, H.C., Herzog, W., & Petzold, E. (1992). The Heidelberg-Mannheim study: Long-term follow-up of anorexia n. patients at the University Medical Center - background and preliminary results. In W. Herzog, H.C. Deter, & W. Vandereycken (Eds.), *The course of eating disorders. Long-term follow-up studies of anorexia and bulimia nervosa* (pp. 71-84). Berlin: Springer.
Deter, H.C., Petzold, E., & Hehl, F.J. (1989). Differenzierung der Langzeitwirkungen einer stationären psychosomatischen Therapie von Anorexia-nervosa-Patienten. *Zeitschrift für psychosomatische Medizin, 35*, 68-91.
Fahy, T., & Russell, G. F. M. (1993). Outcome and prognostic variables in bulimia nervosa. *International Journal of Eating Disorders, 14*, 135-145.
Fairburn, C. G., Jones, R., Peveler, R. C., Carr, S. J., Solomon, R. A., O'Connor, M. E., Burton, J., & Hope, R. A. (1991). Three psychological treatments for bulimia nervosa. *Archives of General Psychiatry, 48*, 463-469.
Fairburn, C. G., Kirk, J., O'Connor, M., Anastasiades, P., & Cooper, P. J. (1987). Prognostic factors in bulimia nervosa. *British Journal of Clinical Psychology, 26*, 223-224.
Fairburn, C. G., Peveler, R. C., Jones, R., Hope, R. A., & Doll, H. A. (1993). Predictors of 12-month outcome in bulimia nervosa and the influence of attitudes to shape and weight. *Journal of Consulting and Clinical Psychology, 61*, 696-698.
Fallon, B. A., Walsh, B. T., Sadik, C., Saoud, J. B., & Lukasik, V. (1991). Outcome and clinical course in inpatient bulimic women: A 2- to 9-year follow-up study. *Journal of Clinical Psychiatry, 52*, 272-278.
Feighner, J. P., Robins, E., Guze, S., Woodruff, R. A., Winokur, G., & Munoz, R. (1972). Diagnostic criteria for use in psychiatric research. *Archives of General Psychiatry, 26*, 57-63.

Fichter, M. M., Quadflieg, N., & Rief, W. (1992). The German longitudinal bulimia nervosa study I. In W. Herzog, H.C. Deter, & W. Vandereycken (Eds.), *The course of eating disorders. Long-term follow-up studies of anorexia and bulimia nervosa* (pp. 133-149). Berlin: Springer.

Frazier, S. H. (1965). Anorexia nervosa. *Diseases of the nervous system* (Vol. 26, pp. 155-159).

Garfinkel, P. E., Moldofsky, H., & Garner, D. M. (1977). The outcome of anorexia nervosa: Significance of clinical features, body image and behavior modification. In R. A. Vigersky (Ed.), *Anorexia Nervosa* (pp. 315-329). New York: Raven Press.

Garner, D. M., & Garfinkel, P. E. (1979). The Eating Attitudes Test: An index of the symptoms of anorexia nervosa. *Psychological Medicine, 9*, 273-279.

Gowers, S. G., & Crisp, A. H. (1990). Anorexia nervosa in an 80-year-old woman. *British Journal of Psychiatry, 157*, 754-757.

Greenfeld, D. G., Anyan, W. R., Hobart, M., Quinlan, D. M., & Plantes, M. (1991). Insight into illness and outcome in anorexia nervosa. *International Journal of Eating Disorders, 10*, 101-109.

Halmi, K. (1988). The course and outcome of eating disorders. *Paper presented at the 3rd International Conference on Eating Disorders, New York.*

Halmi, K. A. (1991). Course of anorexia nervosa: Ten year follow-up. Paper presented at the International Symposium of the "International Society for Adolescent Psychiatry" with the "World Psychiatric Association (WPA) - Section on Eating Disorders", Paris, April 17-19.

Halmi, K. A., Brodland, G., & Loney, J. (1973). Prognosis in anorexia nervosa. *Annals of Internal Medicine, 78*, 907-909.

Halmi, K. A., Brodland, G., & Rigas, C. (1976). A follow-up study of seventy nine patients with anorexia nervosa: An evaluation of prognostic factors and diagnostic criteria. In R. Writ et al. (Ed.), *Life historys research in psychopathology* (pp. 290 - 300). Minneapolis: University of Minnesota Press.

Hawley, R. M. (1985). The outcome of anorexia nervosa in younger subjects. *British Journal of Psychiatry, 146*, 657-660.

Herzog, D. B., Hopkins, J. D., & Burns, C. D. (1993). A follow-up study of 33 subdiagnostic eating disordered women. *International Journal of Eating Disorders, 14*, 261-267.

Herzog, D. B., Keller, M. B., & Lavori, P. W. (1988). Outcome in anorexia nervosa and bulimia nervosa. A review of the literature. *The Journal of Nervous and Mental Disease, 176*, 131-143.

Herzog, D. B., Keller, M. B., Lavori, P. W., Bradburn, I. S., & Ott, I. L. (1990). Course and outcome of bulimia nervosa. In M. M. Fichter (Ed.), *Bulimia nervosa: Basic research, diagnosis and therapy* (pp. 126-141). Chichester: Wiley and Sons.

Herzog, D. B., Keller, M. B., Lavori, P. W., & Ott, I. L. (1988). Short-term prospective study of recovery in bulimia nervosa. *Psychiatry Research, 23*, 45-55.

Herzog, D. B., Keller, M. B., Lavori, P. W., & Sacks, N. R. (1991). The course and outcome of bulimia nervosa. *Journal of Clinical Psychiatry, 52*(Suppl. 10), 4-8.

Herzog, D. B., Sacks, N. R., Keller, M. B., Lavori, P. W., Ranson, K. B. von, & Gray, H. M. (1993). Patterns and predictors of recovery in anorexia nervosa and bulimia nervosa. *Journal of the American Academy of Child and Adolescent Psychiatry.*

Herzog, T., Hartmann, A., Sandholz, A., & Stammer, H. (1991). Prognostic factors in outpatient psychotherapy of bulimia. *Psychotherapie und Psychosomatik, 56*, 48-55.

Herzog, W., Deter, H.C., & Vandereycken, W. (Eds.). (1992). *The course of eating disorders. Long-term follow-up studies of anorexia and bulimia nervosa.* Berlin: Springer.

Higgs, J. F., Goodyer, I. M., & Birch, J. (1989). Anorexia nervosa and food avoidance emotional disorder. *Archives of Disease in Childhood, 64*, 346-351.

Hsu, L. K. G., Crisp, A. H., & Harding, B. (1979). Outcome of anorexia nervosa. *Lancet*, 61-65.

Hsu, L. K. G., & Holder, D. (1986). Bulimia nervosa: Treatment and short-term outcome. *Psychological Medicine, 16*, 65-70.

Hsu, L. K. G., & Sobkiewicz, T. A. (1989). Bulimia nervosa: A four- to six-year follow-up study. *Psychological Medicine, 19*, 1035-1038.

Hsu, L. K. G., & Zimmer, B. (1988). Eating disorders in old age. *International Journal of Eating Disorders, 7*, 133-138.

Jenkins, M. E. (1987). An outcome study of anorexia nervosa in an adolescent unit. *Journal of Adolescence, 10*, 71-81.

Johnson, C., Tobin, D. L., & Dennis, A. (1990). Differences in treatment outcome between borderline and nonborderline bulimics at one-year follow-up. *International Journal of Eating Disorders, 9*, 617-627.

Johnson-Sabine, E., Reiss, D., & Dayson, D. (1992). Bulimia nervosa: A 5-year follow-up study. *Psychological Medicine, 22*, 951-959.
Keller, M. B. (1989). High rates of chronicity and rapidity of relapse in patients with bulimia nervosa and depression. *Archives of General Psychiatry, 46*, 480-481.
Kreipe, R. E., Churchill, B. H., & Strauss, J. (1989). Long-term outcome of adolescents with anorexia nervosa. *American Journal of Diseases in Childhood, 143*, 1322-1327.
Lacey, J. H. (1992). Long-term follow-up of bulimic patients treated in integrated behavioural and psychodynamic treatment programs. In W. Herzog, H.C. Deter, & W. Vandereycken (Eds.), *The course of eating disorders. Long-term follow-up studies of anorexia and bulimia nervosa* (pp. 150-173). Berlin: Springer.
Lacey, J. H., Gowers, S. G., & Bhat, A. V. (1991). Bulimia nervosa: Family size, sibling sex and birth order. A catchment-area study. *British Journal of Psychiatry, 158*, 491-494.
Lesser, L. I., Ashenden, B. J., Debushey, M., & Eisenberg, L. (1960). Anorexia nervosa in children. *American Journal of Orthopsychiatry, 30*, 572-580.
Maddocks, S. E., Kaplan, A. S., Woodside, D. B., Langdon, L., & Piran, N. (1992). Two year follow-up of bulimia nervosa: The importance of abstinence as the criterion of outcome. *International Journal of Eating Disorders, 12*, 133-141.
Maloney, M. J., McGuire, J., Daniels, S. R., & Specker, B. (1989). Dieting behavior and eating attitudes in children. *Pediatrics, 84*, 482-487.
Mitchell, J. E., Hatsukami, D., Pyle, R. L., Eckert, E. D., & Soll, E. (1987). Late onset bulimia. *Comprehensive Psychiatry, 28*, 323-328.
Mitchell, J. E., & Pyle, R. L. (1992). A long-term follow-up study of outpatients with bulimia nervosa treated in a structured group psychotherapy program. In W. Herzog, H.C. Deter, & W. Vandereycken (Eds.), *The course of eating disorders. Long-term follow-up studies of anorexia and bulimia nervosa* (pp. 174 - 181). Berlin: Springer.
Mitchell, J. E., Pyle, R. L., Hatsukami, D., Goff, G., Glotter, D., & Harper, J. (1989). A 2-5 year follow-up study of patients treated for bulimia. *International Journal of Eating Disorders, 8*, 157-165.
Morgan, H. G., & Russell, G. F. M. (1975). Value of family background and clinical features as predictors of long-term outcome in anorexia nervosa: Four-year follow-up study of 41 patients. *Psychological Medicine, 5*, 355-371.
Norman, D. K., & Herzog, D. B. (1986). A 3-year outcome study of normal-weight bulimia: Assessment of psychosocial functioning and eating attitudes. *Psychiatry Research, 19*, 199-205.
Norring, C. E. A., & Sohlberg, S. S. (1993). Outcome, recovery, relapse and mortality across six years in patients with clinical eating disorders. *Acta Psychiatrica Scandinavica, 87*, 437-444.
Nussbaum, M., Shenker, I. R., Baird, D., & Saravay, S. (1985). Follow-up investigation in patients with anorexia nervosa. *Journal of Pediatrics, 106*, 835-840.
Patton, G. C. (1988). Mortality in eating disorders. *Psychological Medicine, 18*, 947-951.
Patton, G. C., Johnson-Sabine, E., Wood, K., Mann, A. G., & Wakeling, A. (1990). Abnormal eating attitudes in london schoolgirls - a prosective epidemiological study: Outcome at twelve-month follow-up. *Psychological Medicine, 20*, 383-394.
Pierloot, R. A., Wellens, W., & Houben, M. E. (1975). Elements of resistance to a combined medical and psychotherapeutic programm in anorexia nervosa. *Psychotherapie-Psychosomatik, 26*, 101-117.
Pope, H. G., Hudson, J. I., Jonas, J. M., & Yurgelun-Todd, D. (1985). Antidepressant treatment of bulimia: A two-year follow-up study. *Journal of Clinical Psychopharmacology, 5*, 320-327.
Pyle, R. L., Mitchell, J. E., Eckert, E. D., Hatsukami, D., Pomeroy, C., & Zimmermann, R. (1990). Maintenance treatment and 6-month outcome for bulimic patients who respond to initial treatment. *American Journal of Psychiatry, 147*, 871-875.
Rammell, M. D., & Brown, N. (1988). Anorexia nervosa in a sixty-seven years old woman. *Postgraduate Medical Journal, 64*, 48-49.
Ratnasuriya, R. H., Eisler, I., Szmukler, G. I., & Russell, G. F. M. (1991). Anorexia nervosa: Outcome and prognostic factors after 20 years. *British Journal of Psychiatry, 158*, 495-502.
Remschmidt, H., & Herpertz-Dahlmann, B. (1990). Bulimia in children and adolescents. In M. Fichter (Ed.), *Bulimia nervosa. Basic research, diagnosis and therapy* (pp. 84-98). Chichester: John Wiley and Sons.
Remschmidt, H., Wienand, F., & Wewetzer, C. (1990). The long-term course of anorexia nervosa. In H. Remschmidt, & M. H. Schmidt (Eds.), *Anorexia nervosa* (pp. 127-136). Toronto: Hogrefe and Huber.

Rosenvinge, J. H., & Mouland, S. O. (1990). Outcome and prognosis of anorexia nervosa. A retrospective study of 41 subjects. *British Journal of Psychiatry, 156*, 92-97.
Russell, G. F. M. (1979). Bulimia nervosa: An ominous variant of anorexia nervosa. *Psychological Medicine, 9*, 429-448.
Russell, G. F. M. (1992). The prognosis of eating disorders: A clinician's approach. In W. Herzog, H.C. Deter, & W. Vandereycken (Eds.), *The course of eating disorders. Long-term follow-up studies of anorexia and bulimia nervosa* (pp. 198-213). Berlin: Springer.
Santonastaso, P., Pantano, M., Panarotto, L., & Silvestri, A. (1991). A follow-up study on anorexia nervosa: Clinical features and diagnostic outcome. *European Psychiatry, 6*, 177-185.
Schmidt, U., Hodes, M., & Treasure, J. (1992). Early onset bulimia nervosa: Who is at risk? A retrospective case-control study. *Psychological Medicine, 22*, 623-628.
Seidensticker, J., & Tzagournis, M. (1968). Anorexia nervosa - clinical features and long-term follow-up. *Journal of Chronic Diseases, 21*, 366-367.
Sohlberg, S., Norring, C., Holmgren, S., & Rosmark, B. (1989). Impulsivity and long-term prognosis of psychiatric patients with anorexia nervosa / bulimia nervosa. *Journal of Nervous and Mental Disease, 177*, 249-258.
Sohlberg, S. S., Norring, C. E. A., & Rosmark, B. E. (1992). Prediction of the course of anorexia nervosa/bulimia nervosa over three years. *International Journal of Eating Disorders, 12*, 121-131.
Spitzer, R. L., Devlin, M., Walsh, B. T., Hasin, D., Wing, R., Marcus, M., Stunkard, A., et al. (1992). Binge eating disorder: A multisite field trial of the diagnostic criteria. *International Journal of Eating Disorders, 11*, 191-203.
Steiner, H., Mazer, C., & Litt, I. F. (1990). Compliance and outcome in anorexia nervosa. *Western Journal of Medicine*.
Steinhausen, H.-C., & Glanville, K. (1983). Follow-up studies of anorexia nervosa: A review of research findings. *Psychological Medicine, 13*, 239-249.
Steinhausen, H.-C., Rauss-Mason, C., & Seidel, R. (1991). Follow-up studies of anorexia nervosa: A review of four decades of outcome research. *Psychological Medicine, 21*, 447-454.
Steinhausen, H.-C., & Seidel, R. (1992). A prospective follow-up study in early-onset eating disorders. In W. Herzog, H.C. Deter, & W. Vandereycken (Eds.), *The course of eating disorders. Long-term follow-up studies of anorexia and bulimia nervosa* (pp. 108-117). Berlin: Springer.
Steinhausen, H.-C., & Seidel, R. (1993a). Outcome in adolescent eating disorders. *International Journal of Eating Disorders, 14*, 487-496.
Steinhausen, H.-C., & Seidel, R. (1993b). Short-term and intermediate-term outcome in adolescent eating disorders. *Acta psychiatrica scandinavica*.
Steinhausen, H.-C., & Seidel, R. (1994a). Die Berliner Verlaufsstudie der Eßstörungen im Jugendalter. II. Die mittelfristige Katamnese nach 4 Jahren. *Nervenarzt, 65*, 26-34.
Steinhausen, H.-C., & Seidel, R. (1994b). Die Berliner Verlaufsstudie der Eßstörungen im Jugendalter. III. Evaluation und Prognose. *Nervenarzt, 65*, 35-40.
Steinhausen, H.-C., Seidel, R., & Vollrath, M. (1993). Die Berliner Verlaufsstudie der Eßstörungen im Jugendalter. I. Der stationäre Verlauf. *Nervenarzt, 64*, 45-52.
Sturzenberger, S., Cantwell, P. D., Burroughs, J., Salkin, B., & Green, J. K. (1977). A follow-up study of adolescent psychiatric inpatients with anorexia nervosa. *Journal of the American Academy of Child Psychiatry, 16*, 703-715.
Swift, W. (1982). The long-term outcome of rarly onset anorexia nervosa - a critical review. *Journal of the American Academy of Child Psychiatry, 21*, 38-58.
Swift, W. J., Ritholz, M., Kalin, N. H., & Kaslow, N. (1987). A follow-up study of thirty hospitalized bulimics. *Psychosomatic Medicine, 49*, 45-55.
Theander, S. (1970). Anorexia nervosa: A psychiatric study of 94 female patients. *Acta Psychiatrica Scandinavica (Suppl), 214*.
Theander, S. (1985). Outcome and prognosis in anorexia nervosa and bulimia: Some results of previous investigations, compared with those of a Swedish long-term study. *Journal of Psychiatric Research, 19*, 493-508.
Tolstrup, K. (1965). Die Charakteristika der jüngeren Fälle von Anorexia nervosa. In J. E. Meyer and H. Feldman (Eds.), *Anorexia nervosa* (pp. 51-58). Stuttgart: Thieme.
Tolstrup, K., Brinch, M., Isagen, T., et al. (1985). Long-term outcome of 151 cases of anorexia nervosa. *Acta Psychologica Scandinavica, 71*, 380-387.
Vandereycken, W., & Pieters, G. (1992). A large-scale longitudinal follow-up study of patients with eating disorders: Methodological issues and preliminary results. In W. Herzog, H.C.

Deter, & W. Vandereycken (Eds.), *The course of eating disorders. Long-term follow-up studies of anorexia and bulimia nervosa* (pp. 182-197). Berlin: Springer.

Walford, G., & McCune, N. (1991). Long-term outcome in early-onset anorexia nervosa. *British Journal of Psychiatry, 159*, 383-389.

Warren, W. A. (1968). A study of anorexia nervosa in young girls. *Journal of Child Psychiatry, 9*, 27-40.

Willi, J., & Hagemann, R. (1976). Langzeitverläufe von Anorexia nervosa. *Schweizerische Medizinische Wochenschrift, 106*, 1459-1465.

Willi, J., Limacher, B., Helbling, P., & Nussbaum, P. (1989). 10-Jahres-Katamnese der 1973 - 1975 im Kanton Zürich erstmals hospitalisierten Anorexie-Fälle. *Schweizer medizinische Wochenschrift, 119*, 147-155.

Yager, J., Landsverk, J., & Edelstein, C. K. (1987). A 20-month follow-up study of 628 women with eating disorders, I: Course and severity. *American Journal of Psychiatry, 144*, 1172-1177.

Yager, J., Landsverk, J., Edelstein, C. K., & Jarvik, M. (1988). A 20-month follow-up study of 628 women with eating disorders: II. Course of associated symptoms and related clinical features. *International Journal of Eating Disorders, 7*, 503-513.

# The Utrecht Prospective Longitudinal Studies on Eating Disorders in Adolescence: Course and the Predictive Power of Personality and Family Variables.

*Herman van Engeland, Thecla van der Ham, Eric F. van Furth, and Din C. van Strien*

## 1 Introduction

In the past 15 years, an increasing number of studies on the course of anorexia nervosa have been published, and a number of excellent review articles is currently available, (Hsu, 1980; Hsu, 1988; Steinhausen & Glanville, 1983; Herzog et al., 1988; Steinhausen et al., 1991). When reading the aforementioned literature, the following points are quite striking: (a) many studies were of a retrospective nature; (b) the studies, for the greater part, reported on patients who had received clinical psychiatric treatment; (c) the studies dealt primarily with adult anorexia nervosa patients; (d) the duration of the follow-up tended to be highly variable; (e) most authors based their report on two reference points only, i.e., the beginning of the hospitalization and the end of the follow-up period; (f) there was often a high attrition rate; and (g) in most studies, relatively little attention had been devoted to the course of the psychosocial and psychosexual development of the anorexia nervosa patients.

Very recently, Herzog, Rathner, and Vandereycken (1992) formulated the criteria that a methodologically sound follow-up study should meet. Follow-up studies should be of a prospective nature. They should include all consecutively treated patients who meet explicit diagnostic criteria within a defined period. The duration of the catamnesis should be at least four years. At least seventy percent of the residents should be examined by means of a direct interview, and Morgan-Russell General Outcome Categories (Morgan & Hayward, 1988) should be used.

In our opinion, only ten of the follow-up studies on the course of eating disorders in adults available at this moment meet these requirements. As far as the course of anorexia nervosa in adolescence is concerned, a maximum of eight studies fulfill the methodological criteria formulated above, (Warren, 1968; Sturzenberger et al., 1977; Martin, 1985; Hawley, 1985; Remschmidt et al., 1988; Jeammet et al., 1991; Jarman et al., 1991, Herpertz-Dahlmann, 1993). In these studies, 391 cases of adolescent eating disorders are evaluated; mean age at admittance was 14.5 years; follow-up periods varied from 3 to 11.7 years; the percentages directly assessed by means of standardized interviews ranged from 43% to 89% and "good outcome" according to the Morgan-Russell criteria, varied between 44% and 77%. All studies except one (Martin, 1985), dealt with clinically treated adolescents. This outpatient study reported the highest percentage of good outcome, namely, 77%.

Since 1983, the Utrecht Department of Child and Adolescent Psychiatry has provided an ambulatory service specialized in young people with eating disorders. The programme focuses on the early detection, diagnosis, assessment, and ambulatory treatment of eating disorders in adolescents. Patients in need of clinical treatment are *excluded* from this programme, which implies that mainly mild cases are accepted.

In the course of years, we noticed that it is not uncommon for patients who meet the DSM-III-R criteria for eating disorders to have a mixed symptomatology that included fasting as well as bingeing. Moreover, over the years, a growing tendency of cross-over in symptomatology has been observed: Initial dieters later develop primarily bulimic problems. There have been repeated references to the mixed nature of eating disorders in the relevant literature (Lowenkopf, 1983; Halmi, 1985; Vandereycken & Meerman, 1984; Mickelide & Anderson, 1985).

These observations have brought us to the hypothesis that what is at issue here is a "spectrum of eating disorders" that is primarily characterized by the triad, (a) pathological fear of getting fat, (b) preoccupation with food, and (c) distorted body-image. This triad, which we feel originates from mainly subconscious, intrapsychological conflicts in the patient concerned, results in fasting and physical hyperactivity, which is often exacerbated later by vomiting, laxative abuse, and bingeing. So, in our opinion, anorexia nervosa is the expression of an underlying personality disturbance, which implies that an integral aspect of the assessment of the outcome of the disease should be focused on the respective personality variables as well. If weight, menstruation, and eating habits improve, but the underlying psychopathological disorder continues, this should be interpreted as a syndrome shift and assessed accordingly.

Following this train of thought, we carried out two prospective longitudinal studies. Minimal duration of the follow-up was four years; repeated assessments and direct, semi-standardized interviews were conducted. We studied the course of adolescent eating disorders, focusing on physical symptoms as well as on psychosexual development and psychosocial adjustment. Because, in our opinion, a "deeper" psychiatric disorder underlies eating disorders, we also decided to examine to what degree personality variables and the family environment influence course and outcome of the disorder.

## 2 The Course of Eating Disorders in Adolescents

The Utrecht follow-up project (van der Ham, van Strien, & van Engeland, 1994) was restricted to the consecutive series of adolescents with eating disorders referred to our outpatient anorexia nervosa programme in the period between 1983-1987. The follow-up period lasted four years. During this period, we saw each patient four times: at intake, one year later, and then two more times at an interval of one and a half year. Treatment was multidimensional and individually tailored to the specific needs of the patients and their families. It included a diet high in calories, supportive psychotherapy, family therapy, and parent counseling. Treatments were carried out partly at our outpatient department and partly by colleagues from other mental health institutions for adolescents. On no occasion was the therapist involved in our follow-up research project.

At entry to the study, information was obtained about sex, age, duration of illness, weight and weight loss, earlier family history, education, work, and socio-economic status of the family. All patients (N=90) were interviewed by a psychiatrist, who used a semi-structured interview method. Information from the interview was used for DSM-III-R diagnosis as well as for Morgan-Russell outcome scores. At the other follow-up assessments, patients were interviewed at our outpatient department by the same psychiatrist. Again, DSM-III-R diagnoses were formulated and Morgan-Russell scales were filled out.

We were obliged to modify the Morgan-Russell Outcome Schedule because a large number of patients in our sample manifested bulimic behavior that is not provided for in the Morgan-Russell scales. For this reason we added a separate bulimia scale. The other scales were also slightly modified. In a reliability analysis of the modified Morgan-Russell Outcome Schedule, Cronbach's alpha proved to be .70 or above except for the psychosocial state scale (van der Ham, et al., 1994). The scales, as we have used them, are as follows:

| Scale | Subscale | Scores poor-good |
|---|---|---|
| A. Anorectic symptoms | A1. Restriction of food intake | 1-4 |
| | A2. Preoccupation with food | 1-3 |
| | A3. Body weight | 1-4 |
| B. Bulimic symptoms | B1. Bingeing | 1-4 |
| | B2. Vomiting | 1-4 |
| C. Menstrual state | C. Menstrual pattern | 1-3 |
| D. Mental state | D. Disturbance of mental state | 1-3 |
| E. Psychosexual state | E1. Sexual attitude | 1-3 |
| | E2. Sexual behavior | 1-3 |
| F. Psychosocial state | F1. Relationship with family | 1-3 |
| | F2. Emancipation from family | 1-3 |
| | F3. Peers | 1-3 |
| | F4. School-/employment record | 1-3 |

The Average Outcome Score = $\frac{A+B+C+D+E+F}{6}$

At the end of the follow-up period, 36% of the patients had dropped out. Post hoc analysis of these patients revealed that the drop-outs differed significantly from the patients who cooperated during the whole follow-up study with respect to their family background, educational background, and personality traits (van Strien, van der Ham, and van Engeland, 1992).

The follow-up study was completed by 56 eating-disordered adolescents, 52 of whom were female. On entry to the study, 47% of the patients met the DSM-III-R criteria for anorexia nervosa; 36% met the criteria for both anorexia nervosa and bulimia nervosa, and 17% met the criteria for the DSM-III-R category "eating disorder not otherwise specified". Scores on Morgan-Russell subscales, measuring mental state, preoccupation with food, body-image distortion, family relations, peer contacts, and school record did not differentiate the anorectic group from the bulimic group or the unspecified eating disorders group.

The average age was 15.7 years (range 12 - 20.8 years); the duration of illness was 1.8 years (range 2 months - 5 years); the average weight was 50 kg (range 34.5 - 79 kg), the average weight loss at intake (corrected in proportion to height) was 16% (range 0 - 43%), and the highest average weight loss ever was 26% (range 9 - 56%). Families from higher social classes predominated, and 90% of the patients lived in an intact family. None of the patients had ever received psychiatric inpatient services; 50% had never sought help before; 30% had been admitted to a pediatric hospital for somatic complaints; and 20% had asked for dietary advice on an ambulatory basis.

After four years, 69% of the entire group functioned well, according to the Average Outcome Score (AOS) of the Morgan-Russell scales; 25% functioned at an intermediate level; and 6% functioned poorly. The outcome of the unspecified eating disorders group was surprising. After an initial recovery, this group turned out to function worst. After four years, only 43% of them functioned well according to Morgan-Russell's criteria. Post hoc analysis revealed that severe psychopathology was found more frequently in the mothers of the patients with unspecified eating disorders than in those of anorectic or bulimic patients. This psychopathology mainly consisted of eating disorders (75%).

Figure 1 gives an overview of Morgan-Russell scale scores for the entire group over the whole follow-up period. Most of the improvement takes place during the first year of our follow-up study. This particularly applies to the bulimic symptoms, anorectic symptoms, and menstrual state. Scores on mental state and psychosexual state hardly improve over time.

Multivariate analysis on Morgan-Russell *sub*scales showed a significant improvement in eating behaviour (fasting and bingeing, but not vomiting), weight, mood, and menstruation pattern. Furthermore, there was a significant improvement on psychosocial variables (family relationships, emancipation from the family, friendships), sexual attitudes and preoccupation with food. However, there is no significant improvement concerning body-image distortion and sexual behaviour.

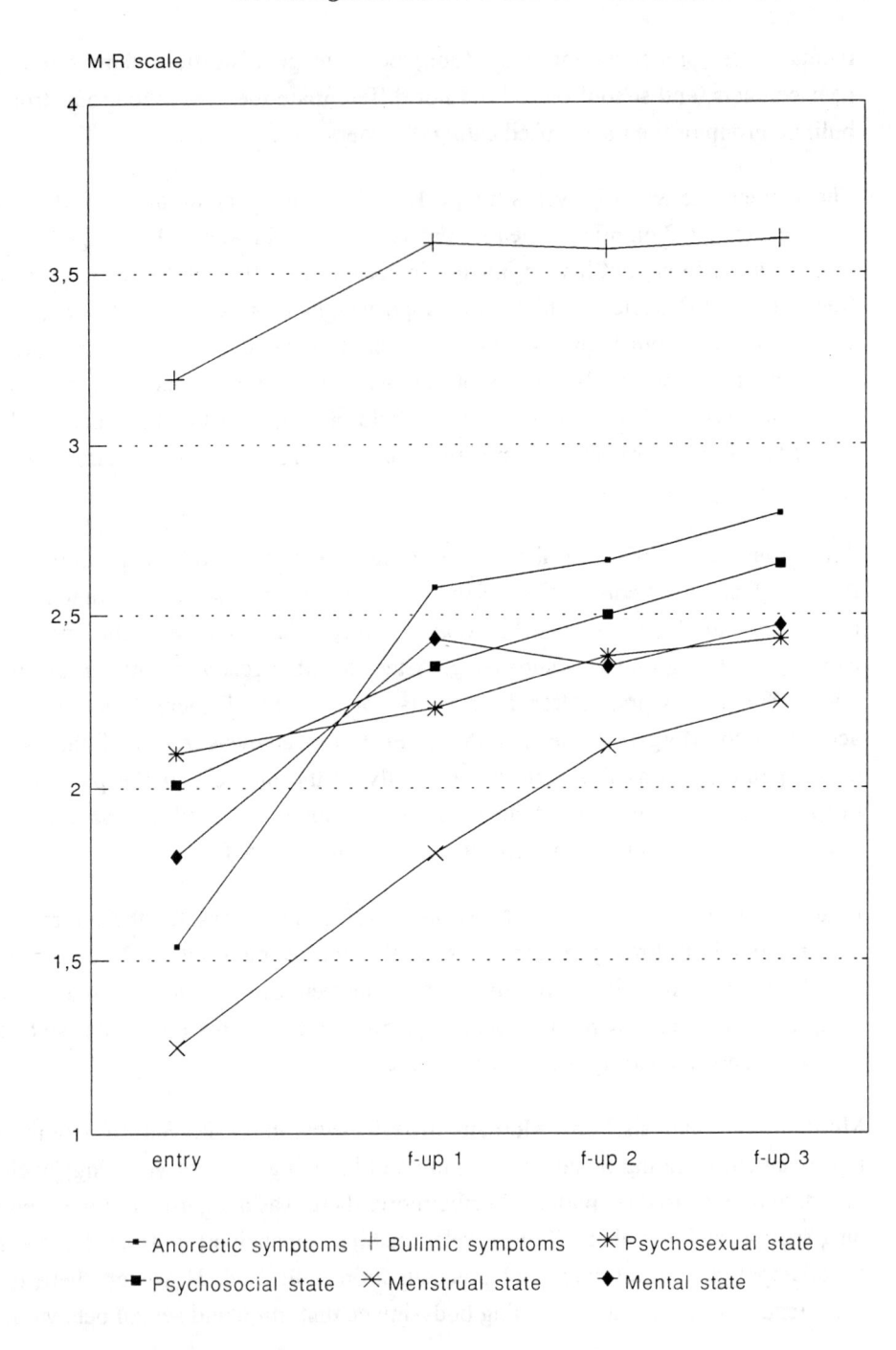

Figure 1. Course of the Average Morgan-Russell scales over the Whole Group

Cross-over of symptomatology actually did occur, but less frequently than expected (14%). This low occurence can perhaps be explained by the relatively short duration of our study and the young age of our patients. From epidemiological research (Hoek, 1991), it appears that the majority of anorectics are under the age of 25, and the majority of bulimics are over the age of 25. Therefore it is quite conceivable that crossover will take place after a long duration of fasting and dieting in older patients.

## 3  The Predictive Power of Psychological Variables

Recently, Steinhausen et al. (1991) and Herzog et al. (1988) reviewed the literature on prognostic factors in eating disorders. These studies mainly concerned retrospective studies on adult patients. Poor outcome was predicted by extreme weight loss, bingeing, vomiting, abuse of laxatives, social isolation, low self-esteem, premorbid personality disorders, and distorted body-image. Good outcome was related to good family relationships and short duration of illness prior to clinical treatment. Conflicting results were found with regard to age at onset and duration of treatment. Most studies reveal a favourable prognosis for both childhood onset as well as adult onset eating disorders.

In adolescent eating disorders, duration of illness, gender, and weight loss were of no predictive value, whereas family variables (single-parent families), number of clinical treatments, duration of treatment, depression, premorbid obesity, distorted body-image, and premorbid behaviour-problems were related to poor outcome (Crisp et al., 1977; Steinhausen & Glanville, 1983; Jarman et al., 1991; Jeammet et al., 1991).

Studies on the predictive power of personality and psychological variables are of recent date. Maddocks and Kaplan (1991) found that depression, ineffectiveness (sense of being ineffective), and low self-esteem in adult bulimics predict a poor prognosis. Sohlberg, Norring, and Rosmark (1992) found a link between lack of ego-strength and interpersonal distrust on the one hand and poor prognosis on the other in adult anorexia nervosa patients. They also found maturity fears to be of significance for prognosis. However, maturity fears were both negatively and positively linked to the prognosis, depending on the time of measurement.

The 90 patients consecutively referred to our outpatient anorexia nervosa programme during the period 1983-1987 filled out the Eating Disorder Inventory (EDI) (Garner et al., 1983) and the Dutch Personality Questionnairre (DPQ) (Luteijn et al., 1985). We studied the predictive power of these instruments in order to compare the predictive value of eating behaviors and demographic variables with psychological and personality factors (van der Ham, van Strien, and van Engeland, in press).

The EDI is a questionnaire with 64 items and consists of 8 subscales representing several psychological constructs that are considered to be essential to eating disorders: drive for thinness, bulimia, body-dissatisfaction, ineffectiveness, perfectionism, interpersonal distrust, interoceptive awareness, and maturity fears. The group of patients who did not fill out the EDI was significantly younger at entry to the study, younger at disease-onset, and had a lower educational level ($p<.05$).

The DPQ examines seven personality traits: neuroticism, social anxiety, rigidity, hostility, egoism, dominance, and self-esteem. Twenty-nine patients were not subjected to the DPQ. These patients were significantly younger at onset of the eating disorder, had suffered larger weight loss, and had achieved a lower educational level. Reliability and validity of the EDI and DPQ for Dutch adolescents are good (van Furth, 1991).

Four different multiple regression analyses (SSPC step-wise method) were performed in order to separately calculate the predictive value of (a) demographic variables, (b) the Morgan-Russell scales, (c) the EDI; and (d) the DPQ in relation to the Morgan-Russell Average Outcome Score (AOS) at Follow-Up 2 (2.5 years after entry) and Follow-Up 3 (4 years after entry). Each analysis was made for the group as a whole, as well as for the anorectic group and the bulimic group separately. We combined all patients with bulimic features ('anorexia combined with bulimia', 'bulimia following anorexia', 'normal-weight bulimia', and 'otherwise unspecified eating disorders with bulimic features') into one group, as suggested by Herzog and Norman (1985). The results of the multiple regression analyses are presented in Table 1.

A.  *Demographic variables*

For bulimics, a short duration of the illness before entry to the study is a predictor of good outcome at Follow-Up 2 and Follow-Up 3. The outcome variance accounted for is 46% and 40%, respectively.

B.  *Morgan-Russell scales*

For the entire group of patients, a distorted body-image is the most important predictive factor of the Morgan-Russell scales. A seriously distorted body-image leads to a poor prognosis, the outcome variance accounted for is 16% and 10% at Follow-Up 2 and 3, respectively. A poor relationship with the parents is a predictor of a poor prognosis. The outcome variance accounted for is 8% and 16% at Follow-Up 2 and 3, respectively.

In the bulimic group, a distorted body-image and a poor relationship with the parents as well as the occurrence of vomiting have a predictive value at Follow-Up 2, but not at Follow-Up 3.

In anorectics, it is primarily poor psychological functioning (variance accounted for 39% and 55%, respectively, at Follow-Up 2 and 3) and inadequate attitude towards sexual matters that are associated with a poor prognosis.

C.  *EDI*

For the entire group, high scores on maturity fears at entry to the study are a predictor for a poor prognosis at Follow-Up 2 and 3. For anorectics in particular, maturity fears have strong predictive power; the outcome-variance accounted for is 42% and 59%, respectively, at Follow-Up 2 and 3. For bulimics, a lack of interoceptive awareness is predictive of a poor prognosis at Follow-Up 2 and at Follow-Up 3. The outcome-variance accounted for is 60% and 45%, respectively.

D.  *DPQ*

For the entire group, low scores in self-esteem predict a poor prognosis. The outcome variance accounted for is 18% at Follow-Up 2 and 19% at Follow-Up 3. For anorectics, low scores on egoism and high scores on social anxiety are predictive for poor outcome at Follow-Up 2.

Table 1. Overview of the Results of Four Multiple Regression Analyses ($p<.05$) for the Whole Group and for the Anorectic and the Bulimic Group. Predictive Value ($R^2$) for the Average Outcome Score (AOS) at Follow-Up 2 and 3.

|  |  | Follow-Up 2 |  |  |  | Follow-Up 3 |  |  |  |
|---|---|---|---|---|---|---|---|---|---|
|  | N | $R^2$ | Beta | T | p | N | $R^2$ | Beta | T | p |
| *Whole group* |  |  |  |  |  |  |  |  |  |  |
| Duration of illness | A 56 | .08 | -.2821 | -2.161 | .0351 | 50 | .16 | -.3946 | -2.975 | .0046 |
| Family relations | B 46 | .08 | .2786 | 2.088 | .0427 | 40 | .16 | .3513 | 2.447 | .0193 |
| Disturbed body image | B 46 | .16 | .3803 | 2.851 | .0067 | 40 | .10 | .3133 | 2.182 | .0355 |
| Maturity fears | C 30 | .19 | -.4406 | -2.597 | .0148 | 31 | .25 | -.7047 | -4.024 | .0004 |
| Perfectionism | C |  |  |  |  | 31 | .12 | .3933 | 2.246 | .0328 |
| Self-esteem | D 40 | .18 | .4213 | 2.864 | .0068 | 41 | .19 | .4338 | 3.007 | .0046 |
| *Anorectics* |  |  |  |  |  |  |  |  |  |  |
| Mood | B 19 | .39 | .5313 | 3.135 | .0064 | 16 | .55 | .5130 | 3.762 | .0027 |
| Peers | B 19 | .17 | .4247 | 2.506 | .0234 |  |  |  |  |  |
| Sexual attitude | B |  |  |  |  | 16 | .18 | .3605 | 2.516 | .0271 |
| Emancipation | B |  |  |  |  | 16 | .09 | .3227 | 2.410 | .0329 |
| Maturity fears | C 14 | .42 | -.6458 | 2.930 | .0216 | 13 | .59 | -.7707 | -4.011 | .0020 |
| Social anxiety | D |  |  |  |  | 15 | .31 | -.6561 | -3.214 | .0074 |
| Egoism | D |  |  |  |  | 15 | .21 | .4693 | 2.299 | .0402 |

Table 1. continued

**Bulimics**

| | | N | Follow-Up 2 $R^2$ | Beta | T | p | N | Follow-Up 3 $R^2$ | Beta | T | p |
|---|---|---|---|---|---|---|---|---|---|---|---|
| Duration of illness | A | 23 | .46 | -.7853 | 5.316 | .0001 | 21 | .40 | -.6284 | 3.521 | .0023 |
| Earlier treatment | A | 23 | .11 | .3482 | 2.277 | .0339 | | | | | |
| Disturbed body image | B | 23 | .31 | .6779 | 4.843 | .0001 | | | | | |
| Vomiting | B | 23 | .22 | .4410 | 3.167 | .0051 | | | | | |
| Fasting | B | 23 | .12 | -.3418 | -2.505 | .0215 | | | | | |
| Family relations | B | 21 | .26 | .5107 | 2.589 | .0180 | | | | | |
| Interoceptive awareness | C | 14 | .60 | -.7762 | -4.264 | .0011 | 14 | .45 | -.6748 | -3.167 | .0081 |
| Self-esteem | D | 21 | .34 | .4401 | 2.397 | .0276 | 21 | .33 | .5748 | 3.062 | .0064 |
| Social anxiety | D | 21 | .13 | -.3923 | -2.137 | .0466 | | | | | |

A = Demographic variables; B = Morgan-Russell scales; C = Eating Disorder Inventory (EDI);
D = Dutch Personality Questionnaire (DPQ)

For bulimics, low scores on self-esteem are predictive of a poor prognosis over the entire follow-up period, the outcome-variance accounted for is 34% and 33%, respectively.

E. *The best predictor*

When examining the variables with the best predictive power in relation to the Average Outcome Score at Follow-Up 2 and 3, we arrived at the results as presented in Table 2. Due to the high drop-out rate, the group numbers in these analyses are small. The respective size of the groups at Follow-Up 2 and 3 are N=24 and N=22. For the entire group, the high scores on maturity fears have a predictive value for both follow-up points. The variance accounted for is 28% and 36%, respectively.

The occurrence of binge eating adds a more or less constant percentage to the variance accounted for, namely, 15% and 14%, respectively. With the anorectics (N=11 at Follow-Up 2 and N=10 at Follow-Up 3), the high predictive value of maturity fears is particularly striking, the variance accounted for is 60% and 66%, respectively.

In bulimic patients (N=10 at both follow-ups), self-esteem, neuroticism, and bingeing have a predictive value for Follow-Up 2 and egoism and ineffectiveness for Follow-Up 3.

We are aware of the fact that our findings are based on a small number of patients, particularly where the question of the best predictor is concerned. This is why these results have to be interpreted cautiously.

The findings reviewed by Steinhausen et al. (1991) and Herzog et al. (1988) are confirmed in this study. A good outcome does indeed correlate with good family relationships and a short duration of the illness. A poor outcome correlates with a high frequency of binges, frequently induced vomiting, and a distorted body-image. However, in our study, these factors only have predictive value for the prognosis of the bulimic group, not for the anorectic group. Psychological factors turn out to have a higher predictive value than the demographic or behavioural variables. Contrary to the findings of Sohlberg et al. (1992), the prognostic value of maturity fears is high and unambiguous in this study.

Table 2. Overview of Best Predictors ($R^2$) for the Average Outcome Score (AOS) at Follow-Up 1, 2 and 3, Analyzed with Stepwise Multiple Regressions.

|  | Follow-Up 1 | | | Follow-Up 2 | | | Follow-Up 3 | | |
|---|---|---|---|---|---|---|---|---|---|
|  | $R^2$ | Beta | T | p | $R^2$ | Beta | T | p | $R^2$ | Beta | T | p |

| | $R^2$ | Beta | T | p | $R^2$ | Beta | T | p | $R^2$ | Beta | T | p |
|---|---|---|---|---|---|---|---|---|---|---|---|---|
| *Whole group* | N=26 | | | | N=24 | | | | N=22 | | | |
| Maturity fears | .14 | -.5054 | -3.962 | .0009 | .28 | -.6368 | -3.725 | .0013 | .36 | -.7329 | -4.300 | .0004 |
| Bulimia | .12 | .4290 | 3.695 | .0017 | | | | | | | | |
| Bingeing | | | | | .15 | -.3989 | -2.334 | .0296 | .14 | -.4008 | -2.351 | .0297 |
| Preoccupation | .17 | .5925 | 4.477 | .0003 | | | | | | | | |
| Menstruation | .13 | .4632 | 4.403 | .0003 | | | | | | | | |
| Peers | .11 | .3797 | 3.561 | .0022 | | | | | | | | |
| Sexual behavior | .10 | -.3526 | -2.588 | .0186 | | | | | | | | |
| Duration illness | .07 | -.2445 | -2.298 | .0337 | | | | | | | | |
| *Anorectics* | N=11 | | | | N=11 | | | | N=10 | | | |
| Maturity fears | .76 | -.5540 | -3.471 | .0084 | .60 | -.7714 | -3.636 | .0054 | .66 | -.8133 | -3.953 | .0042 |
| Sexual behavior | .13 | .4769 | 2.989 | .0174 | | | | | | | | |
| *Bulimics* | N=10 | | | | N=10 | | | | N=10 | | | |
| Dist. body image | .48 | .6940 | 2.727 | .0260 | | | | | | | | |
| Self-esteem | | | | | .46 | .8412 | 6.615 | .0006 | | | | |
| Neuroticism | | | | | .37 | -.7275 | -5.933 | .0010 | | | | |
| Bulimia | | | | | .09 | .3601 | 2.685 | .0363 | | | | |
| Egoism | | | | | | | | | .60 | -.6728 | -6.848 | .0002 |
| Ineffectiveness | | | | | | | | | .33 | -.5857 | -5.961 | .0006 |

## 4 Family Variables and the Prediction of Outcome in Eating Disorders

The interest in the relation between anorexia nervosa and the family of anorexia patients dates back to the first descriptions of the disease by Gull (1874) and Lasègue (1873) where it was suggested that the patient should be separated from the family as a protective measure against family interactions that might perpetuate the disorder. In research, interest in the link between anorexia nervosa and family interactions grew when more reliable methods of measuring family interaction were developed in the 1960's. One of the most well-established methods of measuring family interaction is the expressed emotion (EE) index (Brown and Rutter, 1972).

The index of EE is traditionally rated by means of an audiotaped semi-structured interview — the Camberwell Family Interview (CFI) (Vaughn and Leff, 1976). Based on the content and the tone of the voice, a rating is made of the criticism, hostility, emotional overinvolvement, warmth, and positive remarks of the relatives towards a symptomatic family member. Around the world, EE has proven to be a valuable predictor of the course of psychiatric illness in families with a schizophrenic or a depressed patient (Leff et al., 1990; Hooley et al., 1986). EE has been applied only recently to families of patients suffering from an eating disorder.

Szmukler et al. (1985) found that EE ratings of the parents could predict drop-out from treatment and, recently, evidence was presented showing that EE was related to the outcome of therapy in families with young anorectic patients (Le Grange et al., 1992).

The Utrecht study (van Furth, 1991) examines whether parental EE-ratings based on the CFI can predict the course of illness in a test population of Dutch families with adolescents suffering from an eating disorder. The test population consisted of all consecutive patients and their parents who gave informed consent and who were referred to the eating disorders programme of the Department of Child and Adolescent Psychiatry of the Utrecht University Hospital between January 1987 and June 1989. The subjects met DSM-III-R criteria for anorexia nervosa, bulimia nervosa, or an eating disorder not otherwise specified. In addition, the subjects lived with one or both parents for the three months prior to assessment. The test population consists of 49 families; eight are single-parent, and 41 are two-parent families. Sixteen families (32.7%) dropped out because the patient was unwilling to participate in follow-up assessments. Post hoc analysis revealed that these drop-out families did not differ significantly on any of the demographic, illness, or EE-related variables under research. Five of the 49 patients were male; the average age at the first assessment was 17.3 years (SD=2.4) and the average duration of illness was 23 months (SD=19 months). Eighteen patients met the DSM-III-R criteria for anorexia nervosa, 19 for bulimia nervosa, seven for both anorexia and bulimia nervosa, and five for eating disorders not otherwise specified. Middle class and upper class families dominated in our test population.

Following the initial assessments at admission (T1), treatment was offered to all patients. The formal treatment was not under experimental control but based solely on clinical considerations and carried out partly at other health centres. All treated patients received some form of family therapy or family counseling, combined in 50% of the cases with the most suitable form of individual therapy. Thirty percent of the patients received psychiatric inpatient treatment. The average duration of treatment was 17 months (SD=8 months). As soon as the treatment was concluded, both patients and parents were contacted to make an appointment for an assessment meeting (T2). After a follow-up period of one year, both parents and patients came back for a third assessment (T3). The psychiatric assessment of the patient was conducted by means of a semi-structured interview in which both the patient and the parents served as informants. The information obtained allowed classification of eating disorders according to DSM-III-R criteria. Data were also coded in a manner similar to the Morgan-Russell Outcome Assessments Schedule (Morgan and Hayward, 1988).

Families were interviewed using the CFI. The CFI focuses on the onset and development of the illness, its impact on family life, irritability and quarrelling amongst the family members, the participation of the patient in daily household tasks, the patient's daily activities, and all disease-related symptomatology. The index of EE consists of five variables: (a) critical comments (CC), (b) hostility (HOS), (c) emotional overinvolvement (EOI), (d) warmth (WAR), and (e) positive remarks (POS). The rating was made in accordance with the instructions formulated by Leff and Vaughn (1985). The CFI interrater reliability was very high (Kappa = 1.00 across 12 randomly selected audiotapes). The main question - the predictive value of EE with regard to the outcome of eating disorders - was tackled using a stepwise multiple regression with the Morgan-Russell Average Outcome Score (AOS) as the dependent variable and the parental EE variables as independent variables.

At the first assessment, 35% of the relatives scored `no critical comments', 93% `no hostility', and 26% received a `high emotional overinvolvement' rating. There were no statistical differences between the EE-variable ratings of the father and mother neither at the first assessment nor at the end of treatment. No statistically significant link was found between parental EE ratings and the patient's current body weight, body mass index, lowest body weight during illness, premorbid body weight, age at onset, current age, duration of illness, frequency of bingeing or vomiting, and the father's economic status.

In the first analysis concerning the prediction of outcome, the patient's AOS at the end of treatment (T2) could be predicted by the critical comments rating of the mother at the first assessment (T1) $(F(1.23) = 13.35, p < .005, \beta = -0.61)$. The mothers' critical comments rating accounted for 34% of the AOS variance. A higher number of critical comments was correlated with a poorer outcome. In the second analysis the patients AOS at follow-up (T3) could be significantly predicted by the mothers' critical comments rating at the first assessment (T1). The mothers' critical comments rating accounted for 28% of the AOS variance; a higher number of critical comments was correlated with a poorer outcome.

Thus, EE ratings are predictive of outcome in our test population, but are they the *best* predictors of outcome? In order to investigate this question, other possible predictor variables were introduced and their effectiveness compared to the parental EE variables in the prediction of outcome. These additional variables were: diagnosis, duration of illness, T1 body weight, T1 body mass index, premorbid body weight, age at onset, T1 age, and gender. The results were quite similar to those of the previous analysis: Again, the patients' AOS at T2 could only be predicted by the mothers' critical comments rating at assessment at admission $(F(1.22) = 12.82, p < .005, \beta = -0.61)$. The mothers' critical comments rating accounted for 34% of the AOS variance. The patients' AOS at follow-up (T3) could also be significantly $(p<.005)$ predicted only by the mothers' critical comments rating at T1. The mothers critical comments rating accounted for 28% of the AOS variance.

Summarizing the results, we have shown that a substantial amount of outcome variance (28-34%) could be accounted for by EE variables and, specifically, by maternal critism. A more critical maternal attitude was predictive of a poorer outcome following treatment and at follow-up. We demonstrated that maternal criticism was superior in predicting outcome when compared to other variables such as diagnosis, duration of illness, body weight, body mass index, premorbid body weight, age at onset, and present age and gender.

However, some limitations of our study should be noted. The number of drop-out patients was high (32.7%) and, although these patients and their parents could not be distinguished on any of the variables under research, this may limit the general validity of our results. Another factor that limits the general validity is the dominant number of middle and upper class families in our population. Finally, the diversity of the types of treatment, the duration of treatment, and the different therapists may well have influenced patients' outcome and parental EE levels.

## 5  Discussion and Conclusion

Our premise for setting up these studies was that a spectrum of eating disorders exists that is primarily characterized by a triad of variables that consists of (a) pathological fear of getting fat, (b) preoccupation with food, and (c) distortions in body-image. This triad is generated by underlying psychological problems that lead to aberrant eating behaviour ranging from dieting and fasting to bingeing and induced vomiting. An individual patient can turn to all of these types of eating behaviour at present state or during the course of illness.

We have found no conclusive evidence for a gradual transition from one eating disorder to the other (cross-over), possibly because our patients are too young and because our follow-up period is not long enough to detect such a phenomenon. However, the scores on the Morgan-Russell subscales measuring mental state, preoccupation, body distortion, and peer contacts were deviant for anorectics, bulimics, and patients with unspecified eating disorders. Even the degree of deviation was the same, suggesting that they all fundamentally suffer from the same underlying psychopathology. We consider these findings as supportive of the "spectrum-hypothesis".

When studying the course of disturbed eating behaviour over a longer period of time, one notices that eating behaviour as well as somatic and psychosocial functioning improve strongly in most patients, but that the mental and psychosexual states improve very little, if at all. These findings raise the question of whether it is appropriate to consider these patients as being cured and/or well-functioning as indicated by the Morgan-Russell AOS, or whether one should conclude that these patients will continue to be susceptable to relapse. We feel the latter is the case; however, without a longer follow-up period, we have no empirical material to back this up.

As for the course of eating disorders, the outcome of our outpatient group is comparable with that of Martin's (1985) outpatient-study. The outcome of the group with unspecified eating disorders was particularly striking; after an initially speedy recovery, measured one year after entry to the study, this group turned out to have the worst performance over the entire follow-up period of four years. As far as we know, this has never been reported in the literature before. In our opinion, adolescents with unspecified eating disorders deserve more intensive research interest.

In the prediction of outcome over a longer span of time (three to four years), it turns out that psychological and personality variables in our study are more powerful predictors than the hitherto known predictor variables found in adult anorexia patients. This raises the question whether the predictor variables in adolescents with eating disorders are different from those in adults with disturbed eating behaviour.

This question cannot be easily answered because, in our opinion, not nearly enough attention is being given to the predictive value of psychological and personality variables in the adult contingent of patients with eating disorders.

According to our studies, family factors play an important part in the course of an eating disorder in adolescents. It would be an untenable claim that a high EE score is the cause of eating disorders; it is far more plausible that the adolescent's eating disorder evokes feelings of powerlessness and perplexity on the parents' part, which forms the basis for excessive parental criticism, overinvolvement, and hostility. This reciprocal process eventually results in the persistance of the disturbed eating behaviour. For the clinical practice, this means that it is important to inform the parents about the very nature of the disorder, to assist them in overcoming their powerlessness, criticism, and overinvolvement, and to help them develop a more "favourable" child-rearing attitude towards the patient with the eating disorder.

## References

American Psychiatric Association. (1988). *Diagnostic and Statistical Manual of Mental Disorders* (3rd revised edition). Washington DC: American Psychiatric Association.
Brown, G. W., & Rutter, M. (1966). The measurement of family activities and relationships: a methodological study. *Human Relations, 19*, 241-263.
Crisp, A. H., Palmer, R., & Kalucy, R. S. (1977). The long-term prognosis in anorexia nervosa. Some factors predictive of outcome. In R. A. Vigersky (Ed.), *Anorexia nervosa*. London: Raven Press.
Furth, E. F. van (1991). *Parental expressed emotion and eating disorders*. Utrecht: Elinkwijk.
Garner, D. M., Olmsted, M. P., & Povily J. (1983). Development and validation of a multidimensional eating disorder inventory for anorexia nervosa and bulimia. *International Journal of Eating Disorders, 2*, 15-34.
Gull, W. W. (1964). Anorexia Nervosa. *Transactions of the Clinical Society of London, 7*, 22-28. Reprinted in: R. M. Kaufmann & M. Heimann (Eds.) *Evolution of psychosomatic concepts in anorexia nervosa: a paradigm*. New York: International Universities Press. (Original work published 1874).
Halmi, K. A. (1985). Classification of the eating disorders. *Journal of Psychiatric Research, 19*, 113-119.
Ham, T. van der, Strien, D. C. van, & Engeland H. van (1994). A four-year prospective follow-up study of 49 eating disordered adolescents: differences in course of illness. *Acta Psychiatrica Scandinavica, 90*, 229-235.
Ham, T. van der, Strien, D. C. van, & Engeland H. van (in press). Psychological factors predict outcome of eating disorders in adolescents: a four-year prospective study. *European Child and Adolescent Psychiatry*.
Hawley, R. M. (1985). The outcome of anorexia nervosa in younger subjects. *British Journal of Psychiatry, 146*, 657-660.
Herpertz-Dahlmann, B. (1993). *Eßstörungen und Depression in der Adoleszenz*. Göttingen: Hogrefe.
Herzog, D. B., Keller, M. B., & Lavori, P. W. (1988). Outcome in anorexia nervosa and bulimia nervosa. A review of the literature. *Journal of Nervous and Mental Diseases, 176*, 131-143.
Herzog, D. B., & Norman, D. K. (1985). Subtyping eating disorders. *Comprehensive Psychiatry, 26*, 375-380.
Herzog, W., Rathner, G., & Vandereycken, W. (1992). Longterm course of anorexia nervosa: a review of the literature. In W. Herzog, H. C. Deter, & W. Vandereycken (Eds.), *The course of eating disorders*. Berlin: Springer Verlag.
Hoek, H.W. (1991). The incidence and prevalence of anorexia nervosa and bulimia nervosa in primary care. *Psychological Medicine, 21*, 455-460.
Hooley, J. M., Orley, J., & Teasdale, J. D. (1986). Levels of Expressed Emotion and relapse in depressed patients. *British Journal of Psychiatry, 148*, 642-647.
Hsu, L. K. G. (1990). Outcome of anorexia nervosa: A review of the literature (1954-1978). *Archives of General Psychiatry, 37*, 1041-1046.
Hsu, L. K. G. (1988). Outcome of anorexia nervosa: a reappraisal. *Psychological Medicine, 18*, 807-812.
Jarman, F. C., Rickards, W. S., & Hudson, I. L. (1991). Late adolescent outcome of early onset anorexia nervosa. *Journal of Paediatry and Child Health, 27*, 221-227.
Jeammet, P., Brechon, G., Payan, C., Gorge, A., & Fermanian, J. (1991). Le devenir de l'anorexie mentale: une étude prospective de 129 patients évalués au moins 4 ans après leur première admission. *Psychiatrie de l'enfant, 24*, 381-442.
Lasègue, C. (1964). De l'anorexie hystérique. *Archives Génerales de Médecine, 1*, 385-403. In R. M. Kaufmann & M. Heiman (Eds.), *Evolution of psychosomatic concepts of anorexia nervosa: A paradigm*. New York: International University Press. (Original work published 1873).

Leff, J. P., & Vaughn, C. E. (1985). *Expressed Emotion in families - its significance for mental illness.* New York: The Guilford Press.

Leff, J. P., Wig, N. N., Bedi, A., Menon, D. K., Kuipers, L., Korten, A., Ernberg, G., et al. (1990). Relatives' Expressed Emotion and the course of schizophrenia in Chandigarh - A two year follow-up of a first-contact sample. *British Journal of Psychiatry, 156,* 351-356.

Le Grange, D., Eisler, J., Dare, C., & Russell, G. F. M. (1992). Evaluation of family treatments in adolescent anorexia nervosa: a pilot study. *International Journal of Eating Disorders, 12,* 347-357.

Lowenkopf, E. L. (1983). Anorexia nervosa: some nosological considerations. *Comprehensive Psychiatry, 23,* 233-240.

Luteijn, F. J., Starren, J., & Dijk, H. van (1975, 1985). *Handleiding bij de NPV.* Lisse: Swets & Zeitlinger B.V.

Maddocks, S.E., & Kaplan, A. S. (1991). The prediction of treatment respons in bulimia nervosa; a study of patient variables. *British Journal of Psychiatry, 159,* 846-849.

Martin, F. (1985). The treatment and outcome of anorexia nervosa in adolescents: a prospective study and five year follow-up. *Journal of Psychiatric Research, 19,* 509-514.

Mickelide, A. D., & Anderson, A. E. (1985). Subgroups of anorexia nervosa and bulimia: validity and utility. *Journal of Psychiatric Research, 19,* 121-128.

Morgan, H. G., & Hayward, A. E. (1988). Clinical assessment of anorexia nervosa: the Morgan-Russell Outcome Assessment Schedule. *British Journal of Psychiatry, 152,* 367-371.

Remschmidt, H., Wienand, F., & Wewetzer, C. (1988). Der Langzeitverlauf der Anorexia Nervosa. *Monatschrift für Kinderheilkunde, 136,* 726-731.

Sohlberg, S. S., Norring, C. E. A., & Rosmark, B. E. (1992). Prediction of the course of anorexia nervosa/bulimia nervosa over three years. *International Journal of Eating Disorders, 12,* 121-131.

Steinhausen, H. C., & Glanville, K. (1983). Follow-up studies of anorexia nervosa: a review of research findings. *Psychological Medicine, 13,* 239-249.

Steinhausen, H. C., Rauss-Mason, C., & Seidel, R. (1991). Follow-up studies of anorexia nervosa: a review of four decades of outcome research. *Psychological Medicine, 21,* 447-454.

Strien, D. C. van, Ham, T. van der, & Engeland, H. van (1992). Drop-out characteristics in a follow-up study of 90 eating-disordered patients. *International Journal of Eating Disorders, 12,* 341-343.

Sturzenberger, S., Cantwell, D. P., Burroughs, J., Satkin, B., & Green, J. K. (1977). A follow-up study of adolescent psychiatric inpatients with anorexia nervosa. *Journal of the American Academy of Child Psychiatry, 16,* 703-715.

Szmukler, G. I., Eisler, I., Russell, G. F. M., & Dare, C. (1985) Anorexia nervosa, parental 'Expressed Emotion' and dropping out of treatment. *British Journal of Psychiatry, 147,* 265-271.

Vaughn, C., & Leff, J. (1976). The measurement of Expressed Emotion in the families of psychiatric patients. *British Journal of Social and Clinical Psychology, 15,* 157-165.

Vandereycken, W., & Meermann, R. (1984). *Anorexia nervosa, a clinician's guide to treatment.* Berlin/New York: Walter de Gruyter.

Warren, W. A. (1968). A study of anorexia nervosa in young girls. *Journal of Child Psychology and Psychiatry, 9,* 27-40.

# The Outcome of Adolescent Eating Disorders in Two Different European Regions

*Hans-Christoph Steinhausen, Margret Amstein, Matthias Reitzle, and Reinhold Seidel*

## 1    Introduction

In continuation of extended reviews of 68 outcome studies published in the English and German language psychiatric literature (Steinhausen & Glanville, 1983a; Steinhausen, Rauss-Mason, & Seidel, 1991) and our first long-term outcome study of former adolescent and adult eating-disordered patients (Steinhausen & Glanville, 1983b), we initiated a multi-site collaborative study on the outcome of adolescent patients suffering from eating disorders. It started with a West Berlin sample admitted to a child and adolescent psychiatry department in the 1980's and soon extended to an East Berlin sample at a time when the city was still strictly divided by the wall and two opposing political systems. A comparison of these two samples at the time of admission is described in this volume. A report of follow-up data for these two samples will be available in the near future.

In the meantime, we performed follow-up assessments for a cohort of adolescent eating disorders treated in the same time period in Zurich, Switzerland. Findings derived from a comparison with the West Berlin cohort are the objective of the present report. In the near future, we intend to report on follow-up data obtained from a similar sample that was assessed in Sofia, Bulgaria, and from other sites where further collaboration has started.

## 2    Samples and Methods

The West Berlin sample was comprised of a consecutive series of 60 eating-disordered adolescent patients who received inpatient treatment between

1979 and 1988. These patients were repeatedly assessed in a prospective longitudinal study during inpatient treatment and at follow-up no less than four years later. The Zurich sample was taken from the same time period and consisted of the entire cohort of 64 consecutively admitted eating-disordered adolescent patients. These patients were originally admitted on an outpatient basis. Some patients were later also hospitalized. In contrast with the West Berlin cohort, these patients were studied in a follow-back, catch-up design, i.e., available case-file data were combined with data from a follow-up assessment in 1992.

The participation rate of the two samples at follow-up differed significantly. In the West Berlin sample, four deaths occurred due to the disease, and there were only six patients (10%) who refused to cooperate at follow-up. In contrast, the refusal rate in the Zurich cohort was high, insofar as 28 patients (44%) did not participate in the follow-up assessments. Although there were no deaths of the former patients, the following reasons contributed to non-participation: total unwillingness of the former patients (N=17); living abroad (N=4); and an unwillingness to be involved in a personal interview (N=7).

All patients were systematically interviewed with regard to the current status of the eating disorder at follow-up. The assessment was based on a semi-structured interview that was modified after Sturzenberger et al. (1977) and that we had used previously in an earlier follow-up study (Steinhausen & Glanville, 1983b). In this interview, the rating on a four-point scale of twelve topics dealing with symptoms of the eating disorders, sexuality, and psychosocial outcome is required. Diagnoses were made in accordance with ICD-10 criteria. This more recent scheme, which became available only in the late 1980's, was also retrospectively used for all admission data.

In addition to the interview, the subjects were asked to respond to two questionnaires: (a) the Eating Attitude Test (EAT) (Garner & Garfinkel, 1979) that was translated into German by the first author and used for various samples in the Berlin project (Neumärker, Dudeck, Vollrath, Neumärker, & Steinhausen, 1992; Steinhausen, 1985) and (b) the German version of the Eating Disorders Inventory (EDI) (Garner, Olmsted, & Polivy, 1983) that was also prepared by the first author and used in clinical and in field studies both in West and in East Berlin (Steinhausen, Neumärker, Vollrath, Dudeck, & Neumärker, 1992).

## 3 Results

### 3.1 Patients at Admission

The main clinical features at admission for the two samples are shown in Table 1. Whereas the two cohorts did not differ with regard to weight at admission and BMI, the Zurich sample was characterized by shorter stature, less premorbid weight, less weight loss, younger age at admission, and later menarche (each p=<0.05). However, as Table 2 indicates, the distribution of diagnoses with a preponderance of anorectic patients was very similar. This was also the case when we looked at the defining criteria of the spectrum of eating disorders.

Table 1. Clinical Features

|  | West Berlin (N = 60) Mean | SD | Zurich (N= 64) Mean | SD |
|---|---|---|---|---|
| Weight at admission (kg) | 38.6 | 7.1 | 37.2 | 6.2 |
| Height (cm) | 164.6 | 6.1 | 159.1 | 7.2 |
| BMI | 14.2 | 2.3 | 14.6 | 1.7 |
| Premorbid weight (kg) | 53.4 | 7.8 | 48.0 | 8.2 |
| Weight loss (kg) | 14.8 | 7.4 | 10.8 | 5.6 |
| Age at admission (y) | 15.7 | 1.6 | 14.9 | 2.2 |
| Age at onset (y) | 14.6 | 1.6 | 14.1 | 1.9 |
| Menarche (y) | 12.9 | 1.3 | 13.9 | 2.5 |

Table 2. Diagnostic Classification

|  | West Berlin (N = 60) N | % | Zurich (N= 64) N | % |
|---|---|---|---|---|
| Anorexia nervosa | 48 | 80.0 | 54 | 85 |
| Anorexia nervosa and Bulimia | 6 | 10.0 | 3 | 5 |
| Bulimia nervosa | 5 | 8.3 | 1 | 2 |
| Atypical Anorexia nervosa | 1 | 1.7 | 4 | 6 |
| Atypical Bulimia nervosa | 0 | 0 | 2 | 3 |

## 3.2 Drop-out Analyses

In contrast to the negligible number of 10% refusers in the West Berlin sample, the large drop-out rate of 44% in the Zurich sample calls into question, whether or not the remaining follow-up sample is still representative of the entire cohort. Thus, extensive analyses were carried out. There were no significant differences between participants and refusers with regard to the following variables: (1) age at onset of the disease, (2) age at admission, (3) duration of follow-up, (4) premorbid weight, (5) weight at admission, (6) number of days of inpatient treatment, (7) frequency of hospitalization, (8) mean length of inpatient treatment, and (9) distribution of diagnoses within the spectrum of eating disorders.

In contrast, (a) refusers had more siblings ($p=0.01$), (b) spent less time in outpatient treatment ($p=0.02$), (c) had lower frequencies of outpatient treatment episodes ($p=0.02$) and (d) lower mean duration of outpatient treatment ($p=0.04$) than participants. In a logistic regression analysis, 75.4% of the sample could be correctly classified by showing that refusers came from less harmonious families with a larger number of siblings and less favorable expert ratings of outcome at discharge.

## 3.3 Findings at Follow-up

A total of 50 patients were followed-up in West Berlin after a mean interval of almost five years from admission (Mean=58.1, SD=10.6, range=41-87 months). Due to the follow-back, catch-up character of the Zurich study, the respective 36 patients were reassessed after a more extended mean interval of almost ten years (Mean=118.0, SD=29.3, range=67-167 months).

Findings derived from the follow-up interviews are documented in Table 3. The two samples had very dissimilar rates of former patients who still displayed anorectic behavior, vomited or showed bulimic features. Laxative abuse was almost absent in both samples. Close to 30% of both samples had irregular or absent menstruation. Both the attitude towards sexual matters and the active sexual life were rated as being worse in the Zurich sample, inasmuch as these domains were impaired in half of the sample. The same also applied to the psychosocial domains. Unsatisfying relationships with the family of origin and unsatisfying social contacts outside the family were more common in the Zurich patients.

However, almost the entire cohort, both in West Berlin and in Zurich, was unimpaired in the domain of vocational or school careers.

Table 3. Follow-up Findings

|  | West Berlin (N=50) N | West Berlin (N=50) % | Zurich (N=36) N | Zurich (N=36) % |
|---|---|---|---|---|
| Anorectic |  |  |  |  |
| absent | 34 | 68 | 16 | 44 |
| slight | 7 | 14 | 17 | 47 |
| moderate | 6 | 12 | 2 | 6 |
| severe | 3 | 6 | 1 | 3 |
| Vomiting |  |  |  |  |
| absent | 44 | 88 | 31 | 86 |
| slight | 0 | 0 | 0 | 0 |
| moderate | 2 | 4 | 1 | 3 |
| severe | 4 | 8 | 4 | 11 |
| Bulimia |  |  |  |  |
| absent | 43 | 86 | 27 | 75 |
| slight | 3 | 6 | 3 | 8 |
| moderate | 2 | 4 | 2 | 6 |
| severe | 2 | 4 | 4 | 11 |
| Laxative abuse |  |  |  |  |
| absent | 47 | 94 | 35 | 97 |
| slight | 0 | 0 | 1 | 3 |
| moderate | 1 | 2 | 0 | 0 |
| severe | 2 | 4 | 0 | 0 |
| Amenorrhea (West Berlin: N = 47) |  |  |  |  |
| absent | 33 | 70 | 21 | 58 |
| slight | 1 | 2 | 4 | 11 |
| moderate | 5 | 10 | 7 | 19 |
| severe | 8 | 17 | 4 | 11 |
| Avoidance of sexual matters |  |  |  |  |
| absent | 28 | 56 | 7 | 19 |
| slight | 12 | 24 | 11 | 31 |
| moderate | 6 | 12 | 10 | 28 |
| severe | 4 | 8 | 8 | 22 |
| Avoidance of active sexual behavior |  |  |  |  |
| absent | 22 | 44 | 9 | 25 |
| slight | 9 | 18 | 9 | 25 |
| moderate | 6 | 12 | 9 | 25 |
| severe | 13 | 26 | 9 | 25 |

Table 3.    continued

|  | West Berlin (N=50) N | West Berlin (N=50) % | Zurich (N=36) N | Zurich (N=36) % |
|---|---|---|---|---|
| Unsatisfactory family relationships | | | | |
| absent | 27 | 54 | 16 | 44 |
| slight | 14 | 28 | 8 | 22 |
| moderate | 7 | 14 | 10 | 28 |
| severe | 2 | 4 | 2 | 6 |
| Dependence upon the family | | | | |
| absent | 43 | 86 | 19 | 53 |
| slight | 4 | 8 | 3 | 8 |
| moderate | 3 | 6 | 10 | 28 |
| severe | 0 | 0 | 4 | 11 |
| Unsatisfactory social contacts | | | | |
| absent | 37 | 74 | 27 | 75 |
| slight | 7 | 14 | 2 | 6 |
| moderate | 6 | 12 | 7 | 19 |
| severe | 0 | 0 | 0 | 0 |
| Impaired vocational or school career | | | | |
| absent | 45 | 90 | 33 | 92 |
| slight | 0 | 0 | 0 | 0 |
| moderate | 0 | 0 | 1 | 3 |
| severe | 5 | 10 | 2 | 6 |

The different patterns of diagnoses at follow-up are shown in Table 4. There were less typical cases of anorexia nervosa or a combination of anorexia and bulimia nervosa and more bulimia nervosa and atypical anorectic cases in the Zürich cohort at follow-up than in the West Berlin series. In addition, the rate of recovered patients was lower in the Zurich sample.

Table 4.    Diagnoses at Follow-up

|  | West Berlin (N=50) N | West Berlin (N=50) % | Zurich (N=36) N | Zurich (N=36) % |
|---|---|---|---|---|
| Anorexia nervosa | 5 | 10 | 2 | 5.5 |
| Anorexia and Bulimia nervosa | 2 | 4 | 0 | 0 |
| Bulimia nervosa | 0 | 0 | 4 | 11.0 |
| Atypical Anorexia nervosa | 7 | 14 | 8 | 22.0 |
| Atypical Bulimia nervosa | 2 | 4 | 2 | 5.5 |
| Healthy | 34 | 68 | 20 | 56.0 |

Finally, due to an additional refusal rate in both cohorts, questionnaire data was available only in more limited samples. As Table 5 indicates, the two samples did not differ on any of the scales of the EAT or the EDI with one exception: the Zurich subjects scored significantly higher on a scale measuring 'perfectionism'.

## 4 Discussion

Before addressing the comparison of outcome findings in the two cohorts of differing geographical regions, a comment must be made on the two samples. Although neither of the samples are population-based but, rather, are comprised of consecutive clinical admissions, they should be considered representative due to the specific characteristics of the two institutions in which the data were collected. The West Berlin sample was comprised of the entire admissions to the one and only university department of child and adolescent psychiatry at a time when the city was still surrounded by the wall and there were only two other municipal child and adolescent psychiatric hospitals with differing main obligations and almost no child and adolescent psychiatrist in private practice. Thus, there was a high probability that eating disordered adolescent patients coming from an urban population of two million people would have been referred to the university department where this sample was treated. Due to the political isolation of the city, no referrals came from outside the city. All these patients were treated as inpatients because it was felt that major therapeutic change could only be obtained with a highly controlled therapeutic environment.

The Zurich sample differs in various ways. Although it, too, is a consecutive cohort, it comes from a child and adolescent service with different features. This service has a long-standing tradition of more than seventy years, but since the 1960's, was gradually complemented by a slowly increasing number of child and adolescent psychiatrists who work in private practice. Thus, the present cohort may represent a large but less complete part of the total population of eating-disordered adolescent patients. In addition, the patients came from both rural and urban areas. Due to a lack of inpatient treatment facilities for adolescents, all interventions commenced with outpatient treatment. This was continued in 47% of the follow-up sample for the entire follow-up period, whereas in 53%, additional hospitalization took place. The inpatient treatment usually took place in pediatric and, at a later time of the individual course, in psychiatric hospitals.

Table 5.  Questionnaire Findings at Follow-up

| Scale | West Berlin (N=38/40) Mean | SD | Zurich (N=20) Mean | SD | F | p |
|---|---|---|---|---|---|---|
| EAT - Total Score [1] | 14.0 | 13.7 | 19.9 | 16.1 | 2.15 | n.s. |
| EAT - Diet | 3.9 | 6.0 | 6.2 | 6.9 | 1.71 | n.s. |
| EAT - Bulimia | 0.9 | 2.1 | 1.3 | 2.4 | 0.38 | n.s. |
| EAT - Oral Control | 2.2 | 3.5 | 2.3 | 2.9 | 0.01 | n.s. |
| EDI - Drive for thinness [2] | 3.2 | 4.8 | 3.2 | 5.1 | 0.00 | n.s. |
| EDI - Bulimia | 0.8 | 2.2 | 1.0 | 2.2 | 0.24 | n.s. |
| EDI - Body dissatisfaction | 4.4 | 6.1 | 4.9 | 5.7 | 0.11 | n.s. |
| EDI - Ineffectiveness | 2.9 | 4.7 | 3.5 | 3.8 | 0.22 | n.s. |
| EDI - Perfectionism | 3.4 | 3.9 | 6.3 | 4.1 | 6.99 | 0.01 |
| EDI - Interpersonal distrust | 2.2 | 3.0 | 2.1 | 2.6 | 0.02 | n.s. |
| EDI - Interoceptive awareness | 1.6 | 2.9 | 2.0 | 2.9 | 0.23 | n.s. |
| EDI - Maturity fears | 2.8 | 2.9 | 2.8 | 3.7 | 0.00 | n.s. |

[1] West Berlin: N = 38
[2] West Berlin: N = 40

Besides these different background characteristics, there was one striking difference concerning the admission findings. In comparison to the Berlin cohort, the Zurich cohort was shorter in height, had lower premorbid body weight, had lost less weight prior to admission, was younger at admission, and had later menarche. Not surprisingly, the BMI which takes height and weight into account, did not differ between the two samples. The actual differences between the two samples may reflect real differences in the general population. There is a secular trend in the industrialized western societies for a decrease in the age of menarche and an increase in height and weight. These developmental trends may not only be a consequence of better nutrition, but also a response to stimulation and stress, as hypothesized by Adams (1981). We speculate that these effects are stronger in urban societies than they are in rural or mixed societies. Thus, compared to the Zurich sample, the stress and strain imposed on our entirely urban West Berlin sample may have contributed to the obvious, earlier biological maturation in puberty. This interpretation is corroborated by the finding of our Berlin comparison of the East Berlin and West Berlin cohorts reported in this volume in which the age at menarche was even younger in the East Berlin urban sample.

Another remarkable finding reflects the pronounced differences in drop-out rates. Various factors may account for these differences. One is the design of the study.

The prospective nature and the personal acquaintances of the investigators with the patients from the time of first treatment may have contributed to the high rate of participation in the West Berlin cohort, whereas both these conditions were absent in the Zurich study. Secondly, the longer follow-up period in the Zürich sample may, in addition, have contributed to a higher drop-out rate. Finally, there is some evidence that the refusers in the Zurich study had some rather unfavorable features. Although they did not differ in any of the defining and major clinical symptoms, diagnostic status, or even the amount of inpatient treatment, several indices were retrospectively collected that indicates that this group of refusers was more difficult to treat. They not only received less outpatient treatment, but were also rated as being less improved at discharge. In addition, they came from larger and less harmonious families. In consideration of a large proportion of outcome studies on anorexia nervosa (Steinhausen & Glanville, 1983a; Steinhausen et al., 1991) that have varying and sometimes pronounced drop-out rates and only little or lacking analyses of the causes of drop-out and the consequence of this on the outcome findings, this is an interesting finding.

There is only one further recent study addressing the issue of drop-out characteristics in a follow-up study. In a Dutch study of adolescent patients, it was shown that dropouts came predominantly from the anorectic and atypical group; this finding is not in accord with the present study. On the other hand, the Dutch study parallels to some extent the present study in that it indicates that dropouts had less favorable backgrounds in terms of more psychopathology in the families and lower educational levels. Dropouts also showed more hostile personality traits at admission (van Strien, van der Ham, & van Engeland, 1992).

Before addressing the clinical findings, the difference in age at follow-up between the two samples must be considered. Because of different designs of the investigations, the greater age at follow-up in the Zurich sample has an important consequence for the discussion of the findings. With the higher age, the Zurich patients were developmentally at another step of the life cycle. Whereas the West Berlin sample was to a great extent just at the point of entering early adulthood and leaving adolescence, the Zurich cohort was to a greater extent exposed to the developmental tasks of adulthood, such as vocational careers, partnership, marriage, offspring, and independence from the family of origin. These differences in developmental tasks certainly account for the fact that both the outcome in sexual and psychosocial development were less favorable in the Zurich sample, whereas there were no differences regarding the distribution of symptoms of the eating disorders.

However, when diagnoses based on this distribution of symptoms were compared, there was some indication that the Zurich sample was suffering to a greater extent from bulimic nervosa or bulimic features within the spectrum of the eating disorders. Again, this finding is certainly affected by the more advanced age because bulimia typically has a higher age at onset than anorexia and is manifested at a peak age of 19 years (Steinhausen, 1994)

The slightly lower rate of healthy subjects at follow-up in the Zurich sample also points to an effect of age. There is some evidence coming from other outcome studies that younger age at disease onset is a good prognostic factor (Steinhausen & Glanville, 1983a; Steinhausen & Glanville, 1983b; Steinhausen & Glanville, 1983c; Steinhausen et al., 1991). Whether or not this also applies to age at follow-up has not yet been systematically investigated. Taken together with the other outcome findings, the present study lays some ground to the hypothesis that the increased stress in adulthood as compared to late adolescence and early adulthood may contribute to a less favorable outcome of the eating disorders.

The follow-up findings obtained with two of the most commonly used questionnaires for eating disorders found little differences between the two samples. Amazingly, they did not reflect the differences in the pattern of diagnoses, i.e., the bulimic features, as might have been expected. This adds to some reservation, as delineated from further analyses of the outcome of the West Berlin sample (Steinhausen & Seidel, 1993). There was only little evidence of clinical sensitivity by differentiation of three different outcome groups of either anorexia or bulimia nervosa, partial syndromes, or recovery. The higher score pertaining to perfectionism in the Zurich patients may again reflect the less favorable outcome of this sample. Although we did not observe any obsessive-compulsive disorders in these patients, it may be added that 33% of them fulfilled criteria for affective disorders and 22% for personality disorders. Unfortunately, no data for comparison of co-morbid disorders are available for the West Berlin sample.

In conclusion, the present study of the outcome of two cohorts of patients who were treated during the same time period in two different European regions in differing treatment settings, with different follow-up periods and different participation rates revealed some differences in the status of the eating disorders and the psychosocial functioning of the subjects. Further reports on the outcome of the samples treated in East Berlin and in Sofia will help to clarify whether or not differences in outcome are dependent on age, other sample characteristics, or an interaction of these factors.

## References

Adams, J. F. (1981). Earlier menarche, greater height and weight - a stimulation-stress factor hypothesis. *Genetic Psychology Monograph, 104*
Garner, D. M., & Garfinkel, P. E. (1979). The eating attitude test: An index of the symptoms of anorexia nervosa. *Psychological Medicine, 9*, 273-279.
Garner, D. M., Olmsted, M. P., & Polivy, J. (1983). Development and validation of a multidimensional eating disorder inventory for anorexia nervosa and bulimia. *International Journal of Eating Disorders, 2*, 15-34.
Neumärker, U., Dudeck, U., Vollrath, M., Neumärker, K.-J., & Steinhausen, H. C. (1992). Eating attitudes among adolescent patients and normal school girls in East Berlin and West Berlin. A transcultural comparison. *International Journal of Eating Disorders, 12*, 281-289.
Steinhausen, H.-C. (1985). Eating attitudes in adolescent anorectic patients. *International Journal of Eating Disorders, 4*, 489-498.
Steinhausen, H.-C. (1994). Anorexia and bulimia nervosa. In M. Rutter, L. Hersov & E. Taylor (Eds.), *Child and adolescent psychiatry - modern approaches*. Oxford: Blackwell Scientific Publications. In press.
Steinhausen, H.-C., & Glanville, K. (1983a). Follow-up studies of anorexia nervosa-a review of research findings. *Psychological Medicine, 3*, 239-249.
Steinhausen, H.-C., & Glanville, K. (1983b). A long-term follow-up of adolescent anorexia nervosa. *Acta Psychiatrica Scandinavica, 68*, 1-10.
Steinhausen, H.-C., & Glanville, K. (1983c). Retrospective and prospective follow-up studies in anorexia nervosa. *International Journal of Eating Disorders, 2*, 221-235.
Steinhausen, H.-C., Neumärker, K.-J., Vollrath, M., Dudeck, U., & Neumärker, U. (1992). A transcultural comparison of the Eating Disorder Inventory in former East and West Berlin. *International Journal of Eating Disorders, 12*, 407-416.
Steinhausen, H.-C., Rauss-Mason, C., & Seidel, R. (1991). Follow-up studies of anorexia nervosa: A review of four decades of outcome research. *Psychological Medicine, 21*, 447-451.
Steinhausen, H.-C. & Seidel, R. (1993). Correspondance between the clinical assessment of eating-disordered patients and findings derived from questionnaires at follow-up. *International Journal of Eating Disorders, 14*, 367-374.
Strien van, D. C., van der Ham, T., & van Engeland, H. (1992). Dropout characteristics in a follow-up study of 90 eating-disordered patients. *International Journal of Eating Disorders, 12 (4)*, 341-343.
Sturzenberger, S., Cantwell, D. P., Burroughs, J., Salkin, B., & Green, J. K. (1977). A follow-up study of adolescent psychiatric inpatients with anorexia nervosa: The assessment of outcome. *Journal of the American Academy of Child and Adolescent Psychiatry, 16*, 703-715.

# Subject Index

abuse 36; 41; 84; 85; 87; 88; 89; 90; 92; 115; 116; 120; 121; 123; 124; 125; 161; 162; 163; 164; 165; 166; 167; 169; 170; 226; 227; 233; 243; 247; 264; 279; 306; 315; 323; 324; 326; 340; 345; 362; 363
affective disorder 35; 65; 67; 69; 80; 84; 98; 120; 127; 130; 132; 134; 142; 143; 194; 273; 275; 283; 306; 323; 328; 368
age at onset 4; 7; 40; 43; 44; 87; 147; 301; 302; 303; 304; 324; 327; 328; 331; 332; 345; 354; 355; 362; 368
age at onset, adolescent 69; 71
age at onset, early 84; 85; 87; 88; 90; 301; 302; 303; 304; 306; 322; 323; 324; 327; 328; 331; 332; 333; 357
age at onset, late 301; 302; 304; 306; 314; 322; 323; 324; 327; 328; 332
alcohol abuse 36; 88; 306; 326
amenorrhea 5; 27; 129
amitriptyline 274; 284
anticipation 203; 216
antidepressants 217; 229; 274; 275; 279; 282; 283; 284
anxiety disorders 69; 81; 98; 127; 166; 306; 323
arousal 198; 200; 206; 210; 212; 213; 216; 218
Asperger syndrome 72; 74; 75; 76; 77; 78; 79; 80
assessment 27; 35; 36; 52; 59; 60; 72; 80; 81; 85; 91; 92; 97; 102; 106; 122; 123; 128; 129; 142; 143; 153; 154; 155; 156; 157; 158; 159; 163; 166; 201; 211; 217; 221; 234; 237; 240; 241; 242; 243; 244; 245; 246; 251; 253; 262; 263; 268; 272; 281; 291; 293; 294; 297; 305; 315; 331; 335; 340; 353; 354; 358; 360; 369
attachment 100; 107; 111; 112
attrition 303; 339
auditory evoked potentials 195; 216
autism spectrum disorder (ASD) 74; 75; 76; 77; 78; 79
autistic-like conditions 70; 74; 76; 77; 78; 79; 80
average outcome score 134; 135; 136; 137; 141; 342; 343; 346; 348; 350; 351; 354; 356
Axis I diagnosis 72; 74
Axis II diagnosis 66; 75; 76

behaviour modifications 253; 268
benzodiazepenes 279; 282
binge eating 22; 23; 27; 33; 34; 35; 274; 332; 350
binger 51; 52; 53; 56; 60; 61; 62; 63; 67
binging 129; 315
body image 11; 30; 31; 33; 50; 57; 67; 93; 98; 108; 117; 118; 140; 145; 147; 149; 151; 156; 157; 158; 159; 160; 198; 199; 271; 272; 334
Body Mass Index (BMI) 27; 30; 31; 40; 43; 86; 100; 103; 183; 185; 194; 231; 245; 252; 256; 257; 354; 355; 361; 366
body perception 139; 145; 147; 153; 154; 155; 156; 158
body shape 21; 23; 92; 95; 110; 121; 151; 157; 158; 259; 303
body weight 28; 83; 88; 130; 131; 137; 174; 176; 181; 183; 184; 185; 187; 193; 194; 195; 196; 197; 198; 201; 207; 208; 214; 215; 223; 247; 252; 256; 276; 315; 326; 354; 355; 366
borderline personality disorder 93; 121; 162; 167; 323
bradycardia 209; 212; 223; 232; 237; 239; 250; 252

case histories 11
characterological disturbances 51
childhood trauma 165; 167; 168
chlorpromazine 272; 283
class 56; 85; 86; 90; 118; 353; 355
clinical features 21; 22; 33; 34; 40; 43; 64; 87; 88; 120; 123; 128; 129; 143; 166; 227; 334; 335; 336; 337; 361
clomipramine 233; 277
cognitive processing 110
cognitive therapy 261; 269
comorbid psychopathology 51
comorbidity 51; 53; 66; 80; 124; 130; 132; 143; 165; 166; 167; 281; 305; 306; 323; 324; 326; 328
contingency 203; 216; 284
contingency changes 216
critical comments 60; 90; 206; 293; 353; 354
cyproheptadine 274; 280; 281; 282; 283; 284

day hospital 267; 269
dehydration 224; 227; 232; 236; 239; 241; 252
depression 15; 34; 66; 69; 84; 88; 90; 91; 92; 93; 106; 108; 109; 113; 122; 124; 125; 127; 128; 129; 130; 132; 134; 135; 137; 138; 139; 141; 142; 143; 144; 163; 165; 188; 194; 209; 216; 224; 228; 230; 237; 247; 249; 261; 273; 274; 275; 276; 278; 279; 281; 284; 303; 305; 323; 326; 335; 345
desipramine 274; 275; 282; 283
diagnoses 5; 8; 27; 35; 44; 45; 53; 66; 72; 73; 74; 75; 76; 77; 80; 119; 124; 130; 143; 144; 166; 305; 306; 322; 328; 341; 361; 362; 364; 368
diagnostic classification 41; 361
diagnostic criteria 4; 7; 23; 26; 29; 40; 41; 44; 53; 74; 78; 115; 123; 128; 148; 304; 305; 334; 336; 339
dietary counseling 292
dieting 3; 21; 23; 28; 32; 33; 34; 49; 83; 84; 87; 88; 90; 92; 95; 97; 114; 121; 122; 176; 178; 182; 215; 225; 229; 245; 247; 249; 256; 265; 268; 269; 303; 315; 345; 355
dissociative experiences 163; 165; 167
dissociative symptoms 167
drive for thinness 97; 108; 110; 153; 326; 346
drop-out 22; 128; 293; 315; 350; 352; 353; 355; 362; 366; 367
DSM criteria 5

DSM-III-R  5; 22; 26; 27; 28; 29; 35; 51; 52; 69; 70; 71; 72; 74; 75; 80; 81; 85; 124; 128; 130; 132; 142; 144; 148; 164; 183; 185; 305; 322; 323; 333; 340; 341; 342; 352; 353
duration of illness  88; 129; 185; 293; 301; 304; 324; 326; 332; 341; 343; 345; 353; 354; 355
duration of treatment  244; 251; 345; 353; 355

Eating Attitude Test (EAT)  23; 164; 315; 360; 365; 366
Eating Disorder Inventory (EDI)  46; 151; 153; 162; 163; 164; 165; 346; 347; 360; 365; 366; 369
eating disorder not otherwise specified (NOS)  322; 342; 343 346, 352, 355, 356
eating disturbances  29; 33; 34; 115; 122; 322
ECG  209; 210; 211; 215; 226; 237; 239
EEG  191; 193; 194; 198; 202; 210; 216; 217; 218
electrodermal activity  209; 210; 211; 216
electrolyte imbalance  223; 224
electrolytic disturbance  229; 236
empathy disorders  74; 75; 76; 77; 78; 79
empowering the parents  239
energy expenditure  172; 181; 182; 184; 185; 187; 188; 189
epidemiology  5; 19; 22; 24; 35; 64; 65; 80; 122; 123; 245
ethnicity  118
exercise  11; 21; 110; 183; 186; 189; 209; 217; 230; 232; 233; 242; 245; 249; 250; 251; 258; 259; 260; 268; 270
exercise, excessive  249; 258
Expressed Emotion (EE)  59; 60; 293; 352; 353; 354; 355; 356

familial transmission  55
family assessment  60
family attitudes  39; 100, 102, 111, 114; 144, 164; 169; 296; 334
family background  42; 43; 45; 81; 123; 124; 143; 162; 335; 342
family characteristics  49; 67; 113; 288
family counselling  293; 353
family disturbance  62; 66; 88; 332
family dynamics  57; 58; 61
family features  49; 67; 288
family genetic factors  234
family history  65; 72; 84; 86; 88; 122; 229; 341
family interaction  23; 44; 45; 57; 58; 59; 60; 61; 65; 67; 69; 71; 79; 93; 98; 110; 111; 112; 113; 114; 115; 122; 171; 172; 181; 209; 213; 215; 287; 288; 294; 295; 328; 332; 352; 369
family problems  42; 44; 62; 91; 295
family structure  85; 88; 114; 287
family therapy  61; 66; 93; 121; 124; 243; 252; 262; 269; 287; 288; 289; 290; 291; 292; 293; 294; 296; 341; 353
fat distribution  103; 104
fluoxetine  276; 277; 278; 282; 283; 284
gastrointestinal hormones  172; 178; 181

gender  59; 96; 100; 103; 118; 122; 125; 345; 354; 355
General Outcome Assessment Scale  315
German Anorexia and Bulimia Nervosa Study (GABS)  304; 306; 314; 315; 322; 323; 324; 326; 328; 331; 332
group therapy  255; 275; 289; 291
growth retardation  224

habituation  210
heart rate  209; 210; 215; 216; 232; 237
history  14; 15; 16; 65; 72; 84; 85; 86; 87; 88; 89; 115; 122; 137; 144; 161; 162; 167; 168; 224; 225; 227; 228; 229; 230; 235; 238; 251; 253; 263; 273; 275; 279; 280; 301; 326; 341
hospital  4; 5; 15; 85; 92; 148; 153; 168; 185; 241; 249; 251; 252; 253; 254; 258; 259; 260; 261; 264; 267; 269; 272; 290; 292; 293; 296; 304; 322; 343; 352
hospitalization  15; 27; 228; 239; 240; 241; 242; 247; 248; 252; 269; 339; 362; 365
hypoglycemia  223; 236; 240
hypotension  223; 227; 232; 239; 250; 252; 274

ideal image  151; 154; 155; 157
imipramine  274; 275; 282; 284; 285
incidence  3; 6; 7; 8; 18; 19; 37; 44; 64; 66; 91; 116; 119; 122; 124; 132; 169; 246; 357
individual psychotherapy  242; 289
individual supportive therapy  61
infertility  174; 175; 176; 224
initial interview  221; 238; 249; 251; 268
inpatient treatment  39; 129; 130; 131; 165; 247; 248; 255; 267; 290; 291; 292; 314; 324; 326; 327; 353; 359; 362; 365; 367
intrafamilial discord  85

laboratory investigation  225; 234
laxative abuse  226; 233; 315; 326; 340
laxatives  21; 28; 32; 33; 87; 95; 227; 228; 229; 236; 252; 264; 280; 345
lay theories  290
lithium  279; 280; 282; 283; 284
longitudinal study  63; 80; 92; 96; 246; 360

maturity fears  153; 345; 346; 347; 350; 366
medical assessment  221; 251
menarche  6; 44; 83; 87; 227; 361; 366; 369
metabolic abnormalities  104
mianserin  275
monoamine oxidase inhibitors  278; 279; 282
mood  26; 27; 35; 49; 50; 51; 55; 56; 58; 66; 90; 104; 106; 107; 108; 109; 127; 128; 130; 138; 166; 171; 216; 239; 243; 250; 252; 274; 278; 279; 282; 305; 343
Morgan and Russell's criteria  314
Morgan-Russell Outcome Schedule  342
mortality  96; 221; 224; 240; 302; 315; 322; 328; 331; 333; 335

## Subject Index

multi-impulsive bulimics 162

nasogastric feeding 256
neuroleptics 271; 272; 279; 282; 284
neuronal decoupling 197
neuropsychological functioning 214
non-participants 128
non-participation 28, 360
nutritional counselling 97; 242; 251; 252; 260; 261

obesity 11; 42; 44; 57; 84; 86; 87; 103; 118; 120; 121; 149; 156; 158; 159; 229; 265; 345
obsessive compulsive disorder (OCD) 77; 78; 132
obsessive compulsive personality disorder (OCPD) 69; 74; 75; 76; 77; 78
oligomenorrhea 5
operant programmes 254
orienting 203; 205; 216
osteoporosis 171; 177; 222; 224; 228; 234; 238; 246
outpatient treatment 240; 247; 248; 252; 280; 292; 362; 365; 367

parental care 88; 92
parental characteristics 115
parental neglect (lack of care) 58; 84; 85; 89; 90; 93; 112; 164; 165
parent-child interactions 58
parent-child problems 112
parent-child relationship 288; 324
parents 14; 17; 18; 19; 28; 42; 45; 52; 56; 57; 58; 62; 64; 66; 86; 90; 92; 102; 112; 114; 120; 121; 128; 201; 225; 226; 228; 230; 234; 236; 238; 239; 240; 241; 242; 244; 249; 253; 262; 263; 287; 291; 292; 293; 294; 295; 347; 352; 353; 355; 356
personality 34; 35; 49; 51; 52; 53; 56; 62; 64; 66; 67; 68; 69; 71; 72; 73; 74; 75; 76; 77; 79; 80; 90; 93; 107; 108; 109; 121; 125; 139; 159; 162; 166; 167; 169; 170; 215; 253; 306; 323; 324; 340; 341; 342; 345; 346; 356; 367; 368
personality disorders 52; 53; 68; 69; 71; 73; 74; 75; 76; 77; 79; 80; 90; 93; 121; 162; 166; 167; 169; 170; 306; 323; 324; 345; 368
personality disturbances 51; 62; 139
personality traits 52; 108; 109; 342; 346; 367
physical abuse 163; 164; 165; 166; 167; 169
physical activity 181; 182; 183; 184; 186; 187; 188; 226; 245; 253; 268
physical examination 11; 225; 230; 243
Picture Silhouette Test 149; 151; 154; 155; 157
pimozide 272; 283; 284
population study 70; 80
prandial hyperphagia 29; 34
preadolescent patients 7
predictive value 128; 132; 141; 142; 143; 324; 326; 327; 332; 345; 346; 347; 350; 353; 356
predictor 85; 109; 134; 275; 301; 324; 326; 327; 328; 331; 332; 347; 350; 352; 354; 356

premenarchal 3; 7; 19; 41; 84; 87; 91; 246
premenarchal anorexia 3; 19; 246
premenarchal subjects 7
premorbid features 52
prevalence 6; 7; 21; 22; 23; 26; 28; 30; 33; 35; 36; 37; 44; 70; 93; 102; 115; 118; 119; 123; 127; 132; 134; 142; 144; 162; 169; 212; 223; 275; 278; 357
prognosis 53; 64; 120; 144; 145; 246; 302; 327; 331; 333; 336; 345; 347; 350; 357
prognostic factors 302; 324; 326; 334; 335; 345
Psychiatric Status Rating Scale for Bulimia Nervosa (PSRSB) 315; 328
psychoeducational 224; 225; 245; 265; 269
psychopathology 30; 34; 50; 51; 63; 66; 87; 96; 97; 99; 109; 124; 128; 130; 139; 142; 158; 166; 170; 194; 201; 203; 244; 245; 255; 294; 296; 332; 334; 343; 355; 367
psychopathology, individual 50
psychophysiology 214; 216; 217
psychosexual functioning 139
psychotherapy 165; 242; 253; 254; 265; 266; 276; 279; 282; 283; 284; 289; 292; 296; 297; 314; 322; 333; 334; 335; 341
puberty 3; 6; 13; 50; 100; 103; 117; 122; 172; 234; 302; 366
purging type 21; 51; 129; 168; 226; 229; 231; 232; 236; 237; 271; 275; 276; 277; 278; 279; 304; 306; 322; 323

refeeding 188; 189; 209; 217; 233; 236; 237; 238; 241; 242; 246; 251; 254; 255; 270; 284
refeeding, nasogastric 258
refeeding, tube feeding 257; 258; 332
resting metabolic rate 181; 182; 189
restricter 50; 51; 52; 53; 56; 60; 61; 62; 63; 67
retrospective report 315
risk factors 42; 84; 95; 96; 97; 101; 106; 109; 113; 114; 119
Russell criteria 22; 340

selective serotonin reuptake inhibitors 275; 276; 277; 278; 282
self confidence 153; 156
self image 157
self perception 154; 157
self-harm 84; 87; 90; 91; 303
self-help 266
self-image 50; 54; 62; 149; 154; 159
sexual abuse 84; 85; 89; 115; 116; 121; 123; 161; 162; 163; 164; 165; 166; 167; 169; 170
sexual abuse, childhood 162; 163; 164; 166; 167; 169; 170
Silhouette Selection Method 147; 151; 154; 157
snacking 29; 34
social adaption 137
social interaction 69; 79
sociocultural 37; 43; 45; 46; 118
socioeconomic status 137; 201; 324
standardized outcome measures 331

starvation  5; 6; 14; 45; 66; 97; 122; 124; 132; 142; 143; 171; 174; 177; 188; 189; 215; 222; 223; 224; 229; 237; 246; 248; 250; 253; 265; 296
structural family therapy  291
substance abuse  87; 89; 247; 279; 306; 323; 324
suicide attempts  27; 91; 326
sulpiride  273; 284
supportive therapy, individual  61; 292

target weight  130; 195; 241; 251; 255; 256
temperament  49; 50; 72; 100; 106; 111
transcultural  37; 38; 43; 45; 46; 369
trauma  121; 124; 162; 164; 165; 166; 167; 168; 170; 243
traumatic experiences  115; 161; 164; 165; 166; 167; 168
tricyclic antidepressants  229; 273; 274
tube feeding  257; 258; 332

unspecified eating disorder (NOS)  322; 342; 343 346, 352, 355, 356

vegetarianism  231; 264
violence  85; 166
vomiting  21; 27; 28; 30; 32; 33; 87; 95; 120; 122; 162; 223; 224; 226; 228; 231; 232; 235; 236; 239; 241; 247; 248; 249; 252; 278; 280; 282; 315; 340; 343; 345; 347; 350; 354; 355

weight control strategies  21; 27; 32; 33
weight gain  18; 63; 66; 104; 110; 130; 153; 172; 174; 182; 183; 184; 186; 191; 197; 207; 209; 214; 228; 251; 253; 254; 256; 263; 264; 270; 272; 273; 274; 277; 278; 279; 280; 281; 282; 292; 296
weight loss  5; 6; 7; 16; 40; 79; 117; 132; 142; 148; 156; 174; 176; 221; 222; 223; 228; 247; 259; 341; 343; 345; 346; 361
western culture  116